T0264211

Neurology

Editors

SHARON C. KERWIN
AMANDA R. TAYLOR

VETERINARY CLINICS OF NORTH AMERICA: SMALL ANIMAL PRACTICE

www.vetsmall.theclinics.com

January 2018 • Volume 48 • Number 1

ELSEVIER

1600 John F. Kennedy Boulevard • Suite 1800 • Philadelphia, Pennsylvania, 19103-2899
http://www.vetsmall.theclinics.com

VETERINARY CLINICS OF NORTH AMERICA: SMALL ANIMAL PRACTICE Volume 48, Number 1 January 2018 ISSN 0195-5616, ISBN-13: 978-0-323-56663-6

Editor: Colleen Dietzler
Developmental Editor: Meredith Madeira

Veterinary Clinics of North America: Small Animal Practice (ISSN 0195-5616) is published bimonthly by Elsevier Inc., 360 Park Avenue South, New York, NY 10010-1710. Months of issue are January, March, May, July, September, and November. Business and Editorial Offices: 1600 John F. Kennedy Blvd., Ste. 1800, Philadelphia, PA 19103-2899. Customer Service Office: 3251 Riverport Lane, Maryland Heights, MO 63043. Periodicals postage paid at New York, NY and additional mailing offices. Subscription prices are $325.00 per year (domestic individuals), $622.00 per year (domestic institutions), $100.00 per year (domestic students/residents), $430.00 per year (Canadian individuals), $773.00 per year (Canadian institutions), $469.00 per year (international individuals), $773.00 per year (international institutions), and $220.00 per year (international and Canadian students/residents). To receive student/resident rate, orders must be accompanied by name of affiliated institution, date of term, and the *signature* of program/residency coordinator on institution letterhead. Orders will be billed at individual rate until proof of status is received. Foreign air speed delivery is included in all *Clinics* subscription prices. All prices are subject to change without notice. **POSTMASTER:** Send address changes to *Veterinary Clinics of North America: Small Animal Practice*, Elsevier Health Sciences Division, Subscription Customer Service, 3251 Riverport Lane, Maryland Heights, MO 63043. Customer Service (orders, claims, online, change of address): Elsevier Periodicals Customer Service, Elsevier Health Sciences Division Subscription **Customer Service 3251 Riverport Lane Maryland Heights, MO 63043. Tel: 1-800-654-2452 (U.S. and Canada); 314-447-8871 (outside U.S. and Canada). Fax: 314-447-8029. E-mail: journalscustomerservice-usa@elsevier.com (for print support); journalsonlinesupport-usa@elsevier.com (for online support).**

Reprints. For copies of 100 or more of articles in this publication, please contact the Commercial Reprints Department, Elsevier Inc., 360 Park Avenue South, New York, NY 10010-1710. Tel.: 212-633-3874; Fax: 212-633-3820; E-mail: reprints@elsevier.com.

Veterinary Clinics of North America: Small Animal Practice is also published in Japanese by Inter Zoo Publishing Co., Ltd., Aoyama Crystal-Bldg 5F, 3-5-12 Kitaaoyama, Minato-ku, Tokyo 107-0061, Japan.

Veterinary Clinics of North America: Small Animal Practice is covered in *Current Contents/Agriculture, Biology and Environmental Sciences, Science Citation Index, ASCA, MEDLINE/PubMed (Index Medicus), Excerpta Medica, and BIOSIS.*

Contributors

EDITORS

SHARON C. KERWIN, DVM, MS
Diplomate, American College of Veterinary Surgeons; Diplomate, American College of Veterinary Internal Medicine (Neurology); Professor, Surgery, Department of Small Animal Clinical Sciences, College of Veterinary Medicine & Biomedical Sciences, Texas A&M University, College Station, Texas, USA

AMANDA R. TAYLOR, DVM
Diplomate, American College of Veterinary Internal Medicine (Neurology); Assistant Professor, Neurology and Neurosurgery, Department of Clinical Sciences, Auburn University College of Veterinary Medicine, Auburn, Alabama, USA

AUTHORS

LENORE M. BACEK, DVM, MS
Diplomate, American College of Veterinary Emergency and Critical Care; Assistant Clinical Professor, Emergency and Critical Care, Department of Clinical Sciences, Auburn University College of Veterinary Medicine, Auburn, Alabama, USA

ANDREW K. BARKER, DVM
Diplomate, American College of Veterinary Internal Medicine (Neurology); Staff Neurologist, Toronto Veterinary Emergency Hospital, Scarborough, Ontario, Canada

R. TIMOTHY BENTLEY, BVSc
Diplomate, American College of Veterinary Internal Medicine (Neurology); Associate Professor, Neurology and Neurosurgery, Department of Veterinary Clinical Sciences, Purdue University College of Veterinary Medicine, Purdue University, West Lafayette, Indiana, USA

CHRISTEN ELIZABETH BOUDREAU, DVM, PhD
Diplomate, American College of Veterinary Internal Medicine (Neurology); Assistant Professor, Department of Small Animal Clinical Sciences, Texas A&M University, College Station, Texas, USA

ANNIE V. CHEN, DVM, MS
Diplomate, American College of Veterinary Internal Medicine (Neurology); Department of Veterinary Clinical Sciences, College of Veterinary Medicine, Washington State University, Pullman, Washington, USA

ROBERT C. COLE, DVM
Diplomate, American College of Veterinary Radiology; Assistant Professor of Radiology, Department of Small Animal Clinical Science, Auburn University, Auburn, Alabama, USA

STEVEN DE DECKER, DVM, MVetMed, PhD
Diplomate, European College of Veterinary Neurology; Department of Clinical Science and Services, Royal Veterinary College, University of London, Hatfield, Hertfordshire, United Kingdom

JOE FENN, BVetMed, MVetMed
Diplomate, European College of Veterinary Neurology; Department of Clinical Science and Services, Royal Veterinary College, University of London, Hatfield, Hertfordshire, United Kingdom

MARGARET FOWLER, DVM, MS
Acupuncture and Holistic Veterinary Services, Summerville, South Carolina, USA; Faculty Member, Chi Institute of Traditional Chinese Veterinary Medicine, Reddick, Florida, USA

LAUREN FRANK, DVM, MS, CVA, CVCH, CCRT
Diplomate, American College of Veterinary Sports Medicine and Rehabilitation; Physical Rehabilitation and Acupuncture Service, Long Island Veterinary Specialists, Plainview, New York, USA

PAUL M. FREEMAN, MA, VetMB, CertSAO
Diplomate, European College of Veterinary Neurology; Principal Clinical Neurologist, Department of Veterinary Medicine, University of Cambridge, Cambridge, United Kingdom

TOM R. HARCOURT-BROWN, MA, VetMB
Diplomate, European College of Veterinary Neurology; Chief Clinical Neurologist, Langford Vets, University of Bristol, Bristol, United Kingdom

HEIDI BARNES HELLER, DVM
Diplomate, American College of Veterinary Internal Medicine (Neurology); Clinical Assistant Professor, Neurology/Neurosurgery, Department of Medical Sciences, University of Wisconsin–Madison School of Veterinary Medicine, Madison, Wisconsin, USA

ADRIEN-MAXENCE HESPEL, DVM, MS
Diplomate, American College of Veterinary Radiology; Assistant Professor of Radiology, Department of Small Animal Clinical Science, The University of Tennessee, Knoxville, Tennessee, USA

BIANCA F. HETTLICH, Dr med vet
Diplomate, American College of Veterinary Surgeons; Senior Lecturer, Department of Small Animal Surgery, Vetsuisse Faculty, University of Bern, Bern, Switzerland

NICK D. JEFFERY, BVSc, MSc, PhD, FRCVS
Diplomate, European College of Veterinary Neurology; Diplomate, European College of Veterinary Surgeons; Professor, Neurology and Neurosurgery, Department of Small Animal Clinical Sciences, Texas A&M University, College Station, Texas, USA

SHARON C. KERWIN, DVM, MS
Diplomate, American College of Veterinary Surgeons; Diplomate, American College of Veterinary Internal Medicine (Neurology); Professor, Surgery, Department of Small Animal Clinical Sciences, College of Veterinary Medicine & Biomedical Sciences, Texas A&M University, College Station, Texas, USA

KENDON W. KUO, DVM, MS
Diplomate, American College of Veterinary Emergency and Critical Care; Assistant Clinical Professor, Emergency and Critical Care, Department of Clinical Sciences, Auburn University College of Veterinary Medicine, Auburn, Alabama, USA

JONATHAN M. LEVINE, DVM
Diplomate, American College of Veterinary Internal Medicine (Neurology); Professor and Head, Department of Small Animal Clinical Sciences, Texas A&M University, College Station, Texas, USA

LINDA G. MARTIN, DVM, MS
Diplomate, American College of Veterinary Emergency and Critical Care; Department of Veterinary Clinical Sciences, College of Veterinary Medicine, Washington State University, Pullman, Washington, USA

TINA J. OWEN, DVM
Diplomate, American College of Veterinary Surgeons; Department of Veterinary Clinical Sciences, College of Veterinary Medicine, Washington State University, Pullman, Washington, USA

PATRICK ROYNARD, DVM, MRCVS
Diplomate, American College of Veterinary Internal Medicine (Neurology); Neurology/Neurosurgery Department, Long Island Veterinary Specialists, Plainview, New York, USA; Fipapharm, Mont-Saint-Aignan, France

CATHERINE M. RUOFF, MS, DVM
Diplomate, American College of Veterinary Radiology; Clinical Assistant Professor, Radiology, Department of Large Animal Clinical Sciences, College of Veterinary Medicine & Biomedical Sciences, Texas A&M University, College Station, Texas, USA

AMANDA R. TAYLOR, DVM
Diplomate, American College of Veterinary Internal Medicine (Neurology); Assistant Professor, Neurology and Neurosurgery, Department of Clinical Sciences, Auburn University College of Veterinary Medicine, Auburn, Alabama, USA

STEPHANIE A. THOMOVSKY, DVM
Diplomate, American College of Veterinary Internal Medicine (Neurology); Associate Professor, Neurology and Neurosurgery, Department of Veterinary Clinical Sciences, Purdue University College of Veterinary Medicine, Purdue University, West Lafayette, Indiana, USA

HUISHENG XIE, DVM, PhD, MS
Department of Small Animal Clinical Sciences, University of Florida, Gainesville, Florida, USA

Contents

Erratum xiii

Preface xv

Sharon C. Kerwin and Amanda R. Taylor

Clinical Evaluation of the Feline Neurologic Patient 1

Amanda R. Taylor and Sharon C. Kerwin

Video content accompanies this article at http://www.vetsmall.theclinics.com.

Efficient, gentle, and safe handling of cats can result in complete neurologic evaluations and accurate neuroanatomic localizations. The clinic environment should facilitate the examination by providing a quiet and secure environment for the cat. When direct examination of a cat is not possible, the practitioner should fully use indirect methods of examination and video recordings of cat behavior or clinical signs. Direct examination of a cat should proceed in a logical order, where the most useful tests are performed early on in the examination.

Advances in High-Field MRI 11

Adrien-Maxence Hespel and Robert C. Cole

MRI techniques and systems have evolved dramatically over recent years. These advances include higher field strengths, new techniques, faster gradients, improved coil technology, and more robust sequence protocols. This article reviews the most commonly used advanced MRI techniques, including diffusion-weighted imaging, magnetic resonance spectrography, diffusion tensor imaging, and cerebrospinal fluid flow tracking.

Feline Epilepsy 31

Heidi Barnes Heller

Seizures occur commonly in cats and can be classified as idiopathic epilepsy, structural epilepsy, or reactive seizures. Pursuit of a diagnosis may include a complete blood count, serum biochemistry, brain MRI, and cerebrospinal fluid analysis as indicated. Antiepileptic drugs should be considered if a cat is having frequent seizures, or any 1 seizure longer than 5 minutes. Phenobarbital is often the drug of choice; however, levetiracetam may be more useful for certain types of epilepsy in cats. Long-term prognosis depends on the underlying diagnosis and response to therapy.

An Update on Cerebrovascular Disease in Dogs and Cats 45

Christen Elizabeth Boudreau

This article reviews definitions and normal anatomy and physiology of canine and feline cerebral vasculature. The pathophysiology of cerebrovascular disease (CVD), which results from disturbance of cerebral blood supply, is described, along with its common causes and correlative

findings. The general clinical presentation of companion animals is described, although specific neurologic abnormalities depend on the neuroanatomic location of the disrupted blood supply. Current and future diagnostic approaches are described, including ancillary testing for predisposing factors. Acute and chronic management of patients with CVD is discussed. The prognosis for dogs and cats with acute CVD is generally considered good.

Fungal Infections of the Central Nervous System in Small Animals: Clinical Features, Diagnosis, and Management **63**

R. Timothy Bentley, Amanda R. Taylor, and Stephanie A. Thomovsky

Small animal mycoses vary geographically. Different clinical presentations are seen in animals with infection of the central nervous system (CNS), including multifocal meningoencephalomyelitis, intracranial lesions that accompany sinonasal lesions, rapidly progressive ventriculitis, or solitary granuloma of the brain or spinal cord. Systemic, nasal, or extraneural clinical signs are common but, especially in granuloma cases, do not always occur. Surgery may have a diagnostic and therapeutic role in CNS granuloma. There have been recent advancements in serology. Fluconazole, voriconazole, and posaconazole cross the blood-brain barrier, but voriconazole is neurotoxic to cats. Liposomal and lipid-encapsulated formulations of amphotericin B are preferred.

Diagnostic Imaging of Discospondylitis **85**

Catherine M. Ruoff, Sharon C. Kerwin, and Amanda R. Taylor

Discospondylitis can affect dogs of any age and breed and may be seen in cats. Although radiography remains the gold standard, advanced imaging, such as CT and MRI, has benefits and likely allows earlier diagnosis and identification of concurrent disease. Because discospondylitis may affect multiple disk spaces, imaging of the entire spine should be considered. There is a lengthening list of causative etiologic agents, and successful treatment hinges on correct identification. Image-guided biopsy should be considered in addition to blood and urine cultures and *Brucella canis* screening and as an alternative to surgical biopsy in some cases.

Acute Herniation of Nondegenerate Nucleus Pulposus: Acute Noncompressive Nucleus Pulposus Extrusion and Compressive Hydrated Nucleus Pulposus Extrusion **95**

Steven De Decker and Joe Fenn

Acute herniation of nondegenerate nucleus pulposus material is an important and relatively common cause of acute spinal cord dysfunction in dogs. Two types of herniation of nondegenerate or hydrated nucleus pulposus have been recognized: acute noncompressive nucleus pulposus extrusion (ANNPE) and acute compressive hydrated nucleus pulposus extrusion (HNPE). Spinal cord contusion plays an important role in the pathophysiology of both conditions. Sustained spinal cord compression is not present in ANNPE, whereas varying degrees of compression are present in HNPE. Although affected animals often present with severe neurologic signs, good outcomes can be achieved with appropriate treatment.

VETERINARY CLINICS OF NORTH AMERICA: SMALL ANIMAL PRACTICE

FORTHCOMING ISSUES

March 2018
Immunology and Vaccination
Amy E.S. Stone and Philip Kass, *Editors*

May 2018
Behavior as an Illness Indicator
Liz Stelow, *Editor*

July 2018
Small Animal Theriogenology
Bruce W. Christensen, *Editor*

RECENT ISSUES

November 2017
Wound Management
Marije Risselada, *Editor*

September 2017
Topics in Cardiology
João S. Orvalho, *Editor*

July 2017
Hip Dysplasia
Tisha A.M. Harper and J. Ryan Butler, *Editors*

RELATED INTEREST

Veterinary Clinics: Exotic Animal Practice
January 2018, Volume 21, Issue 1
Exotic Animal Neurology
Susan Orosz, *Editor*
Available at: http://www.vetexotic.theclinics.com

Erratum

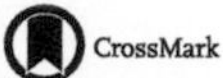

In the July 2017 issue (Volume 47, number 4), in the article on pages 917-934, "Zurich Cementless Total Hip Replacement," by David Hummel, figures 1-8, 14 and 17 should have included the following credit line: From Kyon Inc., with permission. Additionally, figures 9-13, 15 and 16 should have included the following credit line: Courtesy of Aldo Vezzoni, DVM, Dipl. ECVS, Clinica Veterinaria Vezzoni srl, Cremona, Italy.

A corrected version of this article can be found online at http://vetsmall.theclinics.com/.

Vet Clin Small Anim 48 (2018) xiii
https://doi.org/10.1016/j.cvsm.2017.10.009

Preface

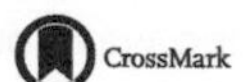

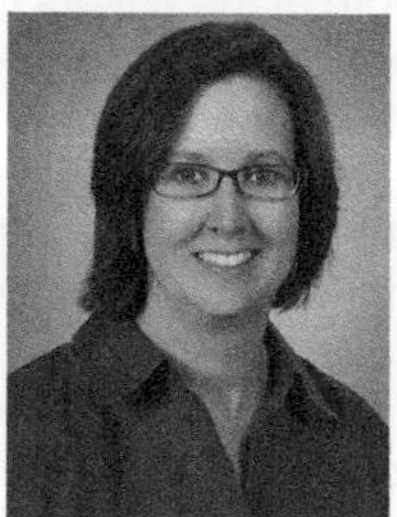

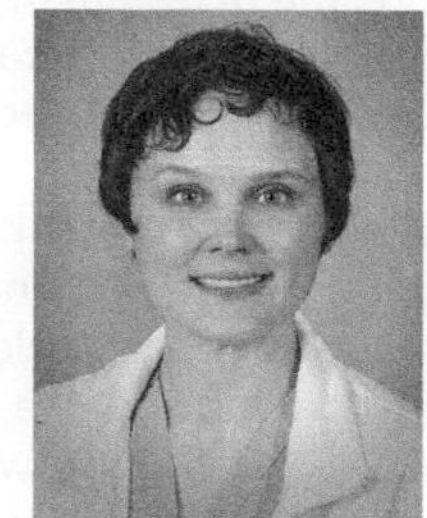

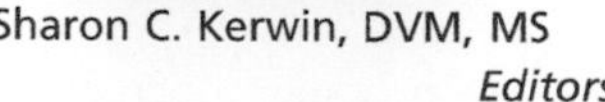

Sharon C. Kerwin, DVM, MS   Amanda R. Taylor, DVM
Editors

This issue of *Veterinary Clinics of North America: Small Animal Practice* is dedicated to neurology. Our diverse and somewhat eclectic choice of topics reflects the diversity of veterinary neurology: a specialty where emergency medicine, internal medicine, imaging, and surgery come together in a unique way unparalleled by any other specialty. We asked each author to give a practical and up-to-date summary of the state-of-the-art in their area of expertise.

Both of us are cat lovers, so we are pleased to have articles on clinical evaluation of the cat with neurologic disease and on seizure management, areas that are important and yet remain underrepresented in the veterinary literature. Moving on to neurologic emergencies, it is our experience that many veterinarians give patients with head trauma a poorer prognosis than is sometimes merited. New advances allow successful management of many of these patients in a general practice setting, despite an often spectacular clinical presentation.

MRI has catapulted our specialty into a new era, so we would be remiss in neglecting any opportunity to continue to delve into new advances. We are grateful to our radiology colleagues for providing a new article on high-field MRI. While even a decade ago, vascular events were thought to be rare in small animals, advances in imaging have dramatically increased our ability to identify these events. Both CNS fungal infections and pituitary hypophysectomy surgery hinge on our ability to make a correct imaging diagnosis, and we are excited about bringing you the latest in these areas.

Leaving the brain, we move on to the spine. As above, imaging allows us to differentiate the many subtleties of intervertebral disc herniation (IVDH). Controversy regarding indications for surgical decompression and new discoveries about acute noncompressive disc extrusion and hydrated nucleus pulposus extrusion challenge our preconceived notions about IVDH. Fenestration continues to be a hot topic...and should we be doing fenestration rather than decompression? If decompression of the spinal cord is elected, is corpectomy better than hemilaminectomy? And can we do it minimally invasively? Access to better technology will pave the way for future surgical breakthroughs. For both specialists and generalists, these articles will certainly change

Vet Clin Small Anim 48 (2018) xv–xvi
https://doi.org/10.1016/j.cvsm.2017.10.001
0195-5616/18/© 2017 Published by Elsevier Inc.

the way you think about surgical intervention for the treatment of intervertebral disk disease.

As imaging has evolved, so has our access to 3D printers, usually using CT scans of our patients. With a turn-around time of less than 24 hours, both of the editors use 3D printed models when we approach challenging cases, and a review of this area is very timely. Discospondylitis, which seems to be becoming more common as we utilize more advanced imaging, continues to present diagnostic and therapeutic challenges. Finally, interest in acupuncture as an adjunct to conventional treatment is growing as more veterinarians gain experience with traditional Chinese veterinary medicine.

Both of us completed our neurology residencies at Texas A&M University, and we are grateful to our mentors, Drs Jonathan Levine (Taylor and Kerwin), Joseph Mankin (Taylor and Kerwin), and Dr Beth Boudreau (Kerwin), all of whom contributed in some way to this publication. Last, a special thank-you to our families, who put up with us during this event!

Sharon C. Kerwin, DVM, MS
Department of Small Animal Clinical Sciences
College of Veterinary Medicine and Biomedical Sciences
Texas A&M University
College Station, TX 77843-4474, USA

Amanda R. Taylor, DVM
Department of Clinical Sciences
Auburn University College of
Veterinary Medicine
Auburn, AL 36849, USA

E-mail addresses:
skerwin@cvm.tamu.edu (S.C. Kerwin)
art0022@auburn.edu (A.R. Taylor)

Clinical Evaluation of the Feline Neurologic Patient

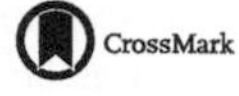

Amanda R. Taylor, DVM[a,*], Sharon C. Kerwin, DVM, MS[b]

KEYWORDS

• Seizures • Myelopathy • Encephalopathy • Cat

KEY POINTS

- Efficient, gentle, and safe handling of cats can result in complete neurologic evaluations and accurate neuroanatomic localizations.
- The clinic environment should facilitate the examination by providing a quiet and secure environment for the cat.
- When direct examination of a cat is not possible, the practitioner should fully use indirect methods of examination and video recordings of cat behavior or clinical signs.
- Direct examination of a cat should proceed in a logical order, where the most useful tests are performed early on in the examination.

 **Video content accompanies this article at http://www.vetsmall.theclinics.com.**

INTRODUCTION

Animals with neurologic disease can be challenging for any practitioner. This task may seem even more daunting when the patient is a cat. As a result, veterinarians' level of stress in dealing with these patients and the emotional environment they create for their patients, themselves, their staff, and clients can set up failure or success. A few accommodations in preparation for cat examinations and adaptations in the neurologic evaluation can result in a successful visit that is defined by low stress, accurate neuroanatomic localization, and appropriate diagnostic plan.

The preparation of the clinic, staff, and doctors involves developing an understanding of the unique qualities of feline behavior and altering the environment, handling, and examination accordingly. Cats with neurologic disease may present additional obstacles due to the relative lack of tolerance for the length of and restraint in classic veterinary neurologic evaluations.

The authors have nothing to disclose.
[a] Department of Clinical Sciences, Auburn University College of Veterinary Medicine, Auburn, AL 36849, USA; [b] Department of Small Animal Clinical Sciences, Texas A&M University, College Station, TX 77843, USA
* Corresponding author.
E-mail address: art0022@auburn.edu

Vet Clin Small Anim 48 (2018) 1–10
http://dx.doi.org/10.1016/j.cvsm.2017.08.001 vetsmall.theclinics.com
0195-5616/18/

In the authors' experience, examination of the neurologic cat has key differences, such as limiting repetition, using tests that are reliable, and focusing the examination on what is most likely to yield results that determine a neuroanatomic localization. The authors' practical steps to preparing for the examination and the indirect and direct components of the examination in the cat are discussed.

GOALS OF THE EXAMINATION

1. Provide an environment and handling techniques that promote a low-stress interaction
2. Using indirect techniques whenever possible
3. Acquiring information from the cat using minimal handling and restraint
4. Localizing the neuroanatomic lesion

PREPARATION STRATEGIES

The Nature of the Cat

The inherent nature of feline patients is that of a solitary hunter that fights as a last resort if flight from a confrontation is unsuccessful or not possible. Veterinarians are in control of many factors in the veterinary clinic that could result in a cat identifying a need to run or confront. These include noise level, odors, quick movements, presence of other species such as dogs, the brightness of a room, brusque or aggressive handling, and agitated handlers. Even when the best prevention strategies are used, cats may still display behavior that indicates they are threatened.[1,2]

Clinic Admission

Although a trip in the car can be a joyous occasion for a dog that could result in a trip to a lake or dog park, cats are unlikely to be in a car at any time other than when they visit a veterinarian. They are not conditioned to being placed in a carrier and transported. By the time cats arrive at a veterinarian's office, they may already be in some state of stress from the car ride to the clinic. The additional stimuli of a visit to the hospital from the noises, smells, and other elements encountered in the lobby of a clinic can be of further threat to a cat.

To limit the negative factors that can detract from the visit, several steps should be taken:

1. Discuss with clients that all cats must be in their own carrier at the hospital and cannot be removed from the carrier until they are moved to the examination room.
2. Allow more time for appointments where the chief complaint is consistent with neurologic disease.
3. Provide a separate waiting area and entrance for cats when possible.
4. Guide the client and cat into an examination room as quickly as possible if a separate waiting area is not available.
5. Maintain 1 or 2 examination rooms that are for feline patients only.
6. Control the light, odor, and noise in the room by providing soft light, synthetic feline facial pheromone analogue, and keep the doors closed.
7. Provide equipment in the examination room to make the cat more comfortable, such as a thick towel on the examination table, catnip, laser pointers, cat treats, and toys.[1–6]

Recognition of Feline Behavior

A well-trained veterinary team can recognize when a cat is fearful or combative and can change an approach when these signs are first identified, rather than reacting after a cat has acted in a defensive and aggressive manner. Experienced cat handlers carefully observe a cat's facial expression, tail movement, and body posture.

When cats identify a threat, they may display mydriasis, whiskers flattened toward the face, wide opening of the eyes, and a general tightening of the muscles of facial expression. The ears change from their normal erect posture to a rostral tilt and to a gradual flattening. The tail may begin to twitch or flick back and forth. A stressed cat has postures, such as arching of the back, bringing the head down toward the ground, and pulling the feet close to the body. Identification of any of these changes in the cat should cause an examiner or handler to either change tactics in handling or take a break in interaction.

If a cat does not display warning signs or if these signs are not recognized, more aggressive behavior from the cat can result. This includes further arching of the back, narrowing of the pupils, and finally vocalization, striking out with the front feet, or attempting to bite the veterinarian or handler. When any of these signs is recognized, the cat should be allowed a respite from the examination or the examination should be concluded.[1,2]

Client Education

Cat owners are often astute and in tune with their pets. Some of the tests performed during neurologic examination can appear strange or even scary to a client, not to mention the negative reactions these tests may elicit from the cat. The authors have been most successful in performing feline examinations for neurologic disease when explaining what will occur to clients prior to performing an examination. The authors explain to the clients that if a cat indicates that the examination is too stressful, the examination will cease and observing the patient will be continued. Open communication with clients prior to examination creates a partnership between client and veterinarian that facilitates the other aspects of a cat's treatment and diagnostics.

INDIRECT PATIENT EVALUATION STRATEGIES

During neurologic examination of a dog, an examiner may repeat tests multiple times and come back to the same test more than once, but cats are often less tolerant of this technique in examination. The order of the examination listed herein is how the authors proceed unless, as they begin to evaluate the case, a cat becomes intolerant of the examination. Should this occur, the order of the examination is changed to prioritize the most helpful tests or a break is taken; for example, cats presenting for seizures indicate they will not tolerate much examination after indirect evaluation. In this case, the authors initially limit the examination to evaluation of cranial nerves followed by postural reactions. If these initial tests were tolerated, other elements of the examination could be completed. The authors attempt to move through the examination with efficiency and safety. If there is an abnormality that needs to be reassessed and the cat is tolerating examination, this portion of the examination is revisited after other tests are complete.

Video Recording

Any cat presenting for a possible neurologic disease should undergo a neurologic examination, but there are some that do not tolerate nor participate. In these cases, it is necessary to base diagnostic and therapeutic plans on historical findings, indirect observations, and, when available, video of the cat in the home environment. One of the most helpful ways to supplement the information gained from the history is to ask owners to video record their observations. Because many clients own smart phones with this capability, this is a practical request. The client can record video before the appointment, or if the examination is unsuccessful the client can send video to the veterinarian at a later time. Even in the most tolerant cats, the changes or problems observed by the client may not be displayed at the clinic. In these cases, video of the cat at home may allow a veterinarian to see the cause of a client's concern. Primary veterinarians seeking consultation with a neurologist or other specialist for assistance with a case can also use video from the client or from the examination in the clinic.

Mentation

Key history questions can enable a veterinarian to learn what a cat's mentation is like at home. These include open-ended questions, such as: How does your cat's temperament now compare to 6 months ago? What does your cat enjoy the most in life? and How does your cat normally interact with you and/or your family/spouse/significant other?

Once a cat has been taken to an examination area, the front of the cage should be opened to allow the cat to exit if it is willing. Alternatively, the top of the carrier can be removed and the cat can explore its surroundings. The history of the cat is discussed while the cat is left alone to allow it time to feel comfortable to exit the carrier. It may take quite some time for the cat to decide to exit the carrier, up to 10 minutes in the authors' experience. In some cases, the cat does not participate in this way. The cat can be gently lifted from the carrier (once the lid has been removed) and placed on the floor away from the carrier to observe its interactions with the environment. Forcing a cat from its carrier by pulling it through the door of the carrier can result in abnormal behavior and unnecessary stress for the patient and is therefore discouraged.[1,2]

Posture

Posture is concurrently assessed with gait and mentation. Common abnormal postures seen include head tilts and turns, ventroflexion of the neck and plantigrade stance (**Fig. 1**). The cat must be carefully observed to determine whether it has low head carriage secondary to fear or weakness. A weak cat does not move the head often and the nose of the cat may point ventrally, whereas a fearful cat pulls the head in toward the body and the nose is pointed away from the tail with the nose pointed forward. Plantigrade stance can be difficult to determine in a cat that is uncomfortable in the clinic and is walking carefully around the room or choosing not to walk. Nervous or scared cats tend to have all 4 feet lowered and pulled in close to the body.

Gait

Challenges with gait evaluation arise when a cat is fearful, because these cats stay as low to the ground as possible when walking or crouch in one place and are reluctant to

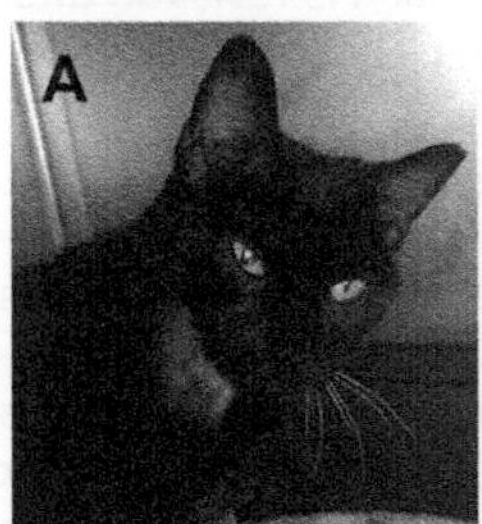

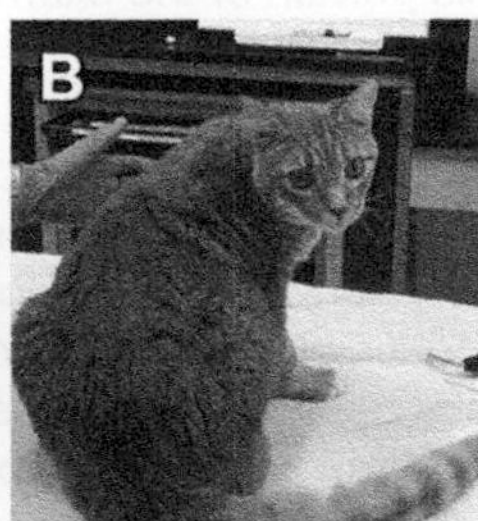

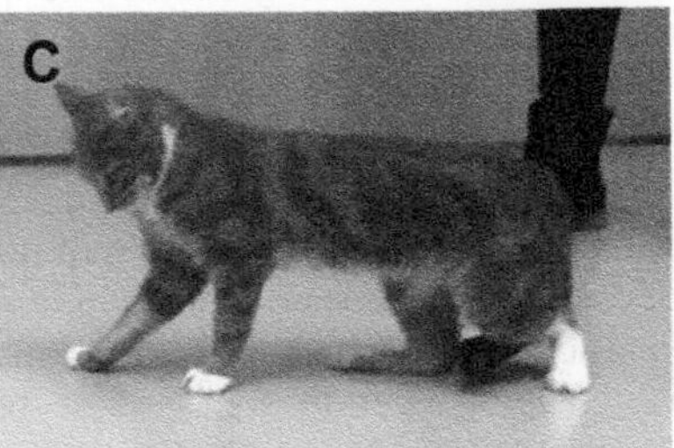

Fig. 1. Cats displaying common abnormal postures: head tilt (*A*), head turn (*B*), and concurrent ventroflexion of the neck with plantigrade stance (*C*).

move. Gait should always be evaluated on a surface with good traction in a room that is closed off to ensure the cat's safety. In cats with abnormal gait, the femoral pulses should always be evaluated if the pelvic limbs are affected (generally done prior to neurologic examination) and an orthopedic examination performed (generally after neurologic examination because direct orthopedic examination may hinder appropriate neuroanatomic localization due to lack of patient compliance with extensive examination).

The following questions should be run through when evaluating the gait to determine if there is a neurologic cause of abnormal gait:

1. Is the cat off-balance (ataxic)? Cats may display proprioceptive (crossing over of the limbs or scuffing of the dorsal surface of the paws), vestibular (circling or falling), or cerebellar ataxia (hypermetria and intention tremors).
2. Does the cat appear weak in a limb (plantigrade or palmigrade stance)?
3. Is there lameness associated with the gait (off-loading of weight seen as a short stride in a limb, head bob, or hike of a hip dorsally when walking)?
4. What is the length of the steps the cat is taking (long strides with a delay in forward movement can indicate proprioceptive deficits; short strides can indicate lameness or a lower motor neuron lesion)?
5. Can you hear scuffing of the dorsal aspect of the paws when you listen to the gait (this is most often an indication of proprioceptive deficits)?

Several techniques can be used to encourage ambulation in the cat in a gentle manner.

1. Laser pointers
   a. A cat's attraction to the light of a laser can cause a previously reluctant cat to follow the light on the floor.
   b. Following a laser pointer may cause a previously unobserved intention tremor to be elicited.
2. Carrier
   a. A cat may think the carrier is a safe place to hide from the examiner.
   b. Place the carrier at the opposite end of the room from the cat on the ground, the cat may walk to it.
   c. Some cats follow a person carrying the carrier across the room.
3. Step stool
   a. A step stool less than two feet tall can cause a cat to move.
   b. Place the cat on top of the stool.
   c. Most cats jump down and walk away from the stool.
   d. If a cat is unwilling to jump down, place a hand over the dorsum or behind it and gently nudge it forward.

DIRECT PATIENT EVALUATION STRATEGIES

Handling and Restraint

A cat cannot be forced into undergoing an examination if the goals are to get accurate results and not harm the cat. The more a cat is made to participate when displaying signs of stress, the more likely a negative or aggressive response is elicited from the cat, resulting in an end to the examination, harm to the cat, or harm to the examiner or handler. Rough handling, such as loudly verbally scolding, scruffing, or muzzling the cat, is likely to result in undesired responses from the cat. Physical contact with a cat during the examination should proceed quietly and slowly, always with the first approach to the cat over the back of the head or the neck and never with a quick approach to the cat's face.

The authors have spent considerable time in investment on the education of their staff in appropriate handling techniques. Implementation of a team approach is the basis for a successful neurologic examination being completed. Acceptable restraint techniques include the use of sturdy Elizabethan collars (the authors prefer reusable collars that snap into place), thick towels, and patience for the cat (**Fig. 2**). If a cat does not tolerate examination, an indirect approach consisting of observation is recommended.

Prioritization of Examination

The order of an examination can be changed and prioritized based on observations made during the indirect examination. If a cat displays signs that direct handling will not be tolerated for long, as discussed previously, the examination can be prioritized by first determining whether or not the gait of the cat is abnormal. Although this method is not failsafe, it can ensure that the most information is gained prior to having to end the examination.

Cranial Nerves

Frightened or stressed cats may not have normal responses to cranial nerve testing, regardless of whether they have neurologic deficits, resulting in false-negative examinations (**Table 1**).[7–12] Therefore, the authors usually test cranial nerves prior to other direct neurologic assessment. A cotton-tipped applicator may be used instead of a finger to perform many of the cranial nerve tests in the cat. All the tests may be performed while a cat is wearing a sturdy Elizabethan collar, should that be necessary for patient and examiner safety. An assessment of facial symmetry is made prior to performing any of the tests discussed later. When possible, the authors recommend performing assessment without touching the cat, because facial expression may change drastically in response to human touch.

In the authors' experience, menace is more reliably assessed when a cat is minimally stressed; therefore, menace is the first direct cranial nerve reflex performed. One eye is covered while the other is assessed as tolerated by the patient. If a cat does not initially respond to a menacing gesture, a gentle tap at the medial and lateral canthus of the eye (which also serves as the palpebral test) may cause a cat to respond to menace testing appropriately. Normal cats often incompletely close their

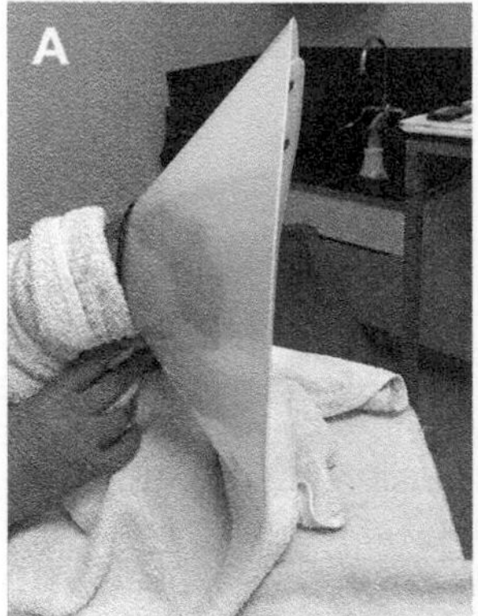

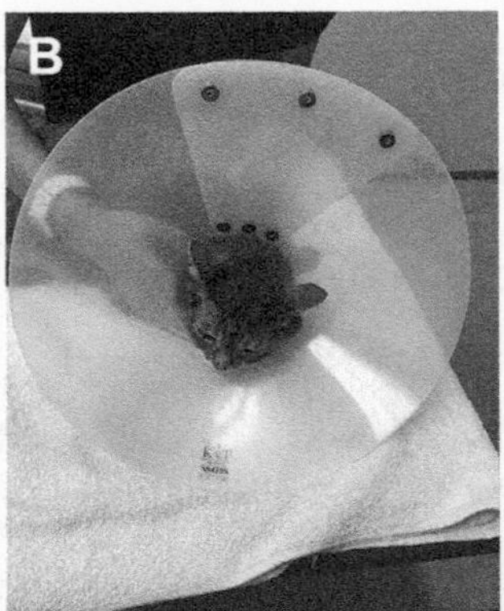

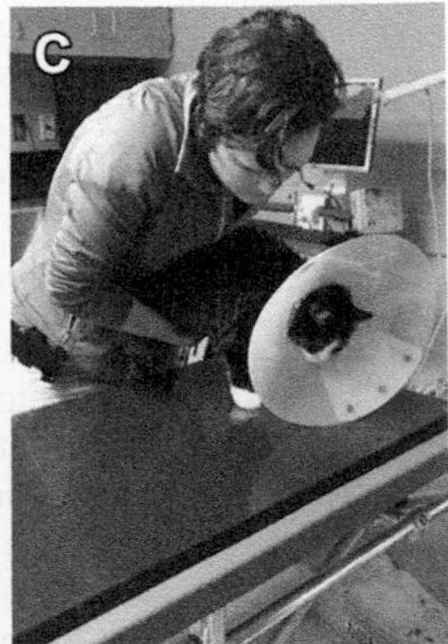

Fig. 2. Profile (*A*) and front view (*B*) of a cat restrained in a reusable Elizabethan collar for examination. Performance of hopping testing in cat with Elizabethan collar (*C*).

Table 1 Cranial nerve tests		
Cranial Nerve Test	**Afferent Arm**	**Efferent Arm**
Menace	CN II	CN VII
Pupillary light reflex	CN II	CN III
Palpebral reflex	CN V	CN VII
Sensation, face	CN V	CN VII
Gag	CN IX	CN X
Physiologic nystagmus	Vestibular apparatus	CNs III and VI

Abbreviation: CN, cranial nerve.

eyes in response to this test. Although a canine patient's reliable interest in cotton balls allows for visual tracking, most cats seem to be less interested in cotton ball testing and the authors have not found this reliable for assessment of vision.

Palpebral reflex is assessed after menace by gently tapping the medial and lateral canthus of each eye to elicit a blink, often with a cotton-tipped applicator for the safety of the examiner. Physiologic nystagmus can be more difficult to elicit and assess in a cat by turning the head from side to side. In cats of calm temperament, it is most helpful for an examiner to pick up a cat, and, with it facing the examiner, the examiner twists his/her body from side to side at the waist, moving the cat with him/her and observing its eyes for movement (Video 1). The cat's eyes should quickly move in the direction the examiner is turning. An evaluation for positional strabismus is performed by swiftly lifting the head and checking the globes for lack of central position of the iris.

Facial sensation is assessed by touching either side of the maxilla, mandible, temporal region, and medial nasal mucosa. The cat should respond by blinking or consciously responding to the sensation with turning the head or body away from the stimulus, vocalization, or other responses.

Assessment of a cat's gag reflex can be performed directly by touching the caudal pharyngeal wall with a finger, generally the index finger. In patients where it is not believed this will be tolerated, pressure can be externally placed on/rub the pharyngeal region and patient observed for swallowing and licking.

Pupillary light reflex is assessed by shining a strong light in 1 pupil and observing both irises for constriction. Fearful cats may have pupils that are mydriatic at rest and less responsive to pupillary light reflex assessment due to increased sympathetic tone; however, direct and indirect responses should still be present.

Postural Reactions

The authors' evaluation of postural reactions begins with utilization of the same step stool that was discussed previously regarding gait evaluation. When a cat jumps down from the stool, if there are deficits in the proprioceptive system, the cat may stumble when it lands. When performing postural reaction testing in dogs, the authors almost always start with knuckling, followed by hopping and other tests, such as wheelbarrowing. In the cat, however, the authors typically perform 1 or 2 methods of postural reaction testing: hopping (most reliable) or tactile placing where the patient is brought to the edge of the table and allowed to place 1 paw at a time on the surface of the table. Knuckling is typically not performed because the reaction in most cats is withdrawal of the limb and inability for an examiner to place the dorsal surface of the paw on the ground. Although some examiners may find knuckling to be a helpful test by observing whether the cat places its paw on the surface normally, the authors find that the cat examined may become agitated by having its feet touched repetitively during knuckling.

Segmental Reflexes

In a classic neurologic examination of a companion animal, the patient is restrained in lateral recumbency to perform segmental reflexes (**Table 2**).[7–12] This technique is often unsuccessful in the cat. To keep a cat in lateral recumbency, the necessary degree of restraint can result in the cat no longer tolerating examination. Therefore, the authors recommend segmental reflexes should be performed with the cat either standing or in extremely tolerant cats on their back in the lap of the examiner. The initial assessment is limited to the flexor withdrawal reflexes of all limbs and patellar reflexes because the authors have found the other reflexes to be unreliable in performance and interpretation. After these initial segmental reflex tests, cutaneous trunci and perineal reflex are assessed in the standing cat. Other reflexes are assessed in some cases, such as cranial tibial, gastrocnemius, triceps, extensor carpi, and biceps reflexes. For example, a cat with monoparesis of a pelvic limb might have all the pelvic limb reflexes assessed.

Nociception Testing

Nociception testing is only performed in cats with absent voluntary motor function.[7–12] If voluntary motor function is present, the degree of dysfunction of the spinal cord or nerves is not severe enough to result in loss of sensation and, therefore, does not warrant nociception testing. The interdigital webbing of the affected limb is tested for superficial nociception by compression with fingers (first) or hemostat forceps (second if no response to digital pressure). The cat is observed for a conscious response to the stimulus, such as turning of the head, vocalization, or attempts to bite. If superficial nociception is absent, deep nociception is tested by cross-clamping a digit of the affected limb with hemostat forceps.

Hyperesthesia Detection and Palpation

While the cat is standing, gentle palpation is performed to detect head pain and paraspinal discomfort. Gentle pressure is placed on head using the thumb and middle finger in the temporal region, as if picking up a 6-pack. Palpation of the paraspinal

Table 2
Segmental reflexes

Reflex	Spinal Cord Segments
Flexor withdrawal, thoracic limb	C6–T2
Biceps	C6–8
Triceps	C7–T2
Extensor carpi radialis	C7–T1
Flexor withdrawal, pelvic limb	L4–S2
Patellar	L4–L6
Gastrocnemius	L6–S2
Cranial tibial	L6–L7
Cutaneous trunci	C8–T1 (efferent), T3–L3
Perineal	S1–S3

musculature is performed with mild pressure placed with the index and middle finger of the dominant hand on the epaxial muscles on dorsal midline proceeding from caudal to cranial. The cervical region is slowly put through a range of motion to detect for resistance or painful reactions from the cat. If initial gentle palpation does not elicit a response, firm pressure is applied and the tests repeated.

Although cessation of panting can be a reliable sign of pain in the dog, cats have other indications. Observed changes include flattening of the ears, lowering of the head, or a sudden contraction of the epaxial muscles tested. Typical responses, such as vocalization, turning of the head, and other behaviors, may also be seen.

SUMMARY

Efficient, gentle, and safe handling of cats can result in complete neurologic evaluations and accurate neuroanatomic localizations. The clinic environment should facilitate the examination by providing a quiet and secure environment for the cat. When direct examination of a cat is not possible, the practitioner should fully use indirect methods of examination and video recordings of cat behavior or clinical signs. Direct examination of a cat should proceed in a logical order where the most useful tests are performed early on in an examination. Should a cat become intolerant of examination, the practitioner should conclude the handling of the cat.

SUPPLEMENTARY DATA

Supplementary data related to this article can be found online at https://doi.org/10.1016/j.cvsm.2017.08.001.

REFERENCES

1. Rodan I, Sundahl E, Carney H, et al. AAFP and ISFM feline-friendly handling guidelines. J Feline Med Surg 2011;13(5):364–75.
2. Rodan I, Heath S. Feline behavioral health and welfare. St. Louis (MO): Elsevier Health Sciences; 2015.
3. Kronen PW, Ludders JW, Erb HN, et al. A synthetic fraction of feline facial pheromones calms but does not reduce struggling in cats before venous catheterization. Vet Anaesth Analg 2006;33(4):258–65.
4. Pereira JS, Fragoso S, Beck A, et al. Improving the feline veterinary consultation: the usefulness of Feliway spray in reducing cats' stress. J Feline Med Surg 2016;18(12):959–64.
5. Frank D, Beauchamp G, Palestrini C. Systematic review of the use of pheromones for treatment of undesirable behavior in cats and dogs. J Am Vet Med Assoc 2010;236(12):1308–16.
6. Gunn-Moore DA, Cameron ME. A pilot study using synthetic feline facial pheromone for the management of feline idiopathic cystitis. J Feline Med Surg 2004;6(3):133–8.
7. De Lahunta A, Glass EN, Kent M. Veterinary neuroanatomy and clinical neurology. Elsevier Health Sciences; 2014.
8. Dewey CW, da Costa RC. Practical guide to canine and feline neurology. John Wiley & Sons; 2015.
9. Garosi L. Neurological lameness in the cat: common causes and clinical approach. J Feline Med Surg 2012;14(1):85–93.
10. Lorenz MD, Coates J, Kent M. Handbook of veterinary neurology. Elsevier Health Sciences; 2010.

11. Fingeroth JM, Thomas WB, editors. Advances in intervertebral disc disease in dogs and cats. John Wiley & Sons; 2015.
12. Garosi L. Neurological examination of the cat: how to get started. J Feline Med Surg 2009;11:340–8.

Advances in High-Field MRI

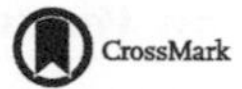

Adrien-Maxence Hespel, DVM, MS[a], Robert C. Cole, DVM[b,*]

KEYWORDS

• MRI • Diffusion-weighted imaging • Magnetic resonance spectrography
• Diffusion tensor imaging • Parallel imaging • CSF flow tracking

KEY POINTS

- Magnetic resonance (MR) is an exciting and ever-expanding imaging modality.
- Advances in MR technology include higher field strengths, new techniques, faster gradients, improved coil technology, and more robust sequence protocols.
- Techniques to move beyond simply generating anatomic images to studying patterns of diffusion, white matter tracking, proton spectrography, and spin labeling for flow tracking are advancing rapidly and are now feasible not only for research but also for clinical use.

INTRODUCTION

This article focuses on advanced modern MRI techniques and sequences. These topics include diffusion-weighted imaging (DWI), magnetic resonance spectroscopy (MRS), diffusion tensor imaging (DTI), and cerebrospinal fluid (CSF) tracking.

MRI is an imaging modality based on the principles of resonance of atomic nuclei (nuclear magnetic resonance).[1–3] Briefly, a magnetic resonance (MR) system is a combination of magnets, coils, gradients, and a computer control station. Using this equipment, a proton (typically hydrogen) can be excited, spatially located, and an image generated.[1,2,4] Most pathologic processes alter the environment of hydrogen protons in tissues, making MR a sensitive tool for imaging disease. When the patient is placed into the MR scanner, the hydrogen protons align with the main magnetic field (B0). An excitatory radiofrequency (RF) pulse is applied, which causes the hydrogen protons to absorb that energy, changing their energy state. When the protons return to their original energy state, a RF energy is produced and released, creating a signal detected in the receiver coil. This signal fades over time as the result of 2 processes, known as T1 and T2 relaxation. The differences in the relaxation times of tissues result in the image contrast. Water has long relaxation times, soft tissues are intermediate, and fat has short relaxation times. By using different MR sequences, these properties can be exploited and tissues differentiated.[1–4]

Disclosure: The authors have nothing to disclose.

[a] Department of Small Animal Clinical Science, University of Tennessee, 2407 River Drive, Knoxville, TN 37991, USA; [b] Department of Small Animal Clinical Science, University of Auburn, 1200 Wire Road, Auburn, AL 36839, USA
* Corresponding author.
E-mail address: rcc0025@auburn.edu

Vet Clin Small Anim 48 (2018) 11–29
http://dx.doi.org/10.1016/j.cvsm.2017.08.002
vetsmall.theclinics.com

Low Versus High Field

At the core of all MR systems is the magnet. The magnet determines signal to noise ratio (SNR) and therefore image quality. The SNR increases approximately linearly with field strength if a similar sequence setup is used.

MR systems are classified as open or closed and as high or low field. High-field MR is usually reserved for systems between 1.5 and 3 T.[3] Most of these systems are closed with a tunnel-like orientation. Low-field scanners are open design and range from 0.2 to 0.3 T. These systems have open sides. The benefits of low-field MR include design and cost as well as easier positioning and monitoring of the patient. Purchase cost is typically much less compared with high-field systems. High field has many advantages that make the cost differential less significant, including greater SNR resulting in improved image quality, thinner slice acquisition, and faster scan times.[3–5]

Ultrahigh Field

Ultrahigh-field MRI operates at a field strength of 7 T and up to 11.4 T. SNR and contrast are the two major contributors to the quality of the MR image, and increase with field strength.[6,7] Higher field means higher potential for lesion localization and characterization. Ultrahigh-field MRI allows the acquisition of higher resolution images with reasonable acquisition times (**Figs. 1** and **2**).[8–15]

ADVANCED TECHNIQUES

Diffusion-Weighted Imaging

DWI is a valuable tool in neuroimaging. Diffusion-weighted imaging and the apparent diffusion coefficient (ADC; calculated from the DWI) provide a quantitative measurement of the brownian motion of water in a three-dimensional space.[2,16–20] Quantification of water diffusion is obtained through the addition of strong gradient pulses that phase encode the location of the hydrogen atoms. An initial diffusion gradient pulse is applied, followed by a second opposing diffusion gradient pulse of equal strength and duration. If the water molecules are stationary, the second diffusion gradient restores the original phase of the hydrogen atoms leading to a coherent signal. If the water molecules are mobile, the phase of the protons following the second gradient will have changed, leading to a decrease in signal. DWI is performed by applying diffusion gradients to T2-weighted sequences and can be performed with a variable parameter called the b value. ADC values are calculated based on the DWI data obtained with at least 2 different b values (diffusion gradient factor). These values represent a

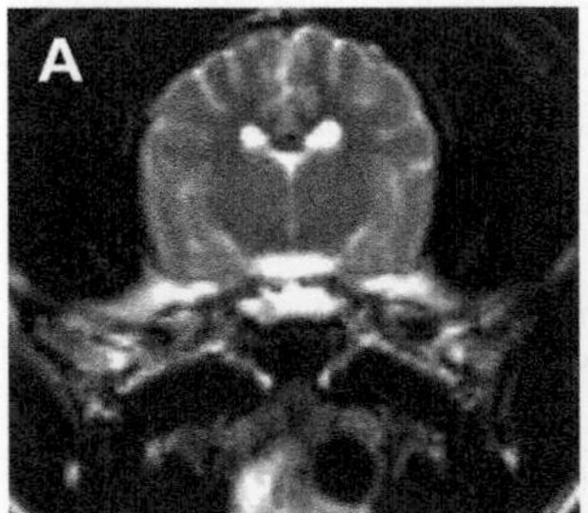

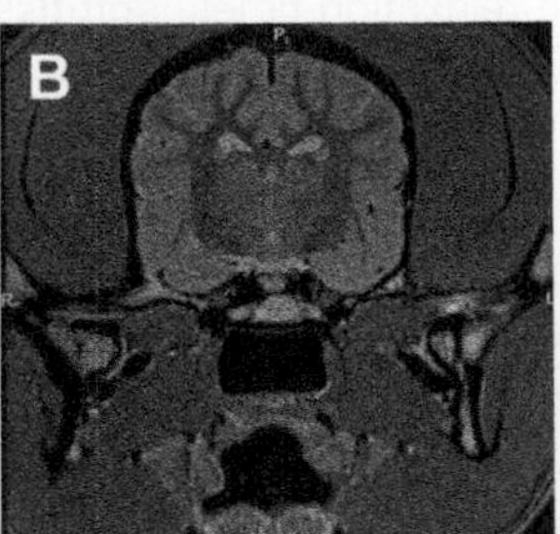

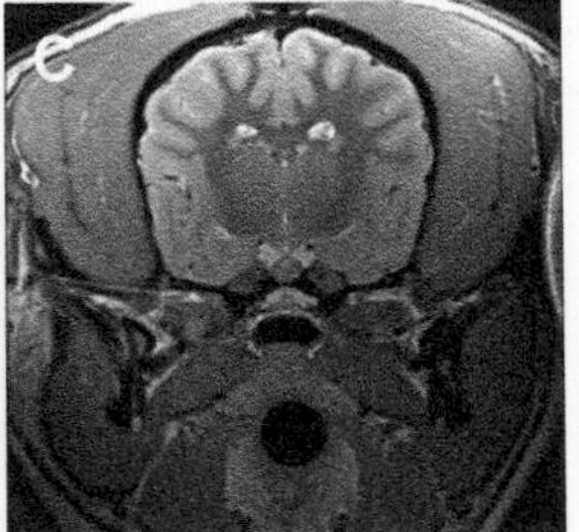

Fig. 1. Transverse T2-weighted images of a mature canine brain at the level of the thalamus. (*A*) 1.5-T turbo spin echo (TSE) T2 at 5-mm slice thickness, (*B*) 3-T TSE T2 at 0.7-mm slice thickness, and (*C*) 7-T TSE T2 0.4-mm slice thickness.

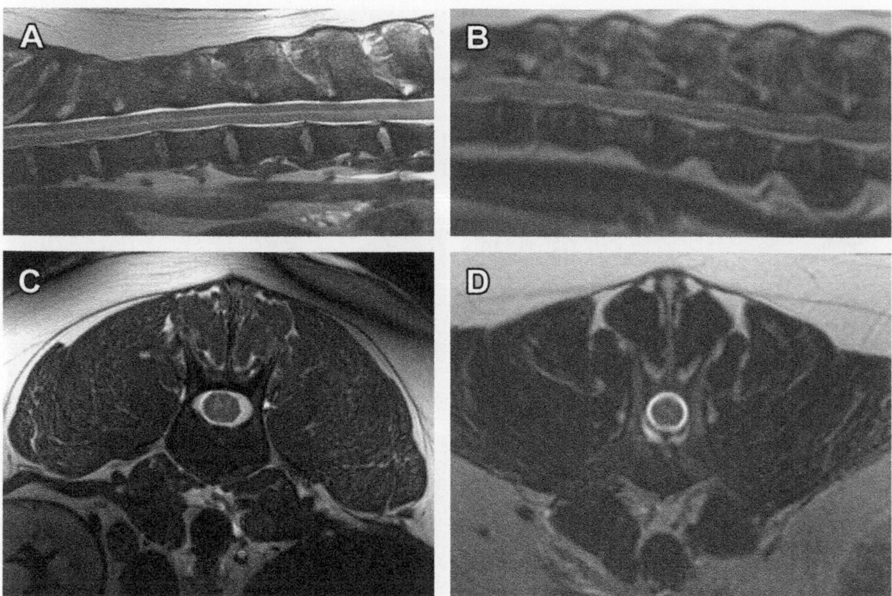

Fig. 2. Sagittal and transverse TSE T2 images of the lumbar vertebral column of canine patients. (*A, C*) 7 T, (*B, D*) similar locations at 1.5 T.

quantitative expression of water diffusion within the voxel and are displayed on an ADC map.[16–20]

Unrestricted diffusion of water (eg, CSF) produces a high signal on DWI (acquired with a high b value) and a high signal on ADC. In contrast, restricted diffusion of water has a high signal on DWI (acquired with a high and low b value) and low signal on ADC (**Table 1**).[16–20]

One of the pitfalls of DWI occurs when the signal from a tissue with a long T2 decay time is visible on DWI. The signal does not occur because of restricted diffusion and is referred to as T2 shine-through. This shine-through can be seen in conditions such as vasogenic edema (**Fig. 3**) or cystic structures.

DWI allows early detection of physiologic changes associated with cerebral ischemia, making it invaluable for identifying cerebrovascular accidents.[17] Acute infarction causes water to become trapped within the cells, resulting in reduced diffusion.[18,19,21,22] Abnormalities on the ADC can be seen within 1 hour of the onset of ischemia with reduction in apparent diffusion seen within 2.5 minutes.[19] An acute infarction is typically hyperintense

Table 1
Summary of the potential changes found on apparent diffusion coefficient and diffusion-weighted imaging with their associated clinical implications

	ADC Map	Low-B-Value DWI	High-B-Value DWI
T2 shine-through	Hyperintense (+)	Hyperintense (+)	Hyperintense (+)
Restricted diffusion	Hypointense (–)	Hyperintense or hypointense (+)/(–)	Hyperintense (+)
Nonrestricted diffusion	Hyperintense (+)	Hyperintense (+)	Hypointense (–)
Loss of signal	Hypointense (–)	Hypointense (–)	Hypointense (–)

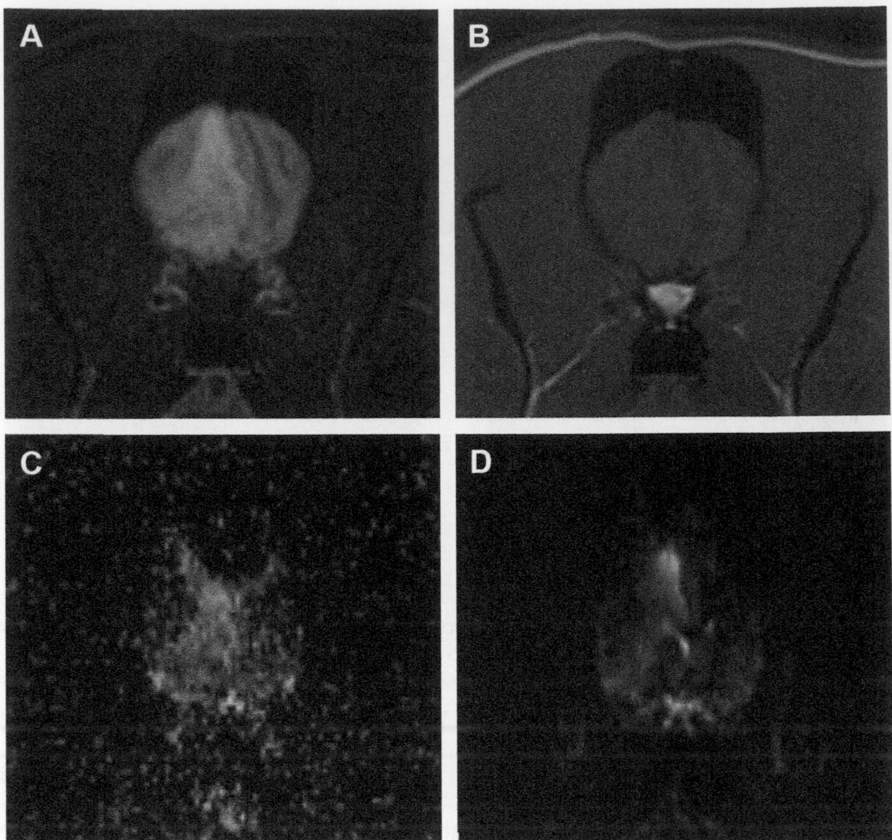

Fig. 3. Transverse images acquired at 1.5 T at the level of the frontal lobes. (*A*) Fluid-attenuated inversion recovery (FLAIR), (*B*) T1 postcontrast, (*C*) ADC map, and (*D*) DWI sequence. The changes seen are those of T2 shine-through. The lesion is hyperintense on FLAIR, DWI, and ADC, whereas it is isointense on T1. This finding was associated with vasogenic edema secondary to an extra-axial mass in the rostral aspect of the cerebrum (likely to be a meningioma).

on DWI and hypointense on ADC (**Fig. 4**). The ADC is less than normal in the first 4 to 10 days and normalizes with chronicity. The ADC goes from reduced diffusion to high (hypointense to hyperintense) after 7 to 10 days, allowing estimation of the age of the lesion.[18,19,21–26] Although this pattern is not unique to ischemic stroke, classic imaging appearance coupled with history is usually sufficient for diagnosis. As with cerebrovascular accidents in the brain, DWI has been used in the spinal cord to identify acute ischemic events. The imaging pattern is similar (hyperintense on DWI and hypointense on ADC) and normalizes after 7 days.[27,28]

Restricted water diffusion can present in disease processes other than ischemia. ADC values may be decreased in highly cellular tumors such as lymphoma, medulloblastoma, and high-grade gliomas.[29–38] ADC values are decreased in highly viscous materials (cerebral abscess).[39–42] Lower ADC values were associated with higher grade tumors and poorer prognosis, and[36,38,43] are used in predicting the progression of intracranial disease in humans. For example, primary central nervous system (CNS) lymphoma with a low pretreatment ADC value was associated with a higher risk of

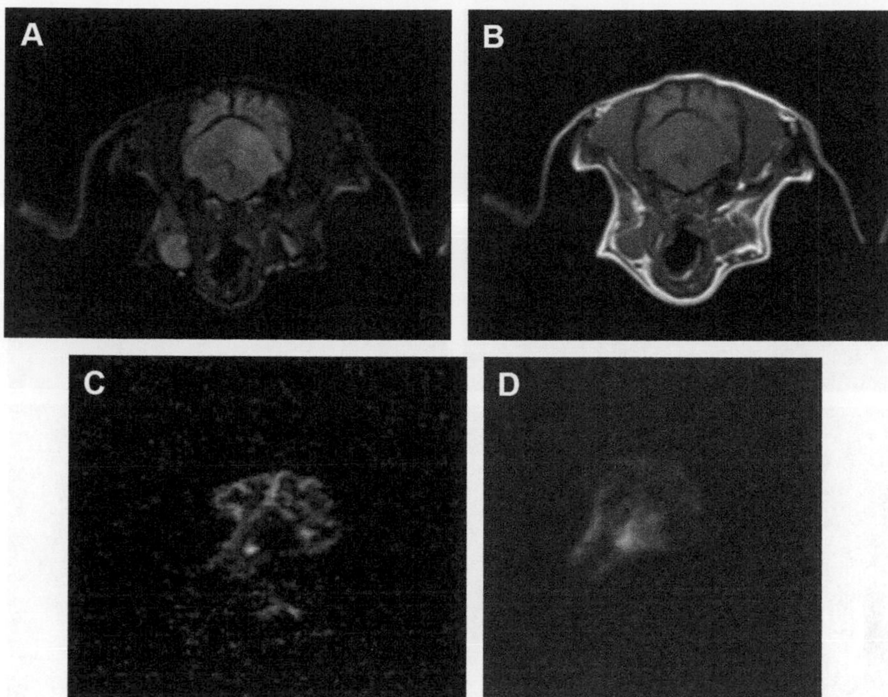

Fig. 4. Transverse images acquired at 1.5 T at the level of the cerebellomedullary angle. (*A*) FLAIR, (*B*) T1 postcontrast, (*C*) ADC map, and (*D*) DWI sequence. The changes are characteristic for a nonhemorrhagic infarct and restricted diffusion. The lesion is hyperintense on FLAIR and DWI, isointense on T1, and hypointense on ADC.

progression and death.[32] Increasing ADC values observed on serial MR examinations may indicate treatment response because responding neoplastic lesions undergo a reduction in cellular integrity with an increase in water mobility.[30,31,43] Although controversial, ADC values may be lower in infiltrative peritumoral edema than in lesions with vasogenic peritumoral edema.[44–46] Veterinary studies using DWI outside of cerebrovascular accidents are limited.[16,18,22,26,47–52] In general, there is a large overlap in ADC values, making a definitive diagnosis based strictly on DWI unlikely.[16,18,22,26,47–52] Future studies of tumor grading, response to treatment, and survival times are warranted.

Magnetic Resonance Spectroscopy

MRS measures the chemical compounds of a sample. The distribution of electrons around an atom's nucleus modifies the magnetic field that the nuclei of different molecules experience. This difference results in different magnetic resonant frequencies, also known as chemical shift, and allows the distinction of different chemicals.[53]

In MRS, the data are collected in the time domain and the resonant frequencies of all the molecules are collected simultaneously. These data undergo a Fourier transformation to separate the signal into the different frequencies and they are displayed in the form of a signal intensity as a function of frequency (**Fig. 5**).[54] The raw data are also processed to suppress the signal arising from water because it would otherwise prevent the visualization of any other frequencies. Two water suppression techniques are available, one being an inversion recovery technique, the other being a chemical shift

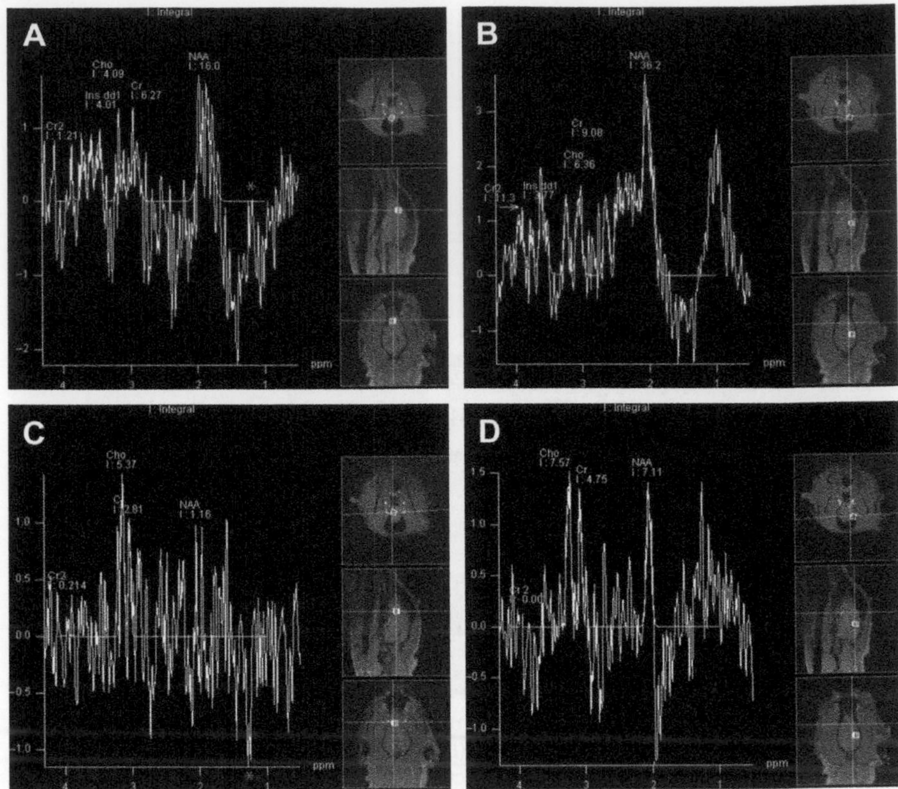

Fig. 5. Magnetic resonance spectroscopy acquired at 1.5 T with a single voxel. (*A, B*) Images acquired at a short echo time (TE) (35 milliseconds), C and D were acquired at a long TE (140 milliseconds). (*A, C*) Images acquired within diseased cerebral parenchyma (suspected meningioma); (*B, D*) Images acquired in healthy white matter. Note the inversion of the double peak of lactate between A and C (*asterisks*).

selective technique.[55] Similarly, if the area to be imaged contains a lot of fat, which cannot be avoided, its signal should also be suppressed. As with conventional MRI technique, the echo time (TE) affects the information obtained. In general, at 1.5 T, long TEs (140 or 280 milliseconds)[56,57] are used. Using such TEs in a normal brain, signals from choline (Cho), creatine (Cr), and *N*-acetyl-aspartate (NAA) can be detected. In pathologic cases, additional chemicals, such as lactate and alanine, can also be detectable if their concentrations are increased.

When using shorter TEs (35 milliseconds or less), chemicals such as glutamine, glutamate, and gamma-aminobutyric acid (GABA) become detectable but cannot be distinguished from one another. Myoinositol and lipids also become detectable. The spectral resolution, or ability to differentiate metabolic peaks, is directly influenced by signal strength of the main magnetic field. The most commonly encountered compounds seen by MRS are reviewed briefly here.

N-acetyl-aspartate

Resonating at 2.01 parts per million (ppm), NAA is the largest signal in a normal adult brain spectrum, and its peak is usually grouped with that of *N*-acetyl-aspartyl glutamate.[56–58] NAA may be a source of acetyl groups used for lipid synthesis, a form of storage for acetyl coenzyme A or aspartate, or a protein synthesis regulator.[59] Most NAA is restricted within the neurons, axons, and dendrites,[60] and is considered a neuronal marker, with disease processes such as brain tumors, infarcts, and multiple sclerosis showing decreased concentrations. However, NAA is also found in non-neuronal cells, including mast cells and oligodendrocytes, therefore changes in its concentration may not be affected solely by neuronal health.[61–63]

Choline

Resonating at 3.20 ppm, Cho is a compound made of trimethylamine, phosphocholine, and glycerophosphocholine, with a small amount of free Cho.[64] The concentration of Cho is highly variable across the brain and is usually lower in the gray matter compared with the white matter. These chemicals are linked to membrane degradation and synthesis, their concentration being increased in disease processes resulting in increased membrane turnover. High levels of Cho are found in glial cells,[65,66] and increase of Cho concentration in cases of active demyelination could be caused by the degradation of myelin[67] or associated inflammation.[68] Cho concentrations may be decreased in cases of hepatic encephalopathy (HE),[69] increased in many types of neoplasms,[54] and can be affected by diet.[70]

Creatine

Resonating at 3.03 ppm, Cr is the summation of the peaks associated with Cr and phosphocreatine. There are large variations of concentration of Cr, with higher amounts in the cerebellum compared with supratentorial regions,[71] and smaller amounts in white matter.

Lactate

Resonating at 1.31 ppm and having a characteristic double peak at long TEs, the lactate concentration is below the detectability threshold in the normal human brain in most studies, except when evaluating the ventricular CSF.[72] The lactate peak can also be difficult to isolate from any overlapping lipid peaks, such as those arising from the brain or scalp. Lactate concentration may be increased in cases of acute ischemia,[73] chronic ischemia,[74] and hypoxia[75]; conditions associated with a lack of oxygen that do not allow the Krebs cycle to be sustained.[76] One of the most peculiar aspects of lactate is its inversion peak when imaged at 140 milliseconds (see **Fig. 5**C).[77]

MRS techniques are beginning to be evaluated in veterinary medicine. In one study, optimization for proton MRS in dogs was investigated.[78] Investigators found that the quality of the spectrum was best using a multivoxel acquisition, with the volume of interest within the brain parenchyma. Metabolite ratios varied among different ages and brain regions in healthy dogs,[79] with an increased Cho/Cr ratio in younger dogs, and decreased NAA/Cho ratio in young and geriatric dogs compared with healthy adults. A similar study[80] showed that there were no metabolite differences between sexes or between cerebral hemispheres in healthy dogs, with significant metabolite concentration variation depending on region of the brain.

Studies have been performed to evaluate the use of MRS in dogs with spontaneous disease. MRS was used to evaluate the brains of dogs with tick-borne encephalitis compared with normal dogs.[81] MRS showed a mild to moderate decrease in the NAA and Cr peaks, and a mild increase in the glutamate-glutamine peak in affected dogs. Because NAA is only found in neurons, it was theorized that damage to neurons caused by flavivirus in affected dogs led to the decreased concentration of NAA.

One study evaluated MRS dogs with noninfectious encephalitis and dogs with intracranial neoplasia compared with healthy controls.[82] In dogs affected with neoplasia or noninfectious meningoencephalitis, there was an increase in Cho concentration and a decrease in NAA, Cr, and myoinositol concentrations. These variations were different from one disease process to another, suggesting that further research may reliably differentiate these diseases based on MRS.

Diffusion Tensor Imaging/Tractography

DTI is a specialized form of DWI used in neuroimaging to visualize white matter fascicles in multiple dimensions.[27,83] Diffusion MRI measures the translational displacement of water molecules,[20,27,83,84] with water molecules moving in all directions equally, called isotropic motion. When diffusion is obstructed, movement is anisotropic or directionally dependent.[2,20,27,83,85,86] Several volumes of data can be obtained during MRI to provide a model of this information, providing a way to measure anisotropic water diffusion occurring at physiologic borders such as axon bundles and myelin sheaths.[2,20,27,83,85,86] By taking diffusion measurements in multiple directions and using tensor decomposition, vector information including fractional anisotropy (FA), ADC, and eigenvalues can be obtained.[20,27,83,85,86] A tensor map is generated and tractography can be performed. Tractography is a method of linking adjacent voxels if the tensors are in the same direction. Colors are assigned to nerve fiber tracts depending on the direction of water displacement, representing the orientation of the white matter fibers (**Fig. 6**).[20,83,86]

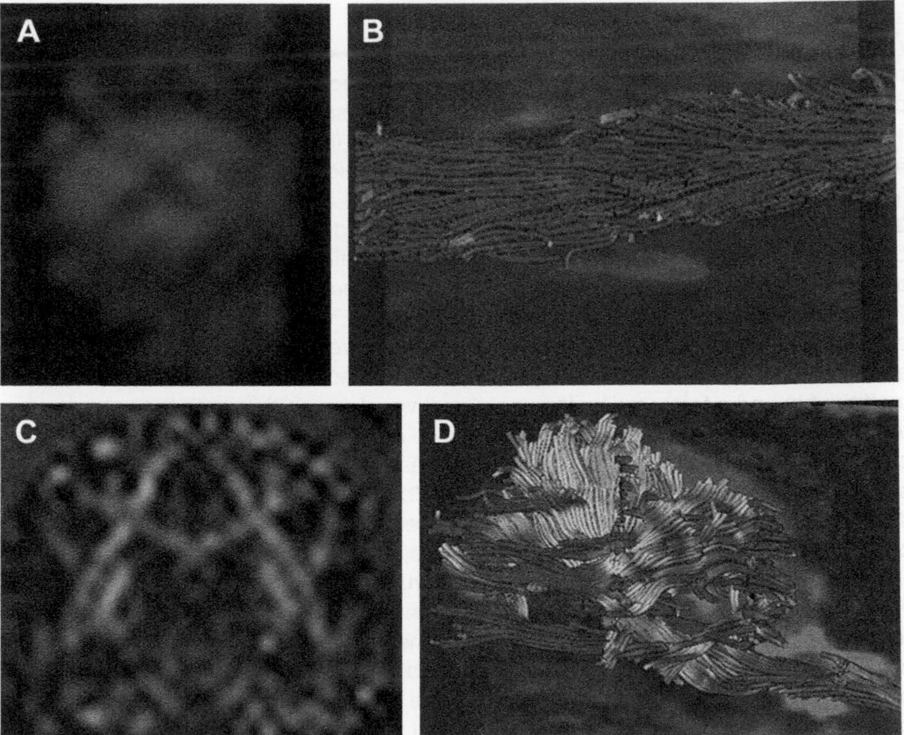

Fig. 6. High-resolution diffusion tensor tractography at 7 T in a normal canine. Transverse and sagittal spinal cord (*A, B*) along with transverse and sagittal brain (*C, D*) delineating white matter tracts.

DTI in neuroimaging has focused on the brain, primarily investigating brain tumor interaction with white matter tracts.[35,36,38,39,43–46,83,84,87] Using DTI, white matter tracts within and surrounding the lesion can be seen, assisting surgical planning to preserve strategic tracts.[35,36,38,39,43–46,83,84,87] DTI is used in people with traumatic brain injury (TBI) and is effective at differentiating TBI from normal brain and may predict outcomes.[84,88] FA derived from DTI may decrease in otherwise normal-appearing white matter on traditional MRI sequences following radiation therapy, providing insight into radiation damage.[89–94] DTI has also been used in degenerative disorders of the CNS, increasing detection of early-onset multiple sclerosis.[84,87,95–100] DTI studies in small animals include a report of normal dogs and a case series of cats with familial spontaneous epilepsy.[50,101] Diseased cats had decreased FA in the amygdala compared with controls.[50]

DTI is used less commonly in the spine, in part because of technical difficulties in acquiring diagnostic images in this region.[27,87,102] DTI is compromised by motion artifacts, local magnetic inhomogeneity, magnetic susceptibility effects from bony structures of the spinal canal, and chemical shift artifacts.[27,102] Some challenges can be overcome with appropriate image parameters and high-field scanners.[87,103,104] Areas in which DTI has shown promise involve both acute and chronic spinal cord injury (SCI).[27,87,95,103–112] In acute SCI, FA and ADC values were decreased at the level of the trauma and in the adjacent normal-appearing spinal cord on MRI, resulting in more accurate assessment of the extent of injury.[27,87,95,97,104,109,111,112] DTI may improve surgical resection of spinal cord tumors by allowing evaluation of the mass and its interaction with the fiber tracts.[87,103,104,106,113,114] DTI, with ADC and FA measurements, may be used in assessing the severity of degenerative myelopathy in humans.[104,105,107,110] Other spinal diseases (eg, multiple sclerosis, inflammatory disorders) have been studied.[27,29,87,104,106] In these conditions, decreased FA values can be seen in areas of the spinal cord that are normal on routine MRI.[104] There is minimal published information regarding DTI in small animal patients apart from studies establishing the technique in normal dogs.[20,85,115]

Cerebrospinal Fluid Tracking

CSF flow studies are phase-contrast studies used in MRI to evaluate qualitatively and quantitatively the pulsatile CSF flow in the CNS.

There are 2 main components to CSF flow: a bulk flow, which is the flow of CSF driven by a pressure gradient between the choroid plexus (production site) and the arachnoid villi (absorption site), and is overall slow and nondetectable with current techniques; and a faster pulsatile flow attributable to the cardiac cycle and the pulsation of the cerebral arteries and choroid plexus.[116,117] Because of this mechanical coupling between the cardiac cycle and the CSF flow, the CSF moves caudally during systole and cranially during diastole.[118–121] The result is a typical waveform depicting the velocity and the amount of CSF flow over time with a nonzero start, biphasic flow, and return to baseline.[118,120,122–124] It is that pulsatile flow that is evaluated with MRI.

The most commonly used technique is a time-resolved, 2-phase–contrast MRI with velocity encoding. This technique is rapid, simple, and noninvasive.[117,125] It does not require any specific hardware, allowing its acquisition on most modern 1.5-T magnets with a standard software and phase-contrast analysis package.[126] This technique is based on the application of a pair of opposite-phase encoding pulses. The static protons receive both opposite pulses, which null each other resulting in no signal. The dynamic protons, having moved between the 2 pulses, do not experience the 2 counteracting pulses. The moving protons receive 2 congruent pulses leading to the creation of signal and their subsequent detectability.[127–130] In order to obtain the optimal signal, the maximum anticipated CSF flow velocity has to be estimated and the velocity encoding (VENC) parameter of the phase-contrast sequence optimized in that regard.[131] If the VENC is set up lower than the velocity of the CSF flow, aliasing results, and if the VENC is set up higher than the velocity of the CSF flow, it creates a weak signal.[128,131] In humans, the expected flow is usually between 5 and 8 cm/s, whereas in hyperdynamic patients this value can reach up to 25 cm/s. Because the pulsatile CSF flow is synchronous with the cardiac cycle, cardiac gating can be used to increase the sensitivity of these studies[132] and can be performed either prospectively or retrospectively.[133]

The reported clinical applications in human medicine include evaluation of Chiari type I malformation, arachnoid cysts, syringomyelia, and ventriculoperitoneal shunts.[127]

In the case of Chiari type I malformation, there is displacement of the cerebellar tonsils through the foramen magnum. Cerebellar displacement alters CSF flow at the level of the craniovertebral junction.[127] The alterations in CSF flow have been associated with clinical status in patients affected by Chiari type I malformation.[120,124,134–137] The evaluation of the CSF flow obstruction can help predict and select the patients who are likely to be most responsive to surgery,[122,138] and restoration of normal CSF flow postsurgery has been linked to an improved postoperative outcome.[134,135]

The evaluation of arachnoid cysts focuses on determining whether the cyst is communicating with the surrounding CSF space, which is an important perioperative factor.[139] It can also help make the distinction between an enlarged, normal, CSF-filled space, and an intracranial cyst in situations in which conventional MRI sequences are insufficient.[140]

Phase-contrast studies are also used to differentiate between syringohydromyelia and cystic myelomalacia.[127] The latter, being caused by obstruction of the spinal CSF pathways,[122,141] does not show evidence of CSF flow, unlike syringohydromyelia. The detection of pulsatile CSF flow in the spinal cord may be predictive of subsequent enlargement.[122,141]

In cases of ventriculoperitoneal shunts, the presence of CSF flow is evaluated to assess the shunt patency. The shunt contains a 1-way valve mechanism resulting in a unidirectional and rhythmic CSF flow. The absence of signal in the shunt represents the absence of CSF flow through it.[142] Because of the very low velocity of the CSF in the shunts, the VENC needs to be adjusted accordingly.

In veterinary medicine, the reported applications are currently sparse[143–145] with, to the author's knowledge, only 1 study focusing on the CSF flow velocity with phase-contrast MRI[143] published to date. That study evaluates the CSF flow of 59 Cavalier King Charles (CKC) spaniels affected with Chiari-like malformation and syringohydromyelia, compared with 5 control, healthy, non-CKC dogs. The sequence was cardiac-gated and CSF flow was evaluated at the mesencephalic aqueduct, the ventral and caudodorsal aspect of the subarachnoid space (1 mm caudal to the foramen magnum), and at the level of the C2-C3 junction. In the CKC group, 70% of dogs had obstruction of the CSF flow through the foramen magnum, primarily dorsally. Of the 10 clinically affected dogs, 9 had signs of CSF obstruction, and, of the 22 dogs with syringomyelia, 17 had signs of obstruction (77%). Turbulent flow and jets were observed at the level of the foramen magnum, C2-C3, and within the syrinxes only in the CKC and not in the control dogs. There was a positive association between the presence of turbulence and jets at the level of C2-C3 and the presence of syringomyelia. However, there was no correlation with the presence of jets or turbulence at any of the locations and the presence or severity of the neurologic signs. In a study evaluating spinal subarachnoid cysts (now called spinal arachnoid diverticula) in 13 dogs,[144] 1 of the dogs was evaluated using phase-contrast MRI. The MRI sequence showed free communication between the subarachnoid space and the subarachnoid lesion.

FUTURE DIRECTIONS

The trend in MRI since its inception has been higher field strengths, faster and more efficient gradients, and more robust sequences. These areas have been targeted to reduce scan times, improve resolution, and to increase SNR. Seven-Tesla clinical scanners are available, but are not currently US Food and Drug Administration (FDA) approved. This approval is anticipated to occur in the very near future. Gradient strengths are currently at the maximum allowed by the FDA. For this reason, technology and research shifted from bigger magnets to better coils. Receiver coils with 32 channels and more are readily available. This increase has the advantage of greater image sampling and improved SNR. One of the most exciting advances involves ways to use the MR system going beyond qualitative imaging and moving into quantitative evaluation. One such technique is known as MR fingerprinting (MRF).

MRF is a recently introduced approach to MR scanning with a different method of data acquisition and evaluation.[146–148] With traditional MR scanning, the tissue of interest is qualitatively evaluated based on the T1 and T2 relaxation properties along with the proton density (PD).[146–148] MR pulse sequences are designed to highlight these various properties, requiring highly trained operators to make appropriate adjustments to the control software during the scan procedure. The signal intensity of the tissue imaged is not quantitative but is relative to the other tissues in the field of view.[148] Hence when describing areas, terms such as hypointense or hyperintense are used. The same material can have different signal intensities in different data sets depending on many variable parameters. Therefore diagnosis is based on comparing signal intensity and the absolute intensity has no real meaning.[146,148] MRF is a technique that is being developed to achieve absolute quantification of T1, T2, and PD tissue parameters while maintaining clinically relevant scan times.[146–148]

MRF uses a pseudorandomized acquisition that causes the signals from different tissues to have a unique signal evolution, termed the fingerprint.[146–148] After acquisition, a pattern recognition algorithm is used to match the fingerprints to an online, predefined dictionary of predicted signal evolutions, which is then converted into a quantitative map of the MR parameter of interest.[146–148] MRF is expected to be much more accurate and reproducible than traditional MRI and less sensitive to motion artifact and field inhomogeneity.[146] With further advances, MRF has the potential to yield studies providing fast quantitative imaging of multiple MR parameters simultaneously (T1, T2, PD, as well as diffusion/perfusion) with a single scan series, in less time than is traditionally used for a clinical scan.[146–148] This technology has the potential to lead to the development of direct imaging identification of tissue or disorder type.[146] Furthermore, imaging would be greatly simplified if 1 scan could yield multiple tissue contrasts.[146] Should the techniques advance, this could ultimately lead to development of a true push-button scanner.

SUMMARY

MR is an exciting and ever-expanding imaging modality. This article discusses some highlights of the recent advances in MR technology as well as potential future trends. These advances include higher field strengths, new techniques, faster gradients, improved coil technology, and more robust sequence protocols. Techniques to move beyond simply generating anatomic images to visualizing patterns of diffusion, white matter tracking, proton spectrography, and spin labeling for flow tracking are advancing rapidly and are now feasible not only for research but also for clinical use.

REFERENCES

1. MacManus D. MRI in practice: Catherine Westbrook and Carolyn Kaut, Blackwell Science. Philadelphia: WB Saunders; 1998. £ 22.50. ISBN 0-632-04205-2. 1999.
2. Hecht S, Adams WH. MRI of brain disease in veterinary patients part 1: basic principles and congenital brain disorders. Vet Clin North Am Small Anim Pract 2010;40(1):21–38.
3. John M. Basic principles. In: Eldelman Robert HJ, Zlatkin M, Crues J, editors. Clincal magnetic resonance imaging, vol. 1, 3rd edition. Philadelphia: Saunders-Elsevier; 2006. p. 23–57.
4. Mitchell Donald CM. MRI principles. Philadelphia: Saunders; 2004.
5. Parizel PM, Dijkstra HAJ, Geenen GJ, et al. Low-field versus high-field MR imaging of the knee: a comparison of signal behaviour and diagnostic performance. Eur J Radiol 1995;19(2):132–8.
6. Duyn JH. The future of ultra-high field MRI and fMRI for study of the human brain. Neuroimage 2012;62(2):1241–8.
7. Kraff O, Fischer A, Nagel AM, et al. MRI at 7 tesla and above: demonstrated and potential capabilities. J Magn Reson Imaging 2015;41(1):13–33.
8. Duvernoy HM. The human hippocampus: functional anatomy, vascularization and serial sections with MRI. New York: Springer Science & Business Media; 2005.
9. Fatterpekar GM, Naidich TP, Delman BN, et al. Cytoarchitecture of the human cerebral cortex: MR microscopy of excised specimens at 9.4 tesla. AJNR Am J Neuroradiol 2002;23(8):1313–21.
10. Kerchner GA. Ultra-high field 7T MRI: a new tool for studying Alzheimer's disease. J Alzheimers Dis 2011;26(s3):91–5.
11. Kollia K, Maderwald S, Putzki N, et al. First clinical study on ultra-high-field MR imaging in patients with multiple sclerosis: comparison of 1.5 T and 7T. Am J Neuroradiol 2009;30(4):699–702.
12. Naidich TP, Duvernoy HM, Delman BN, et al. Vascularization of the cerebellum and the brain stem. New York: Springer; 2009.
13. Prudent V, Kumar A, Liu S, et al. Human hippocampal subfields in young adults at 7.0 T: feasibility of imaging 1. Radiology 2010;254(3):900–6.
14. Thomas BP, Welch EB, Niederhauser BD, et al. High-resolution 7T MRI of the human hippocampus in vivo. J Magn Reson Imaging 2008;28(5):1266–72.
15. Wisse L, Gerritsen L, Zwanenburg JJ, et al. Subfields of the hippocampal formation at 7T MRI: in vivo volumetric assessment. Neuroimage 2012;61(4):1043–9.
16. Kim B, Yi K, Jung S, et al. Clinical applications and characteristics of apparent diffusion coefficient maps for the brain of two dogs. J Vet Sci 2014;15(3):455–8.
17. Bammer Roland LC, Julia PO, Moseley M. Diffusion weighted magnetic resonance imaging. In: Eldelman Robert HJ, Zlatkin M, Crues J, editors. Clinical magnetic resonance imaging third edition, vol. 1. Philadelphia: Saunders-Elsevier; 2006. p. 288–319.
18. Sutherland-Smith J, King R, Faissler D, et al. Magnetic resonance imaging apparent diffusion coefficients for histologically confirmed intracranial lesions in dogs. Vet Radiol Ultrasound 2011;52(2):142–8.

19. McConnell J, Garosi L, Platt S. Magnetic resonance imaging findings of presumed cerebellar cerebrovascular accident in twelve dogs. Vet Radiol Ultrasound 2005;46(1):1–10.
20. Pease A, Miller R. The use of diffusion tensor imaging to evaluate the spinal cord in normal and abnormal dogs. Vet Radiol Ultrasound 2011;52(5):492–7.
21. Garosi LS. Cerebrovascular disease in dogs and cats. Vet Clin North Am Small Anim Pract 2010;40(1):65–79.
22. Hecht S, Adams WH. MRI of brain disease in veterinary patients part 2: acquired brain disorders. Vet Clin North Am Small Anim Pract 2010;40(1):39–63.
23. Rossmeisl JH, Rohleder JJ, Pickett JP, et al. Presumed and confirmed striatocapsular brain infarctions in six dogs. Vet Ophthalmol 2007;10(1):23–36.
24. Xu XQ, Wu CJ, Zu QQ, et al. Temporal evolution of the signal intensity of hyperacute ischemic lesions in a canine stroke model: influence of hyperintense acute reperfusion marker. Jpn J Radiol 2017;35(4):161–7.
25. Xu XQ, Cheng QG, Zu QQ, et al. Comparative study of the relative signal intensity on DWI, FLAIR, and T2 images in identifying the onset time of stroke in an embolic canine model. Neurol Sci 2014;35(7):1059–65.
26. Cervera V, Mai W, Vite CH, et al. Comparative magnetic resonance imaging findings between gliomas and presumed cerebrovascular accidents in dogs. Vet Radiol Ultrasound 2011;52(1):33–40.
27. Tanenbaum LN. Diffusion imaging in the spine. Appl Radiol 2011;40(4):9.
28. Küker W, Weller M, Klose U, et al. Diffusion-weighted MRI of spinal cord infarction. J Neurol 2004;251(7):818–24.
29. Boretius S, Escher A, Dallenga T, et al. Assessment of lesion pathology in a new animal model of MS by multiparametric MRI and DTI. Neuroimage 2012;59(3):2678–88.
30. Theilmann RJ, Borders R, Trouard TP, et al. Changes in water mobility measured by diffusion MRI predict response of metastatic breast cancer to chemotherapy. Neoplasia 2004;6(6):831–7.
31. Padhani AR, Koh DM. Diffusion MR imaging for monitoring of treatment response. Magn Reson Imaging Clin North America 2011;19(1):181–209.
32. Barajas R, Rubenstein J, Chang J, et al. Diffusion-weighted MR imaging derived apparent diffusion coefficient is predictive of clinical outcome in primary central nervous system lymphoma. Am J Neuroradiol 2010;31(1):60–6.
33. Maller VV, Bathla G, Moritani T, et al. Imaging in viral infections of the central nervous system: can images speak for an acutely ill brain? Emerg Radiol 2017;24(3):287–300.
34. Murakami R, Sugahara T, Nakamura H, et al. Malignant supratentorial astrocytoma treated with postoperative radiation therapy: prognostic value of pretreatment quantitative diffusion-weighted MR imaging 1. Radiology 2007;243(2):493–9.
35. Mabray MC, Barajas RF, Cha S. Modern brain tumor imaging. Brain Tumor Res Treat 2015;3(1):8–23.
36. Tien RD, Felsberg G, Friedman H, et al. MR imaging of high-grade cerebral gliomas: value of diffusion-weighted echoplanar pulse sequences. AJR Am J Roentgenol 1994;162(3):671–7.
37. Laothamatas J, Sungkarat W, Hemachudha T. Neuroimaging in rabies. Adv Virus Res 2011;79:309–27.
38. Thoeny HC, Ross BD. Predicting and monitoring cancer treatment response with diffusion-weighted MRI. J Magn Reson Imaging 2010;32(1):2–16.

39. Schaefer PW, Grant PE, Gonzalez RG. Diffusion-weighted MR imaging of the brain 1. Radiology 2000;217(2):331–45.
40. Chang SC, Lai PH, Chen WL, et al. Diffusion-weighted MRI features of brain abscess and cystic or necrotic brain tumors: comparison with conventional MRI. Clin Imaging 2002;26(4):227–36.
41. Ebisu T, Tanaka C, Umeda M, et al. Discrimination of brain abscess from necrotic or cystic tumors by diffusion-weighted echo planar imaging. Magn Reson Imaging 1996;14(9):1113–6.
42. Noguchi K, Watanabe N, Nagayoshi T, et al. Role of diffusion-weighted echo-planar MRI in distinguishing between brain abscess and tumour: a preliminary report. Neuroradiology 1999;41(3):171–4.
43. Kono K, Inoue Y, Nakayama K, et al. The role of diffusion-weighted imaging in patients with brain tumors. AJNR Am J Neuroradiol 2001;22(6):1081–8.
44. Lu S, Ahn D, Johnson G, et al. Diffusion-tensor MR imaging of intracranial neoplasia and associated peritumoral edema: introduction of the tumor infiltration index 1. Radiology 2004;232(1):221–8.
45. Pavlisa G, Rados M, Pavlisa G, et al. The differences of water diffusion between brain tissue infiltrated by tumor and peritumoral vasogenic edema. Clin Imaging 2009;33(2):96–101.
46. Toh CH, Wong AM, Wei KC, et al. Peritumoral edema of meningiomas and metastatic brain tumors: differences in diffusion characteristics evaluated with diffusion-tensor MR imaging. Neuroradiology 2007;49(6):489–94.
47. Vite CH, Cross JR. Correlating magnetic resonance findings with neuropathology and clinical signs in dogs and cats. Vet Radiol Ultrasound 2011; 52(s1):S23–31.
48. Young BD, Fosgate GT, Holmes SP, et al. Evaluation of standard magnetic resonance characteristics used to differentiate neoplastic, inflammatory, and vascular brain lesions in dogs. Vet Radiol Ultrasound 2014;55(4):399–406.
49. MacKillop E, Thrall DE, Ranck RS, et al. Imaging diagnosis—synchronous primary brain tumors in a dog. Vet Radiol Ultrasound 2007;48(6):550–3.
50. Mizoguchi S, Hasegawa D, Hamamoto Y, et al. Interictal diffusion and perfusion magnetic resonance imaging features of cats with familial spontaneous epilepsy. Am J Vet Res 2017;78(3):305–10.
51. DeJesus A, Cohen EB, Galban E, et al. Magnetic resonance imaging features of intraventricular ependymomas in five cats. Vet Radiol Ultrasound 2017;58(3): 326–33.
52. Schmid S, Hodshon A, Olin S, et al. Pituitary macrotumor causing narcolepsy-cataplexy in a dachshund. J Vet Intern Med 2017;31(2):545–9.
53. Proctor W, Yu F. The dependence of a nuclear magnetic resonance frequency upon chemical compound. Phys Rev 1950;77(5):717.
54. Barker PB, Bizzi A, De Stefano N, et al. Clinical MR spectroscopy: techniques and applications. Cambridge: Cambridge University Press; 2010.
55. Hu X, Norris DG. Advances in high-field magnetic resonance imaging. Annu Rev Biomed Eng 2004;6:157–84.
56. Frahm J, Michaelis T, Merboldt KD, et al. On the N-acetyl methyl resonance in localized 1H NMR spectra of human brain in vivo. NMR Biomed 1991;4(4): 201–4.
57. Rémy C, Grand S, Laï ES, et al. 1H MRS of human brain abscesses in vivo and in vitro. Magn Reson Med 1995;34(4):508–14.

58. Pouwels PJ, Frahm J. Differential distribution of NAA and NAAG in human brain as determined by quantitative localized proton MRS. NMR Biomed 1997;10(2): 73–8.
59. Barker PB. N-acetyl aspartate—A neuronal marker? Ann Neurol 2001;49(4): 423–4.
60. Simmons M, Frondoza C, Coyle J. Immunocytochemical localization of N-acetyl-aspartate with monoclonal antibodies. Neuroscience 1991;45(1):37–45.
61. Bhakoo KK, Pearce D. In vitro expression of N-acetyl aspartate by oligodendrocytes. J Neurochem 2000;74(1):254–62.
62. Burlina AP, Ferrari V, Facci L, et al. Mast cells contain large quantities of secretagogue-sensitive N-acetylaspartate. J Neurochem 1997;69(3):1314–7.
63. Urenjak J, Williams SR, Gadian DG, et al. Specific expression of N-acetylaspartate in neurons, oligodendrocyte-type-2 astrocyte progenitors, and immature oligodendrocytes in vitro. J Neurochem 1992;59(1):55–61.
64. Barker PB, Breiter SN, Soher BJ, et al. Quantitative proton spectroscopy of canine brain: in vivo and in vitro correlations. Magn Reson Med 1994;32(2): 157–63.
65. Gill S, Small R, Thomas D, et al. Brain metabolites as 1H NMR markers of neuronal and glial disorders. NMR Biomed 1989;2(5–6):196–200.
66. Gill SS, Thomas DG, Van Bruggen N, et al. Proton MR spectroscopy of intracranial tumours: in vivo and in vitro studies. J Comput Assist Tomogr 1990;14(4): 497–504.
67. Davie C, Barker G, Tofts P, et al. Detection of myelin breakdown products by proton magnetic resonance spectroscopy. Lancet 1993;341(8845):630–1.
68. Brenner R, Munro P, Williams SC, et al. The proton NMR spectrum in acute EAE: the significance of the change in the Cho:Cr ratio. Magn Reson Med 1993;29(6): 737–45.
69. Aboagye EO, Bhujwalla ZM. Malignant transformation alters membrane choline phospholipid metabolism of human mammary epithelial cells. Cancer Res 1999; 59(1):80–4.
70. Stoll AL, Renshaw PF, De Micheli E, et al. Choline ingestion increases the resonance of choline-containing compounds in human brain: an in vivo proton magnetic resonance study. Biol Psychiatry 1995;37(3):170–4.
71. Jacobs MA, Horská A, van Zijl P, et al. Quantitative proton MR spectroscopic imaging of normal human cerebellum and brain stem. Magn Reson Med 2001; 46(4):699–705.
72. Nagae-Poetscher LM, McMahon M, Braverman N, et al. Metabolites in ventricular cerebrospinal fluid detected by proton magnetic resonance spectroscopic imaging. J Magn Reson Imaging 2004;20(3):496–500.
73. Barker PB, Gillard JH, Van Zijl P, et al. Acute stroke: evaluation with serial proton MR spectroscopic imaging. Radiology 1994;192(3):723–32.
74. Petroff O, Graham G, Blamire A, et al. Spectroscopic imaging of stroke in humans Histopathology correlates of spectral changes. Neurology 1992;42(7): 1349–54.
75. Penrice J, Cady E, Lorek A, et al. Proton magnetic resonance spectroscopy of the brain in normal preterm and term infants, and early changes after perinatal hypoxia-ischemia. Pediatr Res 1996;40(1):6–14.
76. Veech RL. The metabolism of lactate. NMR Biomed 1991;4(2):53–8.
77. Kelley DA, Wald LL, Star-Lack JM. Lactate detection at 3T: compensating J coupling effects with BASING. J Magn Reson Imaging 1999;9(5):732–7.

78. Ober CP, Warrington CD, Feeney DA, et al. Optimizing a protocol for 1H-magnetic resonance spectroscopy of the canine brain at 3T. Vet Radiol Ultrasound 2013;54(2):149–58.
79. Ono K, Kitagawa M, Ito D, et al. Regional variations and age-related changes detected with magnetic resonance spectroscopy in the brain of healthy dogs. Am J Vet Res 2014;75(2):179–86.
80. Carrera I, Richter H, Meier D, et al. Regional metabolite concentrations in the brain of healthy dogs measured by use of short echo time, single voxel proton magnetic resonance spectroscopy at 3.0 Tesla. Am J Vet Res 2015;76(2): 129–41.
81. Sievert C, Richter H, Beckmann K, et al. Comparison between proton magnetic resonance spectroscopy findings in dogs with tick-borne encephalitis and clinically normal dogs. Vet Radiol Ultrasound 2017;58(1):53–61.
82. Carrera I, Richter H, Beckmann K, et al. Evaluation of intracranial neoplasia and noninfectious meningoencephalitis in dogs by use of short echo time, single voxel proton magnetic resonance spectroscopy at 3.0 tesla. Am J Vet Res 2016;77(5):452–62.
83. David A. Diffusion tensor MR imaging fundamentals. In: Clinical magnetic resonance imaging, vol. 1. Philadelphia: Saunders-Elsevier; 2006. p. 320–32.
84. Assaf Y, Pasternak O. Diffusion tensor imaging (DTI)-based white matter mapping in brain research: a review. J Mol Neurosci 2008;34(1):51–61.
85. Griffin JF, Cohen ND, Young BD, et al. Thoracic and lumbar spinal cord diffusion tensor imaging in dogs. J Magn Reson Imaging 2013;37(3):632–41.
86. Leandro AW. Temporal characterization and prognostic value determination of severe spinal cord injuries in paraplegic dogs using in vivo diffusion tensor imaging. Hannover: University of Veterinary Medicine Hannover; 2016.
87. Sąsiadek MJ, Szewczyk P, Bladowska J. Application of diffusion tensor imaging (DTI) in pathological changes of the spinal cord. Med Sci Monitor 2012;18(6): RA73–9.
88. Hulkower M, Poliak D, Rosenbaum S, et al. A decade of DTI in traumatic brain injury: 10 years and 100 articles later. AJNR Am J Neuroradiol 2013;34(11): 2064–74.
89. Xing L, Thorndyke B, Schreibmann E, et al. Overview of image-guided radiation therapy. Med Dosimetry 2006;31(2):91–112.
90. Hall DE, Moffat BA, Stojanovska J, et al. Therapeutic efficacy of DTI-015 using diffusion magnetic resonance imaging as an early surrogate marker. Clin Cancer Res 2004;10(23):7852–9.
91. Prabhu SP, Ng S, Vajapeyam S, et al. DTI assessment of the brainstem white matter tracts in pediatric BSG before and after therapy. Childs Nerv Syst 2011;27(1):11–8.
92. Nagesh V, Tsien CI, Chenevert TL, et al. Radiation-induced changes in normal-appearing white matter in patients with cerebral tumors: a diffusion tensor imaging study. Int J Radiat Oncol Biol Phys 2008;70(4):1002–10.
93. Jena R, Price S, Baker C, et al. Diffusion tensor imaging: possible implications for radiotherapy treatment planning of patients with high-grade glioma. Clin Oncol 2005;17(8):581–90.
94. Haris M, Kumar S, Raj MK, et al. Serial diffusion tensor imaging to characterize radiation-induced changes in normal-appearing white matter following radiotherapy in patients with adult low-grade gliomas. Radiat Med 2008;26(3): 140–50.

95. Banaszek A, Bladowska J, Szewczyk P, et al. Usefulness of diffusion tensor MR imaging in the assessment of intramedullary changes of the cervical spinal cord in different stages of degenerative spine disease. Eur Spine J 2014;23(7): 1523–30.
96. Gilli F, Chen X, Pachner AR, et al. High-resolution diffusion tensor spinal cord MRI measures as biomarkers of disability progression in a rodent model of progressive multiple sclerosis. PLoS One 2016;11(7):e0160071.
97. Renoux J, Facon D, Fillard P, et al. MR diffusion tensor imaging and fiber tracking in inflammatory diseases of the spinal cord. Am J Neuroradiol 2006; 27(9):1947–51.
98. Kantarci K, Avula R, Senjem M, et al. Dementia with Lewy bodies and Alzheimer disease neurodegenerative patterns characterized by DTI. Neurology 2010; 74(22):1814–21.
99. Kitamura K, Nakayama K, Kosaka S, et al. Diffusion tensor imaging of the cortico-ponto-cerebellar pathway in patients with adult-onset ataxic neurodegenerative disease. Neuroradiology 2008;50(4):285–92.
100. Douaud G, Jbabdi S, Behrens TE, et al. DTI measures in crossing-fibre areas: increased diffusion anisotropy reveals early white matter alteration in MCI and mild Alzheimer's disease. Neuroimage 2011;55(3):880–90.
101. Anaya García MS, Hernández Anaya JS, Marrufo Meléndez O, et al. In vivo study of cerebral white matter in the dog using diffusion tensor tractography. Vet Radiol Ultrasound 2015;56(2):188–95.
102. Le Bihan D, Poupon C, Amadon A, et al. Artifacts and pitfalls in diffusion MRI. J Magn Reson Imaging 2006;24(3):478–88.
103. Vargas MI, Delavelle J, Jlassi H, et al. Clinical applications of diffusion tensor tractography of the spinal cord. Neuroradiology 2008;50(1):25–9.
104. Hendrix P, Griessenauer CJ, Cohen-Adad J, et al. Spinal diffusion tensor imaging: a comprehensive review with emphasis on spinal cord anatomy and clinical applications. Clin Anat 2015;28(1):88–95.
105. Jones J, Cen S, Lebel R, et al. Diffusion tensor imaging correlates with the clinical assessment of disease severity in cervical spondylotic myelopathy and predicts outcome following surgery. Am J Neuroradiol 2013;34(2):471–8.
106. Thurnher MM, Law M. Diffusion-weighted imaging, diffusion-tensor imaging, and fiber tractography of the spinal cord. Magn Reson Imaging Clin N Am 2009;17(2):225–44.
107. Chatley A, Kumar R, Jain VK, et al. Effect of spinal cord signal intensity changes on clinical outcome after surgery for cervical spondylotic myelopathy: clinical article. J Neurosurg Spine 2009;11(5):562–7.
108. Wang K, Chen Z, Zhang F, et al. Evaluation of DTI parameter ratios and diffusion tensor tractography grading in the diagnosis and prognosis prediction of cervical spondylotic myelopathy. Spine 2017;42(4):E202–10.
109. Chen J, Zhou C, Zhu L, et al. Identifying the injury in demyelinating cervical spinal cord disease: a diffusion tensor imaging and tractography study. Neurol Asia 2016;21(1):73–80.
110. Sąsiadek MJ, Bladowska J. Imaging of degenerative spine disease–the state of the art. Adv Clin Exp Med 2012;21(2):133–42.
111. Kara B, Celik A, Karadereler S, et al. The role of DTI in early detection of cervical spondylotic myelopathy: a preliminary study with 3-T MRI. Neuroradiology 2011; 53(8):609–16.

112. Rindler RS, Chokshi FH, Malcolm JG, et al. Spinal diffusion tensor imaging in the evaluation of pre- and post-operative severity in cervical spondylotic myelopathy: a systematic review of the literature. World Neurosurg 2016;99:150–8.
113. Lowe GM. Magnetic resonance imaging of intramedullary spinal cord tumors. J Neurooncol 2000;47(3):195–210.
114. Mechtler LL, Nandigam K. Spinal cord tumors: new views and future directions. Neurol Clin 2013;31(1):241–68.
115. Hobert MK, Stein VM, Dziallas P, et al. Evaluation of normal appearing spinal cord by diffusion tensor imaging, fiber tracking, fractional anisotropy, and apparent diffusion coefficient measurement in 13 dogs. Acta Vet Scand 2013; 55(1):36.
116. Barkhof F, Kouwenhoven M, Scheltens P, et al. Phase-contrast cine MR imaging of normal aqueductal CSF flow: effect of aging and relation to CSF void on modulus MR. Acta Radiol 1994;35(2):123–30.
117. Stoquart-El Sankari S, Lehmann P, Gondry-Jouet C, et al. Phase-contrast MR imaging support for the diagnosis of aqueductal stenosis. Am J Neuroradiol 2009; 30(1):209–14.
118. Bhadelia RA, Bogdan AR, Wolpert SM. Analysis of cerebrospinal fluid flow waveforms with gated phase-contrast MR velocity measurements. Am J Neuroradiol 1995;16(2):389–400.
119. Enzmann D, Pelc N. Normal flow patterns of intracranial and spinal cerebrospinal fluid defined with phase-contrast cine MR imaging. Radiology 1991;178(2): 467–74.
120. Iskandar BJ, Quigley M, Haughton VM. Foramen magnum cerebrospinal fluid flow characteristics in children with Chiari I malformation before and after craniocervical decompression. J Neurosurg 2004;101(2):169–78.
121. Menick BJ. Phase-contrast magnetic resonance imaging of cerebrospinal fluid flow in the evaluation of patients with Chiari I malformation. Neurosurg focus 2001;11(1):1–4.
122. Brugières P, Idy-Peretti I, Iffenecker C, et al. CSF flow measurement in syringomyelia. Am J Neuroradiol 2000;21(10):1785–92.
123. de Marco G, Idy-Peretti I, Didon-Poncelet A, et al. Intracranial fluid dynamics in normal and hydrocephalic states: systems analysis with phase-contrast magnetic resonance imaging. J Comput Assist Tomogr 2004;28(2):247–54.
124. Haughton VM, Korosec FR, Medow JE, et al. Peak systolic and diastolic CSF velocity in the foramen magnum in adult patients with Chiari I malformations and in normal control participants. Am J Neuroradiol 2003;24(2):169–76.
125. Stadlbauer A, Salomonowitz E, Brenneis C, et al. Magnetic resonance velocity mapping of 3D cerebrospinal fluid flow dynamics in hydrocephalus: preliminary results. Eur Radiol 2012;22(1):232–42.
126. Bhadelia R, Frederick E, Patz S, et al. Cough-associated headache in patients with Chiari I malformation: CSF flow analysis by means of cine phase-contrast MR imaging. Am J Neuroradiol 2011;32(4):739–42.
127. Battal B, Kocaoglu M, Bulakbasi N, et al. Cerebrospinal fluid flow imaging by using phase-contrast MR technique. Br J Radiol 2014;84(1004):758–65.
128. Bradley WG. Neurology in clinical practice: principles of diagnosis and management, vol. 1. Oxford: Taylor & Francis; 2004.
129. Dumoulin CL, Yucel EK, Vock P, et al. Two- and three-dimensional phase contrast MR angiography of the abdomen. J Comput Assist Tomogr 1990; 14(5):779–84.

130. Tsuruda JS, Shimakawa A, Pelc NJ, et al. Dural sinus occlusion: evaluation with phase-sensitive gradient-echo MR imaging. Am J Neuroradiol 1991;12(3): 481–8.
131. Saloner D. The AAPM/RSNA physics tutorial for residents. An introduction to MR angiography. Radiographics 1995;15(2):453–65.
132. Connor S, O'Gorman R, Summers P, et al. SPAMM, cine phase contrast imaging and fast spin-echo T2-weighted imaging in the study of intracranial cerebrospinal fluid (CSF) flow. Clin Radiol 2001;56(9):763–72.
133. Nitz W, Bradley W Jr, Watanabe A, et al. Flow dynamics of cerebrospinal fluid: assessment with phase-contrast velocity MR imaging performed with retrospective cardiac gating. Radiology 1992;183(2):395–405.
134. Armonda RA, Citrin CM, Foley KT, et al. Quantitative cine-mode magnetic resonance imaging of Chiari I malformations: an analysis of cerebrospinal fluid dynamics. Neurosurgery 1994;35(2):214–24.
135. Bhadelia RA, Bogdan AR, Wolpert SM, et al. Cerebrospinal fluid flow waveforms: analysis in patients with Chiari I malformation by means of gated phase-contrast MR imaging velocity measurements. Radiology 1995;196(1): 195–202.
136. Heiss JD, Patronas N, DeVroom HL, et al. Elucidating the pathophysiology of syringomyelia. J Neurosurg 1999;91(4):553–62.
137. Panigrahi M, Reddy BP, Reddy A, et al. CSF flow study in Chiari I malformation. Childs Nerv Syst 2004;20(5):336–40.
138. McGirt MJ, Nimjee SM, Fuchs HE, et al. Relationship of cine phase-contrast MRI to outcome after decompression for Chiari I malformation. Neurosurgery 2006; 59(1):140–6.
139. Yildiz H, Erdogan C, Yalcin R, et al. Evaluation of communication between intracranial arachnoid cysts and cisterns with phase-contrast cine MR imaging. Am J Neuroradiol 2005;26(1):145–51.
140. Yildiz H, Yazici Z, Hakyemez B, et al. Evaluation of CSF flow patterns of posterior fossa cystic malformations using CSF flow MR imaging. Neuroradiology 2006; 48(9):595–605.
141. Ball M, Dayan A. Pathogenesis of syringomyelia. Lancet 1972;300(7781): 799–801.
142. Castillo M, Hudgins PA, Malko JA, et al. Flow-sensitive MR imaging of ventriculoperitoneal shunts: in vitro findings, clinical applications, and pitfalls. Am J Neuroradiol 1991;12(4):667–71.
143. Cerda-Gonzalez S, Olby NJ, Broadstone R, et al. Characteristics of cerebrospinal fluid flow in Cavalier King Charles Spaniels analyzed using phase velocity cine magnetic resonance imaging. Vet Radiol Ultrasound 2009;50(5):467–76.
144. Gnirs K, Ruel Y, Blot S, et al. Spinal sub arachnoid cysts in 13 dogs. Vet Radiol Ultrasound 2003;44(4):402–8.
145. March P, Abramson C, Smith M, et al. CSF flow abnormalities in caudal occipital malformation syndrome. J Vet Intern Med 2005;19(3):418–9.
146. Ma D, Gulani V, Seiberlich N, et al. Magnetic resonance fingerprinting. Nature 2013;495(7440):187–92.
147. Chen Y, Jiang Y, Ma D, et al. Magnetic resonance fingerprinting (MRF) for rapid quantitative abdominal imaging. Paper presented at: Proceedings of the 22nd Annual Meeting ISMRM. Milano, May 10–16, 2014.
148. European Society of Radiology. Magnetic resonance fingerprinting–a promising new approach to obtain standardized imaging biomarkers from MRI. Insights Imaging 2015;6(2):163–5.

Feline Epilepsy

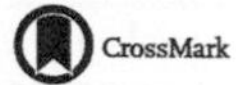

Heidi Barnes Heller, DVM

KEYWORDS

• Feline seizures • Epilepsy • Phenobarbital • Levetiracetam

KEY POINTS

- Seizure disorders can be classified as idiopathic epilepsy, structural epilepsy, or reactive seizures.
- Phenobarbital is commonly the drug of choice.
- Levetiracetam may be more effective for cats with audiogenic seizures.
- Response to treatment is typically favorable, regardless of underlying diagnosis.

INTRODUCTION

Seizures are a common reason cats are presented to a veterinary neurologist. Despite the high prevalence of seizures in cats, debate exists on the correct terminology for seizure classification. Historically, veterinary seizure classification has been based on the human terminology published by the International League Against Epilepsy[1–3]; however, this has been problematic, especially for cats, because etiology and diagnostic investigation differ between human and cat species. The International Veterinary Epilepsy Task Force (IVETF) was formed in 2014 to advance a veterinary seizure classification system, based on the International League Against Epilepsy classification system, with modifications specifically designed for veterinary species. Differences between the International League Against Epilepsy and IVETF classification systems can be found in **Table 1**.

DESCRIPTION OF SEIZURES

The neuroanatomic lesion localization for any animal with seizures is the prosencephalon (the forebrain). Seizures are caused by hypersynchronous neuronal activity that results from an imbalance of excitation and inhibition within the neural network.[4] Animals may have 1 seizure or multiple seizures. After multiple seizures are confirmed, the disorder may be termed epilepsy if a metabolic or toxic cause is not identified. Epilepsy is a neurologic disorder that is defined by recurrent seizures.[5] There are 3

Disclosure Statement: The author has nothing to disclose.
Neurology/Neurosurgery, Department of Medical Sciences, School of Veterinary Medicine, University of Wisconsin-Madison, 2015 Linden Drive, Madison, WI 53706, USA
E-mail address: Heidi.barnesheller@wisc.edu

Vet Clin Small Anim 48 (2018) 31–43
http://dx.doi.org/10.1016/j.cvsm.2017.08.011
vetsmall.theclinics.com
0195-5616/18/

Table 1
Comparison of the International League against Epilepsy (ILAE) and International Veterinary Epilepsy Task Force (IVETF) seizure classification systems

ILAE (2011) Classification	IVETF Classification	Definition
Genetic epilepsy	Idiopathic epilepsy	An intracranial disorder that has a confirmed genetic predisposition in the breed or animal.
Unknown epilepsy	Idiopathic epilepsy	No known genetic predisposition, but no identifiable cause on diagnostic testing (MRI, cerebrospinal fluid, laboratory).
Structural epilepsy	Structural epilepsy	An identifiable cause on diagnostic testing. for example, brain tumor, or encephalitis.
Metabolic seizures	Reactive seizures	Not epilepsy, but is a seizure disorder, for example, hypoglycemia.

phases to a seizure: (1) preictal phase, (2) ictal phase, and (3) postictal phase. The preictal phase is the time before the ictus (ictal phase) in which cats may display behavior or attitudes that owners can recognize as a preamble to a seizure. This activity may include hiding or seeking behavior, nausea, vomiting, or aggression. The preictal phase may last for seconds or hours. The ictus, or "seizure," typically involves both somatic and autonomic systems. Description of the different seizure semiology is discussed elsewhere in this article. Resolution of the ictus leads to the postictal phase, in which neuronal "resetting" occurs. Common clinical signs during the postictal phase may include hiding, blindness, or ataxia.

Seizures may be described as focal, complex focal, or generalized. These descriptions apply to the ictal phase only. Generalized seizures involve bilateral body movements with impaired consciousness. Agreement about the presence or absence of awareness may be difficult, even between veterinarians; therefore, caution should be taken not to overemphasize the state of awareness by practitioners when interrogating owners.[6] Focal seizures may manifest as abnormal movement of 1 part of the body, with or without altered mentation. Complex focal seizures include altered consciousness and are often described as abnormal running behavior, acute changes in mentation with abnormal facial movements, and ptyalism.[7] Complex focal seizures are common in cats. Focal seizures may rapidly generalize therefore a focused, detailed history should be taken to obtain as complete of a description as possible of the seizure event.

Reflex seizures are defined as seizures that occur immediately after a specific, identifiable stimulus.[8] Such stimuli may include visual (eg, photic), auditory (eg, music), or tactile (eg, bathing) stimuli. A reflex seizure may manifest as a generalized or focal seizure; however, they are most often associated with focal seizures.[9,10] Audiogenic reflex seizures have been described in a group of cats in the United Kingdom in which the trigger was a specific, often high-pitched sound.[11] Reflex seizures assume the same lesion localization and differential list as any epileptic seizure phenotype.

SEIZURE ETIOLOGY

The IVETF broadly classifies canine and feline epileptic syndromes by etiology as (1) idiopathic epilepsy (IE) and (2) structural epilepsy (SE).[10] Seizure secondary to metabolic disease or toxin exposure are classified as reactive seizures, but are not considered epileptic events by the IVETF.

Idiopathic Epilepsy

IE (also known as epilepsy of unknown origin), occurs in approximately 30% to 60% of cats.[2,12–16] The diagnosis of IE is achieved through complete metabolic screening, acquisition of a normal brain MRI and cerebrospinal fluid (CSF) analysis. A clinical diagnosis of IE is made in absence of diagnosable etiology in a cat with a history of 2 or more seizures and a normal interictal examination. One study found significantly more cats with IE displayed seizure activity during rest or sleep compared with cats with SE.[13] Spontaneous genetic epilepsy has rarely been documented in cats[17]; however, documentation of inheritance is seldom pursued in clinical practice; therefore, the prevalence may be higher than published data suggest. Age at diagnosis of IE varies widely in cats; therefore, cats with seizure onset greater than 6 years of age should not automatically be given a poor prognosis.[2] Cats diagnosed with IE are typically younger than cats diagnosed with SE.[2,12–14] IE may also be diagnosed in very young cats. IE accounted for approximately 26% of the cats diagnosed with seizures at less than 1 year of age.[18]

Structural Epilepsy

SE is defined by the IVETF as "epileptic seizures which are provoked by intracranial/cerebral pathology."[10] SE is the most common etiologic classification in cats of all ages, and may be caused by neoplastic, inflammatory, infectious, traumatic, vascular, or degenerative causes.[2,13,14,18,19] The diagnosis of SE requires the identification of an intracranial disease in an area of the brain likely to promote seizures. To accomplish this, MRI and CSF analysis may be used. MRI is superior to computed tomography for optimal visualization of intracranial structures.

Neoplasia

Neoplasia and meningoencephalitis (infectious or noninfectious) are the most common causes of SE in adult cats.[2,13,14] Cats with intracranial neoplasia are most frequently diagnosed with meningioma or lymphoma; however, not all cats with intracranial neoplasia develop seizures.[20,21] Tomek and colleagues[21] reported the incidence of seizures was approximately 33% for cats with intracranial neoplasia and the most common anatomic location of the neoplasm was the parietal lobe in these cats. Other types of neoplasia that have been associated with the development of seizures in cats include glial cell neoplasia (astrocytoma, oligodendroglioma), olfactory neuroblastoma, pituitary macroadenoma, and ependymoma.[2,21–23] Treatment options may include surgical treatment, medical treatment, or radiotherapy and are outlined in other resources.

Infectious/noninfectious

The most commonly reported infectious etiologies of meningoencephalitis include feline infectious peritonitis, *Toxoplasma gondii*, and *Cryptococcus* spp. Infection; however, other fungal and bacterial causes may occur.[2,14,24–26] The incidence of seizures is low for cats with feline infectious peritonitis; therefore, the presence of seizures may indicate extensive infection of the prosencephalon and a poorer prognosis.[27] Confirmation of feline infectious peritonitis should be obtained through histopathologic evaluation at necropsy or through brain biopsy. Noninfectious meningoencephalitis, also termed meningoencephalitis of unknown etiology, may be immune-mediated or secondary to a yet unidentified infectious etiology.[2,14,15,24] A diagnosis of meningoencephalitis of unknown etiology is obtained through identification of intracranial inflammation without concurrent evidence of infection. CSF analysis may be more sensitive than MRI for the detection of meningoencephalitis in cats; however, it is a nonspecific test and, therefore, it is not recommended to perform CSF analysis without MRI.[25] Treatment for infectious meningoencephalitis is directed at the infectious etiology, often with concurrent antiinflammatory medication to decrease secondary central nervous system inflammation. Treatment for meningoencephalitis of unknown etiology involves immunosuppression and clinical response is variable. The long-term prognosis depends the clinical response of the cat to treatment.

Traumatic brain injury

Posttraumatic seizures are classified as early if they occur within 7 days of traumatic brain injury or late if they occur after 7 days. Cats sustain crush injuries most commonly; therefore, seizures may result from primary or secondary traumatic brain injury. The incidence of posttraumatic seizures in cats is unknown. Grohmann et al[28] reported no cases of posttraumatic seizures in 52 cats evaluated a minimum of 2 years after mild to moderate traumatic brain injury. Qahwash and colleagues[18] reported 2 of 7 cats (29%) less than 12 months of age at time of first seizure with posttraumatic seizures. Both cats had an abnormal neurologic examination at presentation and were alive at follow-up 13 and 15 months after injury. Hyperglycemia may occur secondary to moderate head trauma in cats; however, no association with prognosis has been identified to date.[29] A diagnosis is made based on historical or physical evidence of trauma paired with advanced brain imaging (MRI or computed tomography scan).

Cerebrovascular disease

Cerebrovascular disease is an uncommon cause of seizures in cats and accounts for 10% to 20% of cats with epilepsy.[14,19] Cerebrovascular disease may be secondary to infarct or hemorrhage. In 1 study, cerebrovascular infarcts were diagnosed in 75% of cats with vascular induced cerebral signs and seizures were reported in 42% of these cats.[30]

Clinical signs reflect the area of the brain affected by poor perfusion. Perfusion to the feline brain differs from the canine brain, which may lead to a different distribution of clinical signs in cats when compared with dogs.[30] Alterations in cerebrovascular perfusion commonly result in acute onset clinical signs. Typically, a cerebrovascular injury results in asymmetric findings on neurologic assessment, however if global ischemia has occurred (eg, anesthetic accident) neurologic examination findings may be symmetric. An underlying etiology has been reported for the majority of cats with cerebrovascular disease; therefore, an investigation into the systemic health of the cat should be pursued after a diagnosis of feline cerebrovascular disease.[30]

Hippocampal sclerosis

Mesial temporal lobe epilepsy with hippocampal sclerosis is a distinct syndrome in human epileptics with common orofacial seizure presentation.[31,32] Hippocampal sclerosis has also been described in cats with a similar seizure semiology.[12,13,33–35] Debate is ongoing in the veterinary literature if this diagnosis is a cause of, or secondary to, seizures in cats. In human epileptics, there are 2 forms of hippocampal sclerosis described. Primary hippocampal sclerosis seems to coincide with seizure onset, thus supporting the hypothesis that it is the underlying seizure etiology. Secondary hippocampal sclerosis occurs after ongoing, long-term seizures, supporting the hypothesis that hippocampal sclerosis occurs as a result of chronic seizures. Secondary hippocampal sclerosis was suggested by the authors of a case report in which 2 cats had a normal brain MRI at seizure onset, and were later diagnosed with hippocampal sclerosis on repeat brain MRI (2 cats) and necropsy (1 cat).[34] Secondary hippocampal sclerosis was considered more likely by others because it is more commonly diagnosed on necropsy in cats with status epilepticus or chronic seizure history.[35] Hippocampal sclerosis may be idiopathic or associated with concurrent intracranial pathology. The majority of cats in 1 report diagnosed with hippocampal sclerosis had concurrent intracranial pathology, including infectious meningoencephalitis, inflammatory meningoencephalitis, vascular disease, or neoplasia.[35] Abnormalities in the temporal lobe on MRI have been described primarily on the fluid-attenuated inversion recovery, T2-weighted and T1-weighted postcontrast sequences for humans diagnosed with mesial temporal lobe epilepsy with hippocampal sclerosis and in cats diagnosed with hippocampal sclerosis. Classen and colleagues[33] reported that hippocampal abnormalities on MRI did not differ significantly among cats with and without seizures. However, when cats with only orofacial seizures, cluster seizures, or a history of status epilepticus were segregated for analysis a significant difference was found in MRI appearance of the hippocampus. Cats with orofacial seizures often have cluster seizures or status epilepticus; therefore, the semiology may be less important than the severity of the seizures to generate MRI-detectable hippocampal pathology; however, further research is needed to evaluate this hypothesis.

Identification of intracranial pathology through evaluation of a brain MRI or CSF analysis may lead to a diagnosis of SE; however, one must exercise caution in this approach. Ictal or interictal electroencephalography is rarely performed in cats and, therefore, the origin of the epileptic focus cannot be documented in most cases. Without identification of the epileptic focus, one is making an assumption that the intracranial pathology identified is associated with the seizure disorder.

Degenerative/Congenital

Reported congenital malformations suspected to cause seizures in cats include hydrocephalus,[18,36,37] porencephaly,[18] occipital arachnoid diverticula,[18] neuronal heterotopia,[38] and a malformation complex in Toyger cats, including commissural malformations, ventriculomegaly, and interhemispheric cysts.[39] Treatment may include surgical or medical management. Surgical correction with a ventriculoperitoneal shunt may improve, or in rare situations eliminate, neurologic abnormalities in young cats with hydrocephalus.[37] Storage disorders have also been reported to cause seizures in cats.[40] A storage disorder should be considered in a young cat with multifocal neurologic abnormalities in which metabolic testing, MRI, and CSF analysis are unremarkable.

Reactive Seizures

Reactive seizures are less common than IE or SE in adult and young cats.[2,13,18,24] Reported causes of reactive seizures in cats include hepatic encephalopathy, hepatic lipidosis, hyperthyroidism, polycythemia, renal disease, hyperosmolality, hypoglycemia, and toxins.[2,13,18,24] Serum bile acids have a high sensitivity and specificity for supporting a diagnosis of portosystemic shunts in cats and should be considered in any young cat presenting with seizures.[41] Additional metabolic testing, including complete blood count, serum biochemistry analysis, and urinalysis, aids in the diagnosis of reactive seizures. A historical exposure to toxins should increase the suspicion of reactive seizures.

DIAGNOSTIC APPROACH

Pursuit of diagnostic testing is recommended for cats presenting with a history of 2 or more seizures within a short time interval. If following the recent IVETF recommendations for dogs, pursuit of testing should be undertaken if 2 or more seizures occur within a 6-month period.[42] Initial blood sampling for a complete blood count, serum biochemistry, and urinalysis may yield a metabolic abnormality, rendering a diagnosis of reactive seizures. If no significant biochemical or hematological abnormalities are detected, advanced imaging of the brain using MRI may be recommended. MRI is the recommended diagnostic imaging tool for the diagnosis of seizures.[43] If no structural abnormalities are identified, removal of CSF via cisternal puncture may be recommended. General anesthesia is recommended for MRI and CSF centesis to minimize risk and allow for immobility during the procedures. Electroencephalography may be used to detect epileptiform patterns in sedated or anesthetized animals, aiding in the identification of interictal activity suggestive of seizures.[44] Routine monitoring with electroencephalography is rarely reported in cats owing to technical difficulties obtaining diagnostic recordings.

The results of the diagnostic testing will lead the clinician to an etiologic classification and confirmed or presumptive diagnosis for the cause of the seizure disorder.

ANTIEPILEPTIC DRUGS

The IVETF published guidelines for initiation of therapy for dogs, which could be extrapolated to cats. Among other parameters, the IVETF recommends starting antiepileptic drugs (AED) when any dog has 2 or more seizures in 6 months and/or any 1 seizure lasting longer than 5 minutes.[42] A secondary reason to begin therapy is the presence of severe (eg, aggression) or long-lasting (eg, longer than 24 hours) clinical signs during the postictal phase. The author also encourages initiation of AED if the cat is at reasonable risk of additional seizures, even if the frequency recommendations are not met, for example, a cat with a brain tumor in the parietal lobe, or a young cat with severe hydrocephalus. Other authors have advocated for more aggressive initiation of treatment and suggested AED treatment should be initiated if 2 or more seizures occur in 6 weeks.[12] A delay in AED initiation may result in a longer time to seizure control, or seizure freedom.[45] Choosing the best AED should be based on the seizure semiology, the cat's health status, and owner considerations (frequency of administration, cost, and liquid vs tablet formulation). A summary of the mechanism of action, dosage, and therapeutic interval for the following AED is in **Table 2**.

Phenobarbital

Phenobarbital is the most commonly used AED in cats.[1,45–47] Rare side effects and no adverse biochemical or hematological events have been reported after use in cats.[48] Side effects may include sedation, ataxia, and weakness, especially during the first 2 weeks of treatment. In a single case report, pseudolymphoma was reported after oral administration of phenobarbital in a cat.[49] Phenobarbital is rapidly absorbed after oral administration, reaching maximal concentration within 1.5 hours. The elimination half-life is similar to what has been reported for dogs and, therefore, a steady state is expected in most cats 10 to 14 days after initiation of treatment.[48] Phenobarbital is lipid soluble, rapidly crosses the blood–brain barrier, and has a high volume of distribution in experimental models. Standard dosing for cats is 2 to 5 mg/kg by mouth every 12 hours (reported ranges, 1.8–10.0 mg/kg/d)[1,12,45,48,50] The therapeutic interval has not been established in cats; however, the dog reference interval of 15 to 45 μg/mL may be used or a more narrow therapeutic window between 23 and 30 μg/mL has been recommended.[1,12,47,50] In 1 study, seizure control was achieved in 93% of cats with a serum phenobarbital concentration between 15 and 45 μg/mL, regardless of underlying etiology.[1] As an alternative to oral administration, topical administration with transdermal phenobarbital has been evaluated in healthy cats using 2 different carrier molecules: pluronic lecithin organogel and Lipoderm Activemax.[51,52] Serum

Table 2
Antiepileptic drugs prescribed for use in cats with seizures

Antiepileptic Drug	Mechanism of Action	Dosage Range	Therapeutic Interval
Phenobarbital	Inhibition of acetylcholine release, norepinephrine and glutamate. Ca^{2+} channel inhibitor, GABA mimetic.	2–5 mg/kg PO q12h[1,12,50] 9 mg/kg transdermal q12h[51]	15–45 μg/mL[c]
Levetiracetam – standard release	Selectively binds SV2A protein thus modulating the release of neurotransmitters.	20 mg/kg PO q8h[53,54]	5–45 μg/mL[a]
Levetiracetam – extended release	Same as above.	500 mg/cat PO q12–24h (in press)	5–45 μg/mL[a]
Zonisamide	Blocks Na and Ca^{2+} channels and may reduce the spread of seizures.	5–10 mg/kg PO q12h[64]	10–40 mg/L[a]
Imepitoin	GABA mimetic.	0–80 mg/kg/d PO[b]	Unknown
Pregablin	Binds voltage-gated Ca channels.	1–2 mg/kg q12h[71]	2.8–8.2 μg/mL[a]
Gabapentin	Same as pregabalin.	10 mg/kg q12h[72]	Unknown

Dosage is based on available literature and clinical studies when applicable.
Abbreviation: PO, by mouth.
[a] Human reference interval. Feline reference interval not established.
[b] Use caution if prescribing this dose because it has not been verified in clinical trials in cats.
[c] Canine reference interval. Feline reference interval not established.

concentrations within the reference interval were not obtained in any cats at standard doses of 3 mg/kg every 12 hours. Dose escalation to 9 mg/kg every 12 hours resulted in serum concentrations of greater than 15 μg/mL for most cats, using both carrier molecules. However, application was easier for owners using Lipoderm Activemax ; therefore, the phenobarbital in Lipoderm Activemax was recommended.[51,52] A clinical trial comparing serum phenobarbital concentrations in epileptic cats on oral therapy and transdermal therapy is currently underway. Midpoint analysis suggests serum concentrations achieved with transdermal phenobarbital are within 20% of serum concentrations achieved with oral phenobarbital, indicating transdermal phenobarbital may be a viable alternative to oral administration for cats.

Levetiracetam

Levetiracetam is an AED that has a novel mechanism of action compared with other common AED.[53,54] The therapeutic interval for levetiracetam is unknown and has been extrapolated from humans for use in dogs and cats (5–45 μg/mL).[53,55,56] Reported side effects in cats receiving levetiracetam include mild transient hypersalivation, inappetance, and mild lethargy.[53,54] There are currently 2 formulations available: (1) standard release levetiracetam and (2) extended-release levetiracetam (XRL). After pharmacokinetic analysis, a dosage of 20 mg/kg by mouth every 8 hours was recommended for cats.[53] A greater than 50% reduction in seizures was noted in 7 of 10 cats after levetiracetam was added to phenobarbital for seizure management.[54] XRL is currently available in 500 mg and 750 mg size tablets. Crushing, splitting, or chewing the tablets is not recommended; therefore, its usefulness in cats has been limited. Single dose pharmacokinetics after 500 mg XRL by mouth were evaluated in healthy cats and a dosing interval of once to twice daily was suggested.[57] A 10-day multidose trial of 500 mg once daily XRL was completed in 9 healthy cats. Seven of 9 cats maintained serum levetiracetam concentrations above the minimum human therapeutic interval at trough samples and minimal side effects were noted (Barnes Heller HL, in progress). Use of XRL in cats allows a decreased frequency of oral administration, thereby improving the quality of life for the cat and client.

Levetiracetam resulted in marked improvement in seizure control, compared with phenobarbital, in cats with suspected audiogenic reflex seizures.[58] This finding is in agreement with a survey of human epileptologists, in which levetiracetam was identified as the first drug of choice for adults and adolescents with seizures involving myoclonus.[59] Further studies are needed to determine if levetiracetam retains greater effectiveness for specific seizure semiology in epileptic cats long term.

Tolerance of levetiracetam has been suggested in dogs; however, this difficulty has yet to be documented in cats.[60,61] The lack of documentation should not exclude the possibility of long-term tolerance (termed the "honeymoon effect" by some authors); rigorous seizure frequency monitoring should be maintained if a cat receives long-term levetiracetam. Administration of intermittent, or pulse, levetiracetam for several days after a seizure has been recommended in dogs to avoid development of long-term tolerance.[62] This approach has not been validated in cats and, therefore, should be used with caution.

Zonisamide

Zonisamide is a sulfa-derived AED developed first in cats and rats in the late 1970s in Japan.[63] The reported half-life of zonisamide in cats (68 hours) is longer than that reported for dogs, which is suspected to be due to the decreased hepatic glucuronide conjugation in cats.[64] Gastrointestinal upset (vomiting, diarrhea, nausea) was reported in one-half of the cats receiving long-term treatment with zonisamide at 20 mg/kg;

therefore, a lower dose may be required to limit these side effects in some cats.[64] Other side effects, including ataxia and sedation, were also noted. Three of 5 cats treated with a mean dose of 11.54 mg/kg/d were reported to have a greater than 50% reduction in seizures in 1 study.[65] Rare, mild side effects were reported and no hematological or biochemical changes were detected after 90 days of administration. Few reports are available discussing the usefulness of zonisamide in cats with naturally occurring epilepsy.[15,65] In 2015, the IVETF did not find sufficient data to recommend using zonisamide either as monotherapy or adjunctive AED therapy in dogs.[42] Given the lesser amount of information available in cats, clients should be counseled on the lack of clinical evidence supporting the use of zonisamide in cats for the treatment of epilepsy before initiation of this medication.

Imepitoin

Imepitoin is licensed in Europe and Australia for use in the management of IE in dogs, and is not approved for use in cats. It is not currently available in the United States. Imepitoin has been used at dosages up to 80 mg/kg/d in healthy cats.[66] Adverse gastrointestinal effects (reduced appetite, vomiting) were noted at the higher dosages; however, it is unclear in the published literature how many of the cats were affected with these side effects. No clinical trials have been published evaluating efficacy of this drug in epileptic cats. Caution should be exercised if prescribing this medication to cats owing to the lack of pharmacokinetic profiling, safety reporting, and clinical efficacy for seizure control.

Bromide

Potassium bromide is not recommended for use in cats owing to the high occurrence of adverse reactions.[67] Most commonly bromide results in coughing and/or dyspnea with resolution in most, but not all, cats after discontinuation of the drug. The respiratory complications are suspected to be secondary to airway hypersensitivity, which is best managed with discontinuation of bromide administration.[68]

Other

Gabapentin, pregablin, and topiramate have been evaluated in limited clinical trials in dogs. To date, no clinical trials have been published evaluating these drugs in cats. There are published dosages for each of these drugs; however, one must be aware of the limited clinical and pharmacokinetic data available when using these drugs in epileptic cats.

Drug Resistance and Recurrence

Drug resistant epilepsy is defined as “a failure of adequate trials of two appropriately chosen and used antiepileptic drug schedules (whether as monotherapies or in combination) to achieve sustained seizure freedom.”[69] Limited data are available for drug resistance in cats; however, because a greater number of cats are diagnosed with IE, this issue may become more prevalent in this population. Current recommendations in humans encourage switching from one monotherapy to another monotherapy, rather than administration of adjunct AED.[59] For cats, poor response to the primary AED warrants trial of a second AED either as addon therapy or a second monotherapy. The pharmacokinetic profile of individual drugs, metabolic state of the cat, and economic situation of the client should be considered before initiation of AED for epileptic cats.

It is well-known that abrupt discontinuation of AED may result in withdrawal seizures and, therefore, this action should be avoided whenever possible. Caution should be exercised when considering reducing or tapering the AED after a period of seizure freedom as well. Six of 8 cats had a recurrence of seizures after reduction of AEDs in 1 study.[45] Given the scarcity of literature addressing recurrent seizures after reduction of AED in cats, owners should be counseled about the risk and benefits of reducing or discontinuing AED before starting a drug tapering protocol.

PROGNOSIS

The prognosis for long-term survival or seizure control depends the underlying etiology, treatment pursued, and response to treatment. The overall long-term survival is good for many cats, regardless of the diagnosis.[70] Similar to dogs, cats with adult-onset seizures secondary to IE have a significantly longer survival compared with cats with adult-onset seizures secondary to SE.[2] In another study evaluating cats less than 12 months of age at seizure onset, cats diagnosed with SE had a slightly longer survival than those diagnosed with IE or reactive seizures.[18] Treatment delay could result in an increased seizure frequency; therefore, AED should be considered if a cat meets the recommendations for initiation of treatment. Given that cat seizures are typically well-controlled with AED, prompt treatment seems to be integral to improved long-term outcome.[12]

ACKNOWLEDGMENTS

The author thanks Dr Helena Rylander for her meticulous review of this article.

REFERENCES

1. Finnerty KE, Barnes Heller HL, Mercier MN, et al. Evaluation of therapeutic phenobarbital concentrations and application of a classification system for seizures in cats: 30 cases (2004-2013). J Am Vet Med Assoc 2014;244(2):195–9.
2. Barnes HL, Chrisman CL, Mariani CL, et al. Clinical signs, underlying cause, and outcome in cats with seizures: 17 cases (1997-2002). J Am Vet Med Assoc 2004; 225(11):1723–6.
3. Mariani CL. Terminology and classification of seizures and epilepsy in veterinary patients. Top Companion Anim Med 2013;28(2):34–41.
4. Fisher RS, Van Emde Boas W, Blume W, et al. Epileptic seizures and epilepsy: Definitions proposed by the International League Against Epilepsy (ILAE) and the International Bureau for Epilepsy (IBE). Epilepsia 2005;46(4):470–2.
5. Fisher RS, Acevedo C, Arzimanoglou A, et al. ILAE official report: a practical clinical definition of epilepsy. Epilepsia 2014;55(4):475–82.
6. Packer RMA, Berendt M, Bhatti S, et al. Inter-observer agreement of canine and feline paroxysmal event semiology and classification by veterinary neurology specialists and non-specialists. BMC Vet Res 2015;11(39):1–11.
7. Pakozdy A, Gruber A, Kneissl S, et al. Complex partial cluster seizures in cats with orofacial involvement. J Feline Med Surg 2011;13:687–93.
8. Koepp MJ, Caciagli L, Pressler RM, et al. Reflex seizures, traits, and epilepsies: from physiology to pathology. Lancet Neurol 2016;15(1):92–105.
9. Engel J, International League Against Epilepsy (ILAE). A proposed diagnostic scheme for people with epileptic seizures and with epilepsy: report of the ILAE task force on classification and terminology. Epilepsia 2001;42(6):796–803.
10. Berendt M, Farquhar RG, Mandigers PJJ, et al. International Veterinary Epilepsy Task Force consensus report on epilepsy definition, classification and terminology in companion animals. BMC Vet Res 2015;11:182–93.

11. Lowrie M, Bessant C, Harvey RJ, et al. Audiogenic reflex seizures in cats. J Feline Med Surg 2015;18(4):328–36.
12. Pakozdy A, Halasz P, Klang A. Epilepsy in cats: theory and practice. J Vet Intern Med 2014;28(2):255–63.
13. Pakozdy A, Leschnik M, Sarchahi AA, et al. Clinical comparison of primary versus secondary epilepsy in 125 cats. J Feline Med Surg 2010;12(12):910–6.
14. Schriefl S, Steinberg TA, Matiasek K, et al. Etiologic classification of seizures, signalment, clinical signs, and outcome in cats with seizure disorders: 91 cases (2000–2004). J Am Vet Med Assoc 2004;233:1591–7.
15. Wahle AM, Brühschwein A, Matiasek K, et al. Clinical characterization of epilepsy of unknown cause in cats. J Vet Intern Med 2014;28(1):182–8.
16. Schwartz-Porsche D, Kaiser E. Feline epilepsy. Probl Vet Med 1989;1(4):628–49.
17. Kuwabara T, Hasegawa D, Ogawa F, et al. A familial spontaneous epileptic feline strain: a novel model of idiopathic/genetic epilepsy. Epilepsy Res 2010;92(1): 85–8.
18. Qahwash M, Barnes Heller HL. Etiology and long-term outcome in feline juvenile onset epilepsy: 15 cases. J Am Vet Med Assoc 2017, in press.
19. Parent JM, Quesnel AD. Seizures in cats. Vet Clin North Am Small Anim Pract 1996;26:811–25.
20. Cameron S, Rishniw M, Miller AD, et al. Characteristics and survival of 121 cats undergoing excision of intracranial meningiomas (1994-2011). Vet Surg 2015;44: 772–6.
21. Tomek A, Cizinauskas S, Doherr M, et al. Intracranial neoplasia in 61 cats: localisation, tumour types and seizure patterns. J Feline Med Surg 2006;8(4):243–53.
22. Woolford L, de Lahunta A, Baiker K, et al. Ventricular and extraventricular ependymal tumors in 18 cats. Vet Pathol 2013;50(2):243–51.
23. Dejesus A, Cohen EB, Galban E, et al. Magnetic resonance imaging features of intraventricular ependymomas in five cats. Vet Radiol Ultrasound 2016;58(3):1–8.
24. Kline KL. Feline epilepsy. Clin Tech Small Anim Pract 1998;13(3):152–8.
25. Negrin A, Lamb CR, Cappello R, et al. Results of magnetic resonance imaging in 14 cats with meningoencephalitis. J Feline Med Surg 2007;9(2):109–16.
26. Singh M, Foster DJ, Child G, et al. Inflammatory cerebrospinal fluid analysis in cats: clinical diagnosis and outcome. J Feline Med Surg 2005;7(2):77–93.
27. Timmann D, Cizinauskas S, Tomek A, et al. Retrospective analysis of seizures associated with feline infectious peritonitis in cats. J Feline Med Surg 2008;10: 9–15.
28. Grohmann KS, Schmidt MJ, Moritz A, et al. Prevalence of seizures in cats after head trauma. J Am Vet Med Assoc 2012;241:1467–70.
29. Syring RS, Otto CM, Drobatz KJ. Hyperglycemia in dogs and cats with head trauma: 122 cases (1997 – 1999). J Am Vet Med Assoc 2000;218:1124–9.
30. Altay UM, Skerritt GC, Hilbe M, et al. Feline cerebrovascular disease: clinical and histopathologic findings in 16 cats. J Am Anim Hosp Assoc 2011;47:89–97.
31. Tatum WO. Mesial temporal lobe epilepsy. J Clin Neurophysiol 2012;29(5): 356–65.
32. Cersósimo R, Flesler S, Bartuluchi M, et al. Mesial temporal lobe epilepsy with hippocampal sclerosis: study of 42 children. Seizure 2011;20(2):131–7.
33. Claßen AC, Kneissl S, Lang J, et al. Magnetic resonance features of the feline hippocampus in epileptic and non-epileptic cats: a blinded, retrospective, multi-observer study. BMC Vet Res 2016;12(1):1–7.

34. Fors S, Van Meervenne S, Jeserevics J, et al. Feline hippocampal and piriform lobe necrosis as a consequence of severe cluster seizures in two cats in Finland. Acta Vet Scand 2015;57:41–50.
35. Wagner E, Rosati M, Molin J, et al. Hippocampal sclerosis in feline epilepsy. Brain Pathol 2014;24:1–13.
36. Dewey CW. External hydrocephalus in two cats. J Am Anim Hosp Assoc 2003; 39(6):567–72.
37. Biel M, Kramer M, Forterre F, et al. Outcome of ventriculoperitoneal shunt implantation for treatment of congenital internal hydrocephalus. J Am Vet Med Assoc 2013;242(7):948–58.
38. DeJesus A, Turek BJ, Galban E, et al. Imaging diagnosis-magnetic resonance imaging of a neuronal heterotopia in the brain of a cat. Vet Radiol Ultrasound 2016;1–5.
39. Keating MK, Sturges BK, Sisó S, et al. Characterization of an inherited neurologic syndrome in Toyger cats with forebrain commissural malformations, ventriculomegaly and interhemispheric cysts. J Vet Intern Med 2016;30(2):617–26.
40. Kuwamura M, Nakagawa M, Nabe M, et al. Neuronal ceroid-lipofuscinosis in a Japanese domestic shorthair cat. J Vet Med Sci 2009;71(5):665–7.
41. Ruland K, Fischer A, Hartmann K. Sensitivity and specificity of fasting ammonia and serum bile acids in the diagnosis of portosystemic shunts in dogs and cats. Vet Clin Pathol 2010;39(1):57–64.
42. Bhatti SFM, De Risio L, Muñana K, et al. International Veterinary Epilepsy Task Force consensus proposal: medical treatment of canine epilepsy in Europe. BMC Vet Res 2015;11(1):176.
43. Hecht S, Adams WH. MRI of brain disease in veterinary patients part 1: basic principles and congenital brain disorders. Vet Clin North Am Small Anim Pract 2010;40(1):21–38.
44. Raith K, Steinberg T, Fischer A. Continuous electroencephalographic monitoring of status epilepticus in dogs and cats: 10 patients (2004-2005). J Vet Emerg Crit Care 2010;20(4):446–55.
45. Pakozdy A, Sarchahi AA, Leschnik M, et al. Treatment and long-term follow-up of cats with suspected primary epilepsy. J Feline Med Surg 2012;15(4):267–73.
46. Smith Bailey K, Dewey CW. The seizuring cat. Diagnostic work-up and therapy. J Feline Med Surg 2009;11(5):385–94.
47. Thomas WB. Idiopathic epilepsy in dogs and cats. Vet Clin North Am Small Anim Pract 2010;40(1):161–79.
48. Cochrane SM, Black WD, Parent JM, et al. Pharmacokinetics of phenobarbital in the cat following intravenous and oral administration. Can J Vet Res 1990;54(1): 132–8.
49. Baho MJ, Hostutler R, Fenner W, et al. Suspected phenobarbital-induced pseudolymphoma in a cat. J Am Vet Med Assoc 2011;238(3):353–5.
50. Platt SR. Feline seizure control. J Am Anim Hosp Assoc 2001;37(6):515–7.
51. Delamaide Gasper JA, Barnes Heller HL, Robertson M, et al. Therapeutic serum phenobarbital concentrations obtained using chronic transdermal administration of phenobarbital in healthy cats. J Feline Med Surg 2014;17(4):359–63.
52. Krull D, Thomovsky SA, Chen-Allen A, et al. Evaluation of transdermal administration of phenobarbital in healthy cats [Abstract ACVIM Forum 2014]. J Vet Intern Med 2014;28:1016.
53. Carnes MB, Axlund TW, Boothe DM. Pharmacokinetics of levetiracetam after oral and intravenous administration of a single dose to clinically normal cats. Am J Vet Res 2011;72(9):7–12.

54. Bailey KS, Dewey CW, Boothe DM, et al. Levetiracetam as an adjunct to phenobarbital treatment in cats with suspected idiopathic epilepsy. J Am Vet Med Assoc 2008;232(6):867–72.
55. Beasley MJ, Boothe DM. Disposition of extended release levetiracetam in normal healthy dogs after single oral dosing. J Vet Intern Med 2015;29:1348–53.
56. Peters RK, Schubert T, Clemmons R, et al. Levetiracetam rectal administration in healthy dogs. J Vet Intern Med 2014;28(2):504–9.
57. Barnard L, Barnes Heller H, Boothe DM. Pharmacokinetic analysis of single dose per os extended release levetiracetam in healthy cats. J Vet Intern Med 2017; 31(4):1260.
58. Lowrie M, Thomson S, Bessant C, et al. Levetiracetam in the management of feline audiogenic reflex seizures: a randomised, controlled, open-label study. J Feline Med Surg 2017;19(2):200–6.
59. Shih JJ, Whitlock JB, Chimato N, et al. Epilepsy treatment in adults and adolescents: expert opinion, 2016. Epilepsy Behav 2017;69:186–222.
60. Charalambous M, Shivapour SK, Brodbelt DC, et al. Antiepileptic drugs' tolerability and safety – a systematic review and meta-analysis of adverse effects in dogs. BMC Vet Res 2016;12(1):79.
61. Volk HA, Matiasek LA, Feliu-Pascual AL, et al. The efficacy and tolerability of levetiracetam in pharmacoresistant epileptic dogs. Vet J 2008;176(3):310–9.
62. Packer RM, Nye G, Porter SE, et al. Assessment into the usage of levetiracetam in a canine epilepsy clinic. BMC Vet Res 2015;11(1):340–8.
63. Ito T, Hori M, Masuda Y, et al. 3-Sulfamoylmethyl-1,2-benzisoxazole, a new type of anticonvulsant drug. Electroencephalographic profile. Arzneimittelforschung 1980;30(4):603–9.
64. Hasegawa D, Kobayashi M, Kuwabara T, et al. Pharmacokinetics and toxicity of zonisamide in cats. J Feline Med Surg 2008;10(4):418–21.
65. Brewer DM, Cerda-Gonzalez S, Dewey CW. Zonisamide for reactive seizures in five cats with presumptive idiopathic epilepsy [Abstract ACVIM Forum 2010]. J Vet Intern Med 2010;24(3):739.
66. Engel O, Mueller J, de Vries F. Imepitoin is well tolerated by healthy cats [abstract ECVN Forum 2016]. J Vet Intern Med 2016;30(1):463.
67. Boothe DM, George KL, Couch P. Disposition and clinical use of bromide in cats. J Am Vet Med Assoc 2002;221(8):1131–5.
68. Bertolani C, Hernandez J, Gomes E, et al. Bromide-associated lower airway disease: a retrospective study of seven cats. J Feline Med Surg 2012;14(8):591–7.
69. Kwan P, Arzimanoglou A, Berg AT, et al. Definition of drug resistant epilepsy: consensus proposal by the ad hoc task force of the ILAE commission on therapeutic strategies. Epilepsia 2010;51(6):1069–77.
70. Quesnel A, Parent J, McDonell W. Clinical management and outcome of cats with seizure disorders: 30 cases (1991-1993). J Am Vet Med Assoc 1997;210:72–7.
71. Dewey CW, Schwark W, Cerda-Gonzalez S, et al. Pharmacokinetics of oral pregablin in cats after single dose administration [Abstract ACVIM Forum 2010]. J Vet Intern Med 2010;24:739.
72. Siao KT, Pypendop BH, Ilkiw JE. Pharmacokinetics of gabapentin in cats. Am J Vet Res 2010;71(7):817–21.

An Update on Cerebrovascular Disease in Dogs and Cats

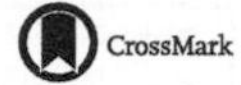

Christen Elizabeth Boudreau, DVM, PhD

KEYWORDS

• Vascular • Brain • Dog • Hemorrhage • Ischemia • Stroke

KEY POINTS

- Cerebrovascular disease (CVD) in dogs and cats can be either ischemic or hemorrhagic. Exclusive of trauma cases, ischemic CVD is more commonly recognized in both species.
- These conditions are often presumptively diagnosed. Exclusion of mimicking brain diseases and identification of predisposing factors are important in animals with suspect CVD.
- Advanced imaging, especially MRI, is the key diagnostic test for making a presumptive diagnosis of either ischemic or hemorrhagic CVD.
- Current standard-of-care treatments are largely supportive and aimed at minimizing secondary brain injury.
- Cases of ischemic CVD and nontraumatic intracranial hemorrhage may have a good prognosis with just supportive care, especially if no underlying cause is identified.

INTRODUCTION

Once thought rare, neurological dysfunction in companion animals due to compromised blood supply is now commonly recognized in veterinary medicine. Terms used to characterize such dysfunction are defined in **Box 1**.[1–3]

VASCULAR ANATOMY IN DOGS AND CATS

Canine arterial cerebrovascular blood supply arises from the basilar and internal carotid arteries, which feed into the cerebral arterial circle. In the cat, blood flow through the basilar artery is predominantly directed craniocaudally, and the external carotid artery (via the maxillary artery) supplies most of the blood to the cerebral arterial circle.

The cerebral arterial circle ensures constant pressure in the end arteries, allowing for collateral perfusion of the parenchyma in the event of arterial occlusion.[5] **Fig. 1** depicts the primary branches of the cerebral arterial circle, other major derivatives, and territories supplied.

Disclosure Statement: The author has nothing to disclose.
Department of Small Animal Clinical Sciences, Texas A&M University, TAMU 4474, College Station, TX 77843-4474, USA
E-mail address: Bboudreau@cvm.tamu.edu

Vet Clin Small Anim 48 (2018) 45–62
http://dx.doi.org/10.1016/j.cvsm.2017.08.009
0195-5616/18/Published by Elsevier Inc.

Box 1
General definitions in cerebrovascular disease

- *Cerebrovascular disease (CVD):* An abnormality of the brain due to disturbance of blood supply[1,2]
- *Stroke:* Rapidly developing clinical signs of focal (or global) disturbance of cerebral function, lasting more than 24 hours or leading to death, with no apparent cause other than that of vascular origin[3]
- *Transient ischemic attack (TIA):* Brief (<24 hours), focal brain dysfunction. The clinical diagnosis of TIA is made when no other cause for the clinical signs is found, and the character of dysfunction implicates a region of the brain served by one vascular supply. TIAs are characterized by complete return of function but often recur.[2,4]

The rostral cerebellar arteries have 3 terminal branches (lateral, intermediate, and medial; shown in **Fig. 2**), which supply overlapping and variable areas of the rostral cerebellar hemispheres and vermis, from lateral to medial, respectively. The rostral cerebellar arteries also supply the dorsal medulla.[6]

The caudal cerebellar arteries are derived from the basilar artery.[7] These arteries supply the caudoventral aspects of the cerebellar hemispheres and vermis, including the flocculus and nodulus, as well as the lateral aspects of the medulla.[8]

Cerebrovascular disease (CVD) results from the disruption of one or more of these vascular territories due to failure of normal regulation, vessel occlusion (ischemic CVD), or vessel rupture (hemorrhagic CVD).

REGULATION OF CEREBRAL BLOOD FLOW

Cerebral arteriolar tone responds to physiologic stimuli to maintain relatively constant blood supply to the brain through autoregulation (**Table 1**). Total cerebral blood flow (CBF) should be constant for mean arterial pressures (MAPs) between 50 and

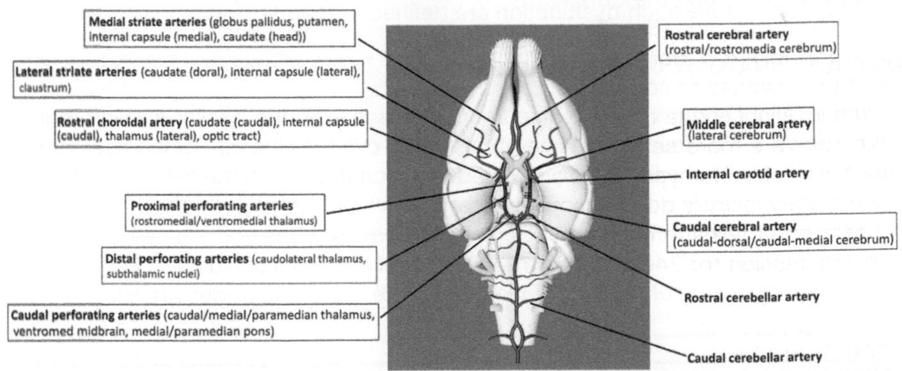

Fig. 1. Schematic of major intracranial arterial supply. The major branches from the cerebral arterial circle to the cerebrum (rostral middle and caudal cerebral arteries) are identified on the right of the diagram. The rostral and caudal cerebellar arteries are identified, branching from the caudal communicating artery and the basilar artery, respectively. On the left side, the major arterial branches to deep structures of the forebrain, midbrain, and pons are labeled, with a summary of the structures they supply presented in the accompanying box for each.

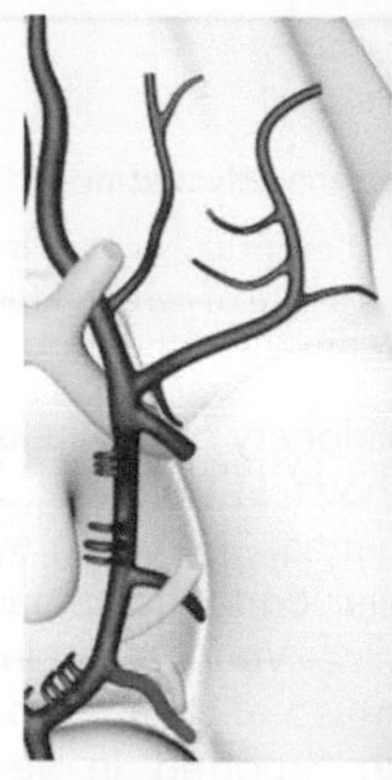

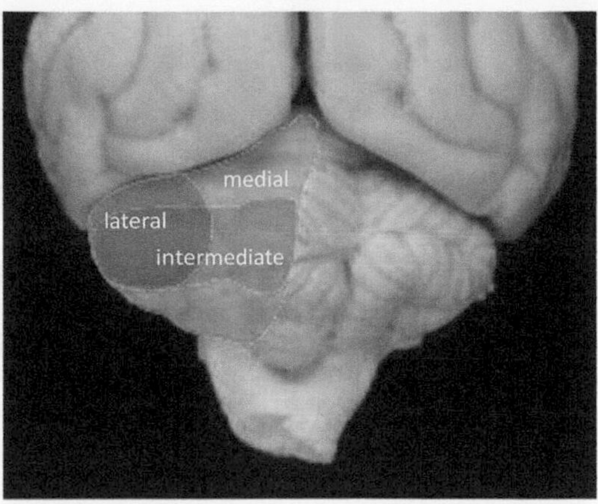

Fig. 2. Regional supply of the 3 main branches of the rostral cerebellar artery. The origin of the rostral cerebellar artery from the caudal communicating artery is identified in the left panel. On the right, the approximate territory supplied by each of its 3 branches (lateral, intermediate, and medial branch of the rostral cerebellar a.) is color-coded as follows: magenta = lateral, teal = intermediate, and green = medial.

150 mm Hg in normal brain. These regulatory responses can be negated in animals with blood-brain barrier (BBB) disruption.[9,10]

CBF and total cerebral vascular resistance (CVR) are related as CBF = CPP/CVR, where CPP is cerebral perfusion pressure. CPP less than 40 mm Hg results in ischemia and loss of autoregulation. CPP is also described by MAP-ICP (intracranial pressure). Severe decreases in MAP or severe increases in ICP may also lead to ischemia.

PATHOPHYSIOLOGY AND CAUSE: ISCHEMIC CEREBROVASCULAR DISEASE

Both the severity and the duration of perfusion reduction influence progression from ischemia to infarction (**Box 2**).[11,12] After 5 hours at less than 40% normal CBF, functional deficits are irreversible.[1,5,13,14] Experimentally, irreversible injury will occur after just 4 to 5 minutes of complete arterial obstruction.[15]

Primary injury is due to energy failure.[16] This process is detailed in **Box 3**.

Neurons are more sensitive than glial cells, which are more sensitive in turn than endothelial cells, to hypoperfusion.[17]

Secondary injury is due to compromise of local vascular endothelium and supporting cells and begins to develop ~4 to 6 hours following the onset of hypoperfusion, with progression for 24 to 48 hours.[18] Secondary injury may be exacerbated where

Table 1
Effect on vascular tone with alteration of physiologic parameters that affect cerebral blood flow

Parameter	Increase	Decrease
MAP	Constriction	Dilation
$Paco_2$	Dilation	Constriction
Pao_2	Constriction	Dilation

Box 2
Definitions for the pathophysiology of ischemic cerebrovascular disease

- *Ischemia:* Perfusion reduction sufficient to induce dysfunction in the affected tissue
- *Infarction:* Perfusion reduction that causes irreversible injury and eventually necrosis

blood flow is still present (eg, during reperfusion, on the periphery of the lesion, or in cases of venous thrombosis[1]).[19,20] These processes are shown in **Box 4**.

Not all areas of the brain are equally susceptible to ischemia. The cerebral cortex (especially the gray matter of the hippocampus), cerebellar cortex, and basal and thalamic nuclei are more prone to ischemic damage.[5,21] Venous occlusion is thought to be less common than arterial occlusion as a cause of cerebral ischemia due to abundant anastomoses; however, it has been reported in veterinary medicine.[22]

DIRECT CAUSES OF ISCHEMIC CEREBROVASCULAR DISEASE

Thromboembolism

Thromboembolism is a local vascular obstruction or obstructive material originating in a distant vascular bed.

1. *Atherosclerosis* is a common cause of thromboembolic CVD in man. It is considered uncommon in dogs,[23] and is unreported in cats,[24] but has been documented, especially in association with dysregulation of lipid metabolism (eg, hypothyroidism[25] or primary hyperlipidemia[25,26]).
2. *Hypercoagulable states* can cause thromboembolic disease. These states include hyperadrenocorticism (HAC), protein-losing nephropathy (PLN), immune-mediated hemolytic anemia, and systemic neoplasia.[27] Cerebrovascular thromboemboli associated with PLN, HAC, and splenic hemangiosarcoma have been documented in dogs with evidence of ischemic CVD.[28] Sepsis and infective endocarditis can also cause hypercoagulability,[29] and the latter has been implicated in ischemic CVD in dogs.[30]
3. Diseases such as neoplasia and heartworm disease have been implicated in hypercoagulable states[27] and direct production of cerebrovascular emboli.[31]
4. *Cardiomyopathy* is a major cause of thromboembolic disease in cats and has been reported in association with feline CVD.[32]
5. *Fibrocartilaginous embolism* has been reported as a cause of cerebrovascular disease in the dog.[33]
6. *Leishmania*[34] and intravascular lymphoma[35] have been implicated in cases of multiple cerebral infarcts.

Box 3
Key processes in primary injury in ischemic cerebrovascular disease

- Failure of Na+/K+ ATPase pumps → cytotoxic edema
- Failure of aerobic metabolism → lactic acidosis → cytotoxicity
- Loss of ionic gradients → depolarization of resting potential → increased Ca^{2+} release → activation of proteases and phospholipases → membrane damage and free radical formation[16]

Box 4
Key processes in secondary injury in ischemic cerebrovascular disease

- Damage to the BBB → vasogenic edema[19] and inflammatory cell infiltrate[20]
- In very severe endothelial injury, hemorrhagic conversion occurs (extravasation of all blood components, including RBCs, through compromised capillaries)[19]

Hemodynamic

Anesthesia-related accidents may result in CVD.[2,32,36] Although cardiogenic cerebral ischemia has been investigated in dogs with ischemic CVD, this association is rarely seen.[12]

Local Vasospasm

Focal vascular injury may occur in cats because of aberrant cerebral *Cuterebra* larval migrans (feline ischemic encephalopathy),[37,38] although vascular lesions may not be found.[1] Vasospasm of the middle cerebral artery has been implicated in this disease.[18]

INDIRECT PREDISPOSITIONS TO ISCHEMIC CEREBROVASCULAR DISEASE (CORRELATIVE)

Chronic hypertension is a major risk factor for CVD in man because of its induction of atherosclerosis and lipohyalinosis in small penetrating arteries of the brain.[5] Similar changes have been documented in the brains of cats with renal dysfunction, hypertension, and suspected hypertensive encephalopathy.[39]

In companion animals, secondary hypertension seems more common than primary hypertension.[40] Causes are shown in **Box 5**.[41–47]

Certain dog breeds, including the Cavalier King Charles spaniel[48] and greyhound,[49] may be more predisposed to ischemic CVD.

PATHOPHYSIOLOGY AND CAUSE: INTRACRANIAL HEMORRHAGE

Primary injury[1,5,50,51] occurs because of direct damage from the growing hematoma (**Box 6**).

Secondary injury[50,52] peaks ~3 to 5 days after onset, but may persist for up to 7 days (**Box 7**).

HEMORRHAGE: CAUSE

- Intracranial hemorrhage (ICH) can be classified according to location.
- *Subdural:* Following trauma in dogs,[53,54] or chronically, associated with hydrocephalus or storage disease.[55,56]

Box 5
Common causes of secondary endocrine hypertension in dogs and cats

- Chronic renal disease (dogs and cats)
- Hyperadrenocorticism (dogs)
- Hyperthyroidism (cats)
- Primary hyperaldosteronism (cats)
- Pheochromocytoma (dogs)

Box 6
Processes in primary injury in intracranial hemorrhage

- Compression of tissue occurs primarily during the first 6 hours following clinical onset[50]
- Elastic resistance of the surrounding parenchyma and increasing ICP limit hematoma expansion[1]
- Once expansion ceases, the hematoma organizes and resolves within days to weeks[5]
- Hematoma resolution includes breakdown of blood products. Heme is damaging to neuronal parenchyma through several mechanisms, including proinflammatory and pro-oxidant activities, and stimulation of excessive glutamate release[13,30,51]

- *Epidural:* Uncommon, may be seen with trauma.[53]
- *Subarachnoid:* Often modeled in dogs, but rarely clinically reported.[57–59]
- *Intraventricular:* May occur alone or in conjunction with ICH into other spaces. It is reported infrequently in dogs.[60–64]
- *Parenchymal:* Most common location for nontraumatic ICH in dogs,[65] although it can also occur following trauma.[53,66] Other causes include both primary and secondary causes[50] (**Table 2**). In many cases, especially those of a single hemorrhagic area ≥ 5 mm, no cause is identified.[65]

Primary ICH due to hypertension is thought to be relatively rare in animals. Published associations between hypertension and ICH in dogs and cats are limited to cases with one or more <5 mm T2*-weighted signal voids,[65,74,75] sometimes termed microbleeds, which have unknown clinical significance. The other main primary cause of ICH in humans, cerebral amyloid angiopathy, has been reported in aged dogs in association with hemorrhage.[76]

Secondary causes of ICH can be divided into several subcategories,[13] as shown in **Box 8**.

Vascular malformations: 4 main recognized types are arteriovenous,[82,83] venous,[84] cavernous, and capillary malformations or telangiectases.[85] Clinical signs of vascular malformations usually manifest upon vessel rupture. Some benign cerebrovascular lesions are proliferative and can cause mass effect in the absence of rupture, including vascular hamartoma[86–89] and meningioangiomatosis.[90]

Neoplasia Associated with Intracranial Hemorrhage

Pituitary apoplexy, or sudden neurologic impairment due to acute hemorrhage or infarction of the pituitary gland, has been described in a dog and cat[62,91] with pituitary tumors. Intracerebral hemangioblastoma[92] and nonneoplastic hemorrhagic masses, such as cavernous hemangioma,[93–95] have also been reported in the canine brain.

Box 7
Processes in secondary injury in intracranial hemorrhage

- Perihemorrhagic edema may occur due to thrombin-induced activation of inflammatory cascades, and overexpression of matrix metalloproteases.[52] Hematoma and edema can cause increased ICP and risk of brain herniation, ± obstructive hydrocephalus
- Ischemia (eg, compression of vascular supply by increased ICP or loss of perfusion from the ruptured vessel)

Table 2
Intracranial neoplasms reported to have intratumoral hemorrhage

Metastatic/Multicentric Tumors	Primary Brain Tumors
Hemangiosarcoma[59,65] (may also cause ischemic necrosis[67])	Pituitary tumors[68]
Other metastatic tumors[69]	Gliomas[68,70,71]
Histiocytic sarcoma[69]	Meningiomas[65,72]
Intravascular lymphoma[35,65]	Choroid plexus tumors[68]
	Others[69,73]

CLINICAL SIGNS

By definition, stroke (or transient ischemic attack [TIA]) has an acute to peracute onset. Ischemic strokes may be nonprogressive or have limited progression over days if secondary vasogenic edema or hemorrhagic conversion develops. Hemorrhagic strokes likewise may have a slightly more gradual onset and longer progression.[1] More recently, clinical neurologic abnormalities have been documented in patients with evidence of chronic CVD.[39,74,96,97] These cases may have a preceding history of TIA-like events. TIA-like events are rarely reported in dogs and cats; however, one case was reported in association with apparent primary hypertension.[98]

Signs are consistent with an intracranial lesion localization, but will differ depending on the region of the brain affected. The relative anatomic incidence of CVD has been variably reported, with cortical, telencephalic, or forebrain structures the majority in some studies[4,7,99,100] but not others.[28,49,101] Hemorrhage may be more commonly identified in the cerebrum than brainstem.[4,65,100] The reported intracranial lesion distributions seem similar in cats.[32,102] Although focal signs are more common than diffuse or multifocal intracranial signs, exceptions exist.[36,74,101,103,104]

Initial clinical evaluation in cases of suspect CVD should also include a thorough review of medical history and current systemic health for predisposing causes.

DIAGNOSIS

Imaging

Advanced brain imaging is indicated to rule out other causes of neurologic clinical signs, to define the extent of the affected area, and to distinguish ischemic from hemorrhagic vascular events.

Box 8
Categories of secondary causes of intracranial hemorrhage

Coagulopathy (*Angiostrongylus vasorum*,[60,65,77–79] von Willebrand factor deficiency[80])

Vascular malformation (see text)

Vasculopathy[13,14,32]

Neoplasia (see **Table 2**)

Bacterial/septicemia[4,30,65]

Postprocedural[81]

Hemorrhagic conversion of ischemic insult[30]

Computed Tomography

Imaging of ischemic change may show only mild focal edema with mild mass effect and minimal contrast enhancement that is subtle and nonspecific.

Acute Hemorrhage

Acute hemorrhage results in relatively conspicuous changes on computed tomography (CT):

- Hyperattenuation due to globin (56–76 HU),[100] relative to 39 HU for gray matter or 32 HU for white matter, is initially seen.
- Hyperattenuation increases for 72 hours after onset, then gradually decreases to isoattenuation at ~1 month posthemorrhage, beginning from the periphery and extending inward.
- Peripheral contrast enhancement may be seen from 6 days to 6 weeks postevent and is thought to be associated with neovascularization.[18]

MRI

MRI is considered more sensitive for ischemic CVD compared with standard CT techniques and is currently recommended for presumptive diagnosis of CVD in veterinary cases.

ISCHEMIA

- Visible within hours of clinical onset[18,100]; initial signs (<6 hours) may be subtle[105]
- Canonically well demarcated, often with one or more linear or curvilinear borders[48,101,106]
- Should correspond to a known vascular territory[105]
- Hypointense to surrounding parenchyma on T1-weighted sequences
- Hyperintense to surrounding tissues on T2-weighted sequences
- Mass effect may develop in hours to days and then decrease over days to weeks
- Contrast enhancement, associated with reperfusion, develops over days and is reported to be maximal ~7 to 10 days after clinical onset[5]
- Changes with global ischemia include mild diffuse T2 hyperintensity in the gray matter of the cerebrum, thalamus, and cerebellum, with mild contrast enhancement of the same regions[36,104]

Diagnostic accuracy for distinguishing ischemic CVD from other intra-axial lesions, especially glial tumors, is variable between observers and studies.[107–109]

Diffusion-weighted imaging (DWI) uses paired dephasing and rephasing gradients to identify areas of restricted diffusion (ie, cytotoxic edema). DWI can be used in the calculation of apparent diffusion coefficient (ADC) maps. DWI and ADC maps improve discrimination between ischemic CVD and glial tumors,[109] but ADC values alone are poorly discriminatory for ischemic, neoplastic, or inflammatory brain lesions.[110] DWI showed ischemic change earlier than conventional MRI sequences in an experimental feline model.[111] A recent experimental study of middle cerebral arterial infarction in the dog shows evolution of MRI changes on conventional sequences and DWI from 24 hours to 14 days after occlusion.[112]

HEMORRHAGE

Gradient echo (GRE) images (such as T2*-weighted images) can identify ICH.[69,105] This technique exploits the sensitivity of GRE sequences to small magnetic field inhomogeneities, like those produced by paramagnetic intracellular deoxyhemoglobin or methemoglobin in the hours to days after ICH. GRE images will show a blooming, hypointense artifact in the region of such substances. This artifact must be distinguished from signal voids caused by bone-air interfaces or calcium salts. If paramagnetic globin derivatives are widely distributed in a larger background of weakly diamagnetic substance (eg, following red blood cell [RBC] lysis in the breakdown of blood products), this artifact will be lost. Superparamagnetic blood breakdown products (eg, hemosiderin) may produce GRE artifacts for months or years.[113]

Differentiating benign ICH from hemorrhagic neoplasm may be challenging. Intratumoral hemorrhage may appear more heterogeneous on T1- and T2-weighted images due to the presence of hemoglobin at various stages of degradation, whereas nonrecurrent spontaneous ICH may appear more uniform.[105] In many cases, hemorrhagic masses also exhibit a nonhemorrhagic component. Hemorrhagic vascular malformations may also appear as hemorrhagic masses on MRI.[83,84,92]

CEREBROSPINAL FLUID

- Cerebrospinal fluid is often nonspecific and may be normal.[5] Mild increases in protein content, reflecting disruption of the BBB, or increases in neutrophilic and mononuclear populations, may be seen.[5]
- With hemorrhagic CVD that involves the meninges, frank hemorrhage may be seen and must be distinguished from blood contamination. Xanthochromia is considered consistent with preexisting hemorrhage.[114] Erythrophagocytosis may be observed in association with preexisting hemorrhage,[114] but can occur ex vivo with delays in sample processing.[115]
- In canine models and clinical cases of ischemic stroke, elevations in interleukin-6[112,116] have been observed.

Table 3
Ancillary testing for suspected cerebrovascular disease in dogs and cats

Ischemia	Hypertension	NIBP, Fundic Examination, Chemistry, UA, T4 (Cats) ± AUS
	Hypercoagulable state	Complete blood count (CBC), chemistry, UA, ± UPC ratio, ± serum ATIII, ± TEG
	Hyperlipidemia	Serum cholesterol, thyroid panel, serum triglycerides
	Sepsis	CBC, CXR, AUS, echo, ± blood culture
	Neoplasia	Palpation, CXR, AUS, ± aspirates
	Endoparasitism	*Dirofilaria immitis* serology
	Cardiomyopathy (cats)	Auscultation, CXR, echo, ± ECG
Hemorrhage	Coagulopathy	CBC, PT/PTT, ± PIVKA, BMBT
	Endoparasitism	*A vasorum* serology (available in UK from IDEXX)
	Neoplasia	See above
	Sepsis	See above
	Hypertension	See above

Abbreviations: ATIII, antithrombin III level; AUS, abdominal ultrasound; BMBT, buccal mucosal bleeding time; CXR, thoracic radiographs; NIBP, noninvasive blood pressure; PIVKA, protein induced by vitamin K absence test; PT/PTT, prothrombin time/partial thromboplastin time; TEG, thromboelastography; UA, urinalysis; UPC, urine protein/creatinine ratio.

ANCILLARY TESTING AND JUSTIFICATION

Additional testing for patients with suspected CVD should focus on identification of direct or indirect risk factors or underlying causes, as shown in **Table 3**.

TREATMENT AND MANAGEMENT STRATEGIES

Acute Management

Acute management is largely supportive and focuses on minimizing secondary damage and preventing complications. Key components are listed in **Box 9**.

Aggressive intervention for hypertension may worsen CPP. Systemic blood pressure should not be pharmacologically lowered in the setting of acute CVD unless there is concern for end-organ damage (eg, clinical signs of hypertensive damage to retina or kidney, or persistent systolic blood pressures >180 mm Hg and unresponsive to other management).[117–119]

Fibrinolytic therapy

Fibrinolytic therapy has not been evaluated in cases of acute ischemic brain events in dogs or cats. In humans, thrombolytic therapy with tissue plasminogen activator has been shown to improve outcomes when administered within 4.5 hours of the onset of clinical signs,[120] but should only be used when hemorrhagic CVD has been ruled out.

Neuroprotective agents

Neuroprotective agents are aimed at decreasing secondary injury, such as the development of vasogenic edema, hemorrhagic conversion, or inflammation. Agents under investigation are shown in **Table 4**.

Surgical evacuation of hematomas

Surgical evacuation of hematomas for severe nontraumatic ICH associated with worsening neurologic status may be considered,[54,119] but has not been proven to affect outcome in humans[121] and has not been evaluated in a controlled manner in veterinary medicine. Surgical intervention for traumatic extra-axial hemorrhage is appropriate for cases that deteriorate in the face of aggressive medical therapy, but may result in rebleeding after surgery.[122] Surgical treatment of hemorrhagic intracerebral masses in dogs has been reported.[83,123]

Hemostatic therapies

Hemostatic therapies may be considered for emergency use in cases with underlying hemostatic abnormalities. In humans, these most often include chronic antiplatelet therapy and exposure to vitamin K antagonists. In the former, platelet transfusions may be indicated if surgical intervention is planned. In the latter, prothrombin complex

Box 9
Key components of acute management of cerebrovascular disease

- Maintenance of good CPP focuses on maintaining MAP $\pm$ normalizing ICP, if it is elevated. If increased ICP is suspected clinically, treatment with osmotic agents (eg, mannitol or hypertonic saline) and head elevation is warranted.
- If hypoxia is present, O_2 supplementation should be instituted.
- If seizures occur, they should be aggressively controlled.
- Glucocorticoid therapy has no proven benefit in either ischemic or hemorrhagic cerebrovascular insult.

Table 4
Investigational neuroprotective agents for ischemic cerebrovascular disease

Pharmacologic	Nonpharmacologic
Free radical scavengers	Hypothermia
Excitotoxicity blockers	Hyperbaric O_2
Immunomodulators	Near-infrared laser
	Stem cell therapies

Current guidelines in human medicine indicate that no neuroprotectives have demonstrated clinical efficacy.

Adapted from Rajah GB, Ding Y. Experimental neuroprotection in ischemic stroke: a concise review. Neurosurg Focus 2017;42:E2; with permission.

concentrate transfusion is preferred to fresh-frozen plasma (FFP) transfusion.[121] FFP transfusion in hypocoagulable dogs and cats remains controversial.[124]

CHRONIC MANAGEMENT AND RISK REDUCTION

Current recommendations for long-term recurrence reduction for humans with ischemic stroke include management of risk factors combined with antiplatelet therapy.[125] In cases of ischemic stroke due to atherosclerosis, antiplatelet therapies are considered standard of care over anticoagulant therapies, because of increased risk of ICH with the latter.[126,127] Neither anticoagulant nor antiplatelet therapy has been evaluated in companion animals for reduction in risk of CVD. Management of risk factors, if identified, is recommended.

PROGNOSIS

Ischemia

Recovery within weeks with only supportive care is commonly reported in dogs with acute ischemic CVD.[12,28,48,99,101,128] Cases with severe or progressive neurologic dysfunction, thought to be associated with secondary injury, have a more guarded prognosis.[1,4,15] In a recent study of ischemic CVD in dogs, 23% died within the first 30 days of the onset of signs, but those that survived greater than 30 days had a median survival time of 505 days.[99] The presence of concurrent medical conditions in dogs with ischemic CVD is associated with shorter survival times and increased frequency of subsequent infarcts.[12,99]

Hemorrhage

Hemorrhagic stroke is associated with higher mortality than ischemic stroke in humans.[129] In dogs with single nontraumatic ICH $\geq$ 5 mm, long-term outcome was good in 60%.[65] In dogs with multiple nontraumatic ICH $\geq$ 5 mm, outcome was poor in 70%.[65] In both cases, most poor outcomes were death or euthanasia related to neurologic signs shortly after identification of ICH. Intraventricular hemorrhage is associated with higher mortality in humans[130] but has not been systematically evaluated in veterinary medicine.

Population information about outcomes in cats with presumed or confirmed CVD is not currently available.

In people with stroke, most of the early deaths following stroke is related to worsening neurologic status. After ~1 week beyond clinical diagnosis, mortality is more likely a result of cardiopulmonary complications, rather than neurologic injury.[131,132]

SUMMARY

Although the incidence of CVD in companion animals is unknown, presumptive diagnoses of CVD have increased with the increasing availability of clinical veterinary MRI and, in particular, imaging sequences with increased sensitivity for vascular disruptions. For both ischemic and hemorrhagic CVD, patient evaluation is aimed at ruling out other possible causes of neurologic signs and identifying underlying causes, if possible. Treatment goals are largely supportive, and general prognosis is good for long-term survival.

ACKNOWLEDGMENTS

The author would like to thank Peter J. Dickinson, DVSc, PhD, DACVIM (Neurology) for his assistance with creating the figures for this article.

REFERENCES

1. Thomas WB. Cerebrovascular disease. Vet Clin North Am Small Anim Pract 1996;26:925–43.
2. Special report from the national institute of neurological disorders and stroke. Classification of cerebrovascular diseases III. Stroke 1990;21:637–76.
3. Sacco RL, Kasner SE, Broderick JP, et al. An updated definition of stroke for the 21st century: a statement for healthcare professionals from the American Heart Association/American Stroke Association. Stroke 2013;44:2064–89.
4. Joseph RJ, Greenlee PG, Carrillo JM, et al. Canine cerebrovascular disease: clinical and pathological findings in 17 cases. J Am Anim Hosp Assoc 1988;24:569–76.
5. Wessmann A, Chandler K, Garosi L. Ischaemic and haemorrhagic stroke in the dog. Vet J 2009;180:290–303.
6. Guo J, Liao JJ, Preston JK, et al. A canine model of acute hindbrain ischemia and reperfusion. Neurosurgery 1995;36:986–92 [discussion: 992–83].
7. Gredal H, Skerritt GC, Gideon P, et al. Spontaneous ischaemic stroke in dogs: clinical topographic similarities to humans. Acta Neurol Scand 2013;128:e11–6.
8. Negrin A, Gaitero L, Anor S. Presumptive caudal cerebellar artery infarct in a dog: clinical and MRI findings. J Small Anim Pract 2009;50:615–8.
9. Bouma GJ, Muizelaar JP, Bandoh K, et al. Blood pressure and intracranial pressure-volume dynamics in severe head injury: relationship with cerebral blood flow. J Neurosurg 1992;77:15–9.
10. Tidwell AS, Mahony OM, Moore RP, et al. Computed tomography of an acute hemorrhagic cerebral infarct in a dog. Vet Radiol Ultrasound 1994;35:290–8.
11. Heiss WD, Rosner G. Functional recovery of cortical neurons as related to degree and duration of ischemia. Ann Neurol 1983;14:294–301.
12. Garosi LS, McConnell JF. Ischaemic stroke in dogs and humans: a comparative review. J Small Anim Pract 2005;46:521–9.
13. Sasaki M, Pool R, Summers BA. Vasculitis in a dog resembling isolated angiitis of the central nervous system in humans. Vet Pathol 2003;40:95–7.
14. Swann JW, Priestnall SL, Dawson C, et al. Histologic and clinical features of primary and secondary vasculitis: a retrospective study of 42 dogs (2004-2011). J Vet Diagn Invest 2015;27:489–96.
15. Victor M, Ropper AH. Cerebrovascular diseases. In: Wonsiewicz MJ, Medina MP, Navrozov M, editors. Adams and Victor's principles of neurology. New York: McGraw-Hill; 2001. p. 821–924.
16. Adams HP, Hachinski V, Norris JW. Ischemic cerebrovascular disease. New York: Oxford University Press; 2001.

17. Summers BA, Cummings JF, de Lahunta A. Degenerative diseases of the central nervous system. In: Veterinary neuropathology. St Louis (MO): Mosby - Year - Book; 1995. p. 237–49.
18. Garosi LS. Cerebrovascular disease in dogs and cats. Vet Clin North Am Small Anim Pract 2010;40:65–79.
19. Simard JM, Kent TA, Chen M, et al. Brain oedema in focal ischaemia: molecular pathophysiology and theoretical implications. Lancet Neurol 2007;6:258–68.
20. Amantea D, Nappi G, Bernardi G, et al. Post-ischemic brain damage: pathophysiology and role of inflammatory mediators. FEBS J 2009;276:13–26.
21. Vandevelde M, Higgins RJ, Oevermann A. Veterinary neuropathology: essentials of theory and practice. Ames (IA): Wiley-Blackwell; 2012.
22. Swayne DE, Tyler DE, Batker J. Cerebral infarction with associated venous thrombosis in a dog. Vet Pathol 1988;25:317–20.
23. Detweiler DK. Spontaneous and induced arterial disease in the dog: pathology and pathogenesis. Toxicol Pathol 1989;17:94–108.
24. Clark M, Hoenig M. Metabolic effects of obesity and its interaction with endocrine diseases. Vet Clin North Am Small Anim Pract 2016;46:797–815.
25. Hess RS, Kass PH, Van Winkle TJ. Association between diabetes mellitus, hypothyroidism or hyperadrenocorticism, and atherosclerosis in dogs. J Vet Intern Med 2003;17:489–94.
26. Manning PJ. Thyroid gland and arterial lesions of Beagles with familial hypothyroidism and hyperlipoproteinemia. Am J Vet Res 1979;40:820–8.
27. Hackner SG, Schaer BD. Thrombotic disorders. In: Weiss DJ, Wardrop KJ, editors. Schalm's veterinary hematology. 6th edition. Ames (IA): Wiley-Blackwell; 2010.
28. Garosi L, McConnell JE, Platt SR, et al. Results of diagnostic investigations and long-term outcome of 33 dogs with brain infarction (2000-2004). J Vet Intern Med 2005;19:725–31.
29. Sykes JE, Kittleson MD, Chomel BB, et al. Clinicopathologic findings and outcome in dogs with infective endocarditis: 71 cases (1992-2005). J Am Vet Med Assoc 2006;228:1735–47.
30. Cook LB, Coates JR, Dewey CW, et al. Vascular encephalopathy associated with bacterial endocarditis in four dogs. J Am Anim Hosp Assoc 2005;41:252–8.
31. Patton CS, Garner FM. Cerebral infarction caused by heartworms (Dirofilaria immitis) in a dog. J Am Vet Med Assoc 1970;156:600–5.
32. Altay UM, Skerritt GC, Hilbe M, et al. Feline cerebrovascular disease: clinical and histopathologic findings in 16 cats. J Am Anim Hosp Assoc 2011;47:89–97.
33. Axlund TW, Isaacs AM, Holland M, et al. Fibrocartilaginous embolic encephalomyelopathy of the brainstem and midcervical spinal cord in a dog. J Vet Intern Med 2004;18:765–7.
34. Jose-Lopez R, la Fuente CD, Anor S. Presumed brain infarctions in two dogs with systemic leishmaniasis. J Small Anim Pract 2012;53:554–7.
35. Kent M, Delahunta A, Tidwell AS. MR imaging findings in a dog with intravascular lymphoma in the brain. Vet Radiol Ultrasound 2001;42:504–10.
36. Timm K, Flegel T, Oechtering G. Sequential magnetic resonance imaging changes after suspected global brain ischaemia in a dog. J Small Anim Pract 2008;49:408–12.
37. Williams KJ, Summers BA, de Lahunta A. Cerebrospinal cuterebriasis in cats and its association with feline ischemic encephalopathy. Vet Pathol 1998;35: 330–43.

38. Glass EN, Cornetta AM, deLahunta A, et al. Clinical and clinicopathologic features in 11 cats with Cuterebra larvae myiasis of the central nervous system. J Vet Intern Med 1998;12:365–8.
39. Brown CA, Munday JS, Mathur S, et al. Hypertensive encephalopathy in cats with reduced renal function. Vet Pathol 2005;42:642–9.
40. Reusch CE, Schellenberg S, Wenger M. Endocrine hypertension in small animals. Vet Clin North Am Small Anim Pract 2010;40:335–52.
41. Dukes J. Hypertension: a review of the mechanisms, manifestations and management. J Small Anim Pract 1992;33:119–29.
42. Ortega TM, Feldman EC, Nelson RW, et al. Systemic arterial blood pressure and urine protein/creatinine ratio in dogs with hyperadrenocorticism. J Am Vet Med Assoc 1996;209:1724–9.
43. Goy-Thollot I, Pechereau D, Keroack S, et al. Investigation of the role of aldosterone in hypertension associated with spontaneous pituitary-dependent hyperadrenocorticism in dogs. J Small Anim Pract 2002;43:489–92.
44. Novellas R, de Gopegui RR, Espada Y. Determination of renal vascular resistance in dogs with diabetes mellitus and hyperadrenocorticism. Vet Rec 2008; 163:592–6.
45. Taylor SS, Sparkes AH, Briscoe K, et al. ISFM consensus guidelines on the diagnosis and management of hypertension in cats. J Feline Med Surg 2017;19: 288–303.
46. Gilson SD, Withrow SJ, Wheeler SL, et al. Pheochromocytoma in 50 dogs. J Vet Intern Med 1994;8:228–32.
47. Barthez PY, Marks SL, Woo J, et al. Pheochromocytoma in dogs: 61 cases (1984-1995). J Vet Intern Med 1997;11:272–8.
48. McConnell JF, Garosi L, Platt SR. Magnetic resonance imaging findings of presumed cerebellar cerebrovascular accident in twelve dogs. Vet Radiol Ultrasound 2005;46:1–10.
49. Kent M, Glass EN, Haley AC, et al. Ischemic stroke in greyhounds: 21 cases (2007-2013). J Am Vet Med Assoc 2014;245:113–7.
50. Sutherland GR, Auer RN. Primary intracerebral hemorrhage. J Clin Neurosci 2006;13:511–7.
51. Righy C, Bozza MT, Oliveira MF, et al. Molecular, cellular and clinical aspects of intracerebral hemorrhage: are the enemies within? Curr Neuropharmacol 2016; 14:392–402.
52. Babi MA, James ML. Peri-hemorrhagic edema and secondary hematoma expansion after intracerebral hemorrhage: from benchwork to practical aspects. Front Neurol 2017;8:4.
53. Yanai H, Tapia-Nieto R, Cherubini GB, et al. Results of magnetic resonance imaging performed within 48 hours after head trauma in dogs and association with outcome: 18 cases (2007-2012). J Am Vet Med Assoc 2015;246:1222–9.
54. Adamo PF, Crawford JT, Stepien RL. Subdural hematoma of the brainstem in a dog: magnetic resonance findings and treatment. J Am Anim Hosp Assoc 2005; 41:400–5.
55. Nykamp S, Scrivani P, DeLahunta A, et al. Chronic subdural hematomas and hydrocephalus in a dog. Vet Radiol Ultrasound 2001;42:511–4.
56. Asakawa MG, MacKillop E, Olby NJ, et al. Imaging diagnosis–neuronal ceroid lipofuscinosis with a chronic subdural hematoma. Vet Radiol Ultrasound 2010; 51:155–8.

57. Yu CH, Yhee JY, Kim JH, et al. Pro- and anti-inflammatory cytokine expression and histopathological characteristics in canine brain with traumatic brain injury. J Vet Sci 2011;12:299–301.
58. Packer RA, Bergman RL, Coates JR, et al. Intracranial subarachnoid hemorrhage following lumbar myelography in two dogs. Vet Radiol Ultrasound 2007; 48:323–7.
59. Dennler M, Lange EM, Schmied O, et al. Imaging diagnosis–metastatic hemangiosarcoma causing cerebral hemorrhage in a dog. Vet Radiol Ultrasound 2007; 48:138–40.
60. Garosi LS, Platt SR, McConnell JF, et al. Intracranial haemorrhage associated with Angiostrongylus vasorum infection in three dogs. J Small Anim Pract 2005;46:93–9.
61. Dunn KJ, Nicholls PK, Dunn JK, et al. Intracranial haemorrhage in a Dobermann puppy with von Willebrand's disease. Vet Rec 1995;136:635–6.
62. Long SN, Michieletto A, Anderson TJ, et al. Suspected pituitary apoplexy in a German shorthaired pointer. J Small Anim Pract 2003;44:497–502.
63. de Stefani A, de Risio L, Platt SR, et al. Surgical technique, postoperative complications and outcome in 14 dogs treated for hydrocephalus by ventriculoperitoneal shunting. Vet Surg 2011;40:183–91.
64. Muhle AC, Kircher P, Fazer R, et al. Intracranial haemorrhage in an eight-week-old puppy. Vet Rec 2004;154:338–9.
65. Lowrie M, De Risio L, Dennis R, et al. Concurrent medical conditions and long-term outcome in dogs with nontraumatic intracranial hemorrhage. Vet Radiol Ultrasound 2012;53:381–8.
66. Kitagawa M, Okada M, Kanayama K, et al. Traumatic intracerebral hematoma in a dog: MR images and clinical findings. J Vet Med Sci 2005;67:843–6.
67. Waters DJ, Hayden DW, Walter PA. Intracranial lesions in dogs with hemangiosarcoma. J Vet Intern Med 1989;3:222–30.
68. Kraft SL, Gavin PR, DeHaan C, et al. Retrospective review of 50 canine intracranial tumors evaluated by magnetic resonance imaging. J Vet Intern Med 1997; 11:218–25.
69. Hodshon AW, Hecht S, Thomas WB. Use of the T2*-weighted gradient recalled echo sequence for magnetic resonance imaging of the canine and feline brain. Vet Radiol Ultrasound 2014;55:599–606.
70. Rodenas S, Pumarola M, Gaitero L, et al. Magnetic resonance imaging findings in 40 dogs with histologically confirmed intracranial tumours. Vet J 2011;187: 85–91.
71. Young BD, Levine JM, Porter BF, et al. Magnetic resonance imaging features of intracranial astrocytomas and oligodendrogliomas in dogs. Vet Radiol Ultrasound 2011;52:132–41.
72. Martin-Vaquero P, Da Costa RC, Aeffner F, et al. Imaging diagnosis–hemorrhagic meningioma. Vet Radiol Ultrasound 2010;51:165–7.
73. Wisner ER, Dickinson PJ, Higgins RJ. Magnetic resonance imaging features of canine intracranial neoplasia. Vet Radiol Ultrasound 2011;52:S52–61.
74. O'Neill J, Kent M, Glass EN, et al. Clinicopathologic and MRI characteristics of presumptive hypertensive encephalopathy in two cats and two dogs. J Am Anim Hosp Assoc 2013;49:412–20.
75. Fulkerson CV, Young BD, Jackson ND, et al. MRI characteristics of cerebral microbleeds in four dogs. Vet Radiol Ultrasound 2012;53:389–93.

76. Uchida K, Miyauchi Y, Nakayama H, et al. Amyloid angiopathy with cerebral hemorrhage and senile plaque in aged dogs. Nihon Juigaku Zasshi 1990;52:605–11.
77. Denk D, Matiasek K, Just FT, et al. Disseminated angiostrongylosis with fatal cerebral haemorrhages in two dogs in Germany: a clinical case study. Vet Parasitol 2009;160:100–8.
78. Glaus T, Sigrist N, Hofer-Inteeworn N, et al. Unexplained bleeding as primary clinical complaint in dogs infected with Angiostrongylus vasorum. Schweiz Arch Tierheilkd 2016;158:701–9.
79. Wessmann A, Lu D, Lamb CR, et al. Brain and spinal cord haemorrhages associated with Angiostrongylus vasorum infection in four dogs. Vet Rec 2006;158:858–63.
80. Whitley NT, Corzo-Menendez N, Carmichael NG, et al. Cerebral and conjunctival haemorrhages associated with von Willebrand factor deficiency and canine angiostrongylosis. J Small Anim Pract 2005;46:75–8.
81. Rossmeisl JH, Andriani RT, Cecere TE, et al. Frame-based stereotactic biopsy of canine brain masses: technique and clinical results in 26 cases. Front Vet Sci 2015;2:20.
82. Hause WR, Helphrey ML, Green RW, et al. Cerebral arteriovenous malformation in a dog. J Am Anim Hosp Assoc 1982;18:601–7.
83. Thomas WB. Surgical excision of a cerebral arteriovenous malformation in a dog. Prog Vet Neurol 1995;6:20–3.
84. Thomas WB, Adams WH, McGavin MD, et al. Magnetic resonance imaging appearance of intracranial hemorrhage secondary to cerebral vascular malformation in a dog. Vet Radiol Ultrasound 1997;38:371–5.
85. McCormick WF. Pathology of vascular malformations of the brain. In: Wilson CB, Stein BM, editors. Intracranial arteriovenous malformations. Baltimore (MD): Williams and Wilkins; 1984. p. 44–63.
86. Sakurai M, Morita T, Kondo H, et al. Cerebral vascular hamartoma with thrombosis in a dog. J Vet Med Sci 2011;73:1367–9.
87. Smith SH, Van Winkle T. Cerebral vascular hamartomas in five dogs. Vet Pathol 2001;38:108–12.
88. Martin-Vaquero P, Moore SA, Wolk KE, et al. Cerebral vascular hamartoma in a geriatric cat. J Feline Med Surg 2011;13:286–90.
89. Stalin CE, Granger N, Jeffery ND. Cerebellar vascular hamartoma in a British shorthair cat. J Feline Med Surg 2008;10:206–11.
90. Bishop TM, Morrison J, Summers BA, et al. Meningioangiomatosis in young dogs: a case series and literature review. J Vet Intern Med 2004;18:522–8.
91. Beltran E, Dennis R, Foote A, et al. Imaging diagnosis: pituitary apoplexy in a cat. Vet Radiol Ultrasound 2012;53:417–9.
92. Liebel FX, Summers BA, Lowrie M, et al. Imaging diagnosis-magnetic resonance imaging features of a cerebral hemangioblastoma in a dog. Vet Radiol Ultrasound 2013;54:164–7.
93. Woods JP, Cuddon PA. Prefrontal cortical and diencephalic cavernous hemangioma in a dog. Prog Vet Neurol 1992;3:126–30.
94. Eichelberger BM, Kraft SL, Halsey CH, et al. Imaging diagnosis–magnetic resonance imaging findings of primary cerebral hemangioma. Vet Radiol Ultrasound 2011;52:188–91.
95. Schoeman JP, Stidworthy MF, Penderis J, et al. Magnetic resonance imaging of a cerebral cavernous haemangioma in a dog. J S Afr Vet Assoc 2002;73:207–10.

96. Bowman CA, Witham A, Tyrrell D, et al. Magnetic resonance imaging appearance of hypertensive encephalopathy in a dog. Ir Vet J 2015;68:5.
97. Major AC, Caine A, Rodriguez SB, et al. Imaging diagnosis–magnetic resonance imaging findings in a dog with sequential brain infarction. Vet Radiol Ultrasound 2012;53:576–80.
98. Bentley RT, March PA. Recurrent vestibular paroxysms associated with systemic hypertension in a dog. J Am Vet Med Assoc 2011;239:652–5.
99. Gredal H, Toft N, Westrup U, et al. Survival and clinical outcome of dogs with ischaemic stroke. Vet J 2013;196:408–13.
100. Paul AE, Lenard Z, Mansfield CS. Computed tomography diagnosis of eight dogs with brain infarction. Aust Vet J 2010;88:374–80.
101. Garosi L, McConnell JF, Platt SR, et al. Clinical and topographic magnetic resonance characteristics of suspected brain infarction in 40 dogs. J Vet Intern Med 2006;20:311–21.
102. Rylander H, Eminaga S, Palus V, et al. Feline ischemic myelopathy and encephalopathy secondary to hyaline arteriopathy in five cats. J Feline Med Surg 2014; 16:832–9.
103. Salger F, Stahl C, Vandevelde M, et al. Multifocal ischemic brain infarctions secondary to spontaneous basilar artery occlusion in a dog with systemic thromboembolic disease. J Vet Intern Med 2014;28:1875–80.
104. Panarello GL, Dewey CW, Barone G, et al. Magnetic resonance imaging of two suspected cases of global brain ischemia. J Vet Emerg Crit Care 2004;14: 269–77.
105. Tidwell AS, Robertson ID. Magnetic resonance imaging of normal and abnormal brain perfusion. Vet Radiol Ultrasound 2011;52:S62–71.
106. Berg JM, Joseph RJ. Cerebellar infarcts in two dogs diagnosed with magnetic resonance imaging. J Am Anim Hosp Assoc 2003;39:203–7.
107. Wolff CA, Holmes SP, Young BD, et al. Magnetic resonance imaging for the differentiation of neoplastic, inflammatory, and cerebrovascular brain disease in dogs. J Vet Intern Med 2012;26:589–97.
108. Young BD, Fosgate GT, Holmes SP, et al. Evaluation of standard magnetic resonance characteristics used to differentiate neoplastic, inflammatory, and vascular brain lesions in dogs. Vet Radiol Ultrasound 2014;55:399–406.
109. Cervera V, Mai W, Vite CH, et al. Comparative magnetic resonance imaging findings between gliomas and presumed cerebrovascular accidents in dogs. Vet Radiol Ultrasound 2011;52:33–40.
110. Sutherland-Smith J, King R, Faissler D, et al. Magnetic resonance imaging apparent diffusion coefficients for histologically confirmed intracranial lesions in dogs. Vet Radiol Ultrasound 2011;52:142–8.
111. Moseley ME, Cohen Y, Kucharczyk J, et al. Diffusion-weighted MR imaging of anisotropic water diffusion in cat central nervous system. Radiology 1990;176: 439–45.
112. Jeon JH, Jung HW, Jang HM, et al. Canine model of ischemic stroke with permanent middle cerebral artery occlusion: clinical features, magnetic resonance imaging, histopathology, and immunohistochemistry. J Vet Sci 2015;16:75–85.
113. Lee B, Newberg A. Neuroimaging in traumatic brain imaging. NeuroRx 2005;2: 372–83.
114. Parent J. Neurologic disorders. In: Willard MD, Tvedten H, editors. Small animal clinical diagnosis by laboratory methods. St. Louis (MO): Elsevier Saunders; 2012. p. 304–15.

115. Moore AR, Barger AM. Central nervous system cytology. In: Barger AM, MacNeill AL, editors. Small animal cytologic diagnosis. New York: CRC Press; 2017. p. 95–148.
116. Gredal H, Thomsen BB, Boza-Serrano A, et al. Interleukin-6 is increased in plasma and cerebrospinal fluid of community-dwelling domestic dogs with acute ischaemic stroke. Neuroreport 2017;28:134–40.
117. Brown S, Atkins C, Bagley R, et al. Guidelines for the identification, evaluation, and management of systemic hypertension in dogs and cats. J Vet Intern Med 2007;21:542–58.
118. Cruz-Flores S. Acute stroke and transient ischemic attack in the outpatient clinic. Med Clin North Am 2017;101:479–94.
119. Garosi L. Cerebrovascular accidents. In: Platt S, Garosi L, editors. Small animal neurological emergencies. London: Manson Publishing/The Veterinary Press; 2012. p. 319–32.
120. Emberson J, Lees KR, Lyden P, et al. Effect of treatment delay, age, and stroke severity on the effects of intravenous thrombolysis with alteplase for acute ischaemic stroke: a meta-analysis of individual patient data from randomised trials. Lancet 2014;384:1929–35.
121. Hemphill JC 3rd, Greenberg SM, Anderson CS, et al. Guidelines for the management of spontaneous intracerebral hemorrhage: a guideline for healthcare professionals from the American Heart Association/American Stroke Association. Stroke 2015;46:2032–60.
122. Freeman C, Platt S. Head trauma. In: Platt S, Garosi L, editors. Small animal neurological emergencies. London: Manson Publishing/The Veterinary Press; 2012. p. 363–82.
123. Shihab N, Summers BA, Benigni L, et al. Novel approach to temporal lobectomy for removal of a cavernous hemangioma in a dog. Vet Surg 2014;43:877–81.
124. Beer KS, Silverstein DC. Controversies in the use of fresh frozen plasma in critically ill small animal patients. J Vet Emerg Crit Care (San Antonio) 2015;25:101–6.
125. Hoak DA, Lutsep HL. Management of symptomatic intracranial stenosis. Curr Cardiol Rep 2016;18:83.
126. Kwon SU, Kim JS. Antithrombotic therapy. Front Neurol Neurosci 2016;40:141–51.
127. Chimowitz MI, Lynn MJ, Howlett-Smith H, et al. Comparison of warfarin and aspirin for symptomatic intracranial arterial stenosis. N Engl J Med 2005;352:1305–16.
128. Goncalves R, Carrera I, Garosi L, et al. Clinical and topographic magnetic resonance imaging characteristics of suspected thalamic infarcts in 16 dogs. Vet J 2011;188:39–43.
129. Andersen KK, Olsen TS, Dehlendorff C, et al. Hemorrhagic and ischemic strokes compared: stroke severity, mortality, and risk factors. Stroke 2009;40:2068–72.
130. Subramaniam S, Hill MD. Controversies in medical management of intracerebral hemorrhage. Can J Neurol Sci 2005;32(Suppl 2):S13–21.
131. Freeman WD, Dawson SB, Flemming KD. The ABC's of stroke complications. Semin Neurol 2010;30:501–10.
132. Bamford J, Dennis M, Sandercock P, et al. The frequency, causes and timing of death within 30 days of a first stroke: the oxfordshire community stroke project. J Neurol Neurosurg Psychiatry 1990;53:824–9.

Fungal Infections of the Central Nervous System in Small Animals

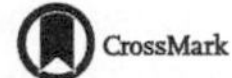

Clinical Features, Diagnosis, and Management

R. Timothy Bentley, BVSc[a,*], Amanda R. Taylor, DVM[b], Stephanie A. Thomovsky, DVM[a]

KEYWORDS

• Dog • Cat • Brain • *Aspergillus* • *Blastomyces* • *Cladophialophora* • *Coccidioides* • *Cryptococcus*

KEY POINTS

- Central nervous system (CNS) fungal infections in small animals often present as multifocal meningoencephalomyelitis, intracranial lesions that accompany sinonasal lesions, ventriculitis, or a solitary brain or spinal cord granuloma.
- Systemic clinical signs vary; there is often no detectable extraneural involvement in CNS granuloma cases.
- Surgery may have a diagnostic and therapeutic role in CNS granuloma cases.
- Recent advances have occurred in serology for the systemic mycoses, but for the rarer fungi demonstration of the organism remains obligatory for definitive diagnosis (eg, cytology, histology or culture).
- Fluconazole, voriconazole, and posaconazole cross the blood-brain barrier, but voriconazole is neurotoxic to cats. Liposomal and lipid-encapsulated formulations of amphotericin B improve renal safety and the distribution to the CNS.

INTRODUCTION

Mycotic infections of the central nervous system (CNS) of dogs and cats are, depending on geographic location, a very rare to sporadic but severe cause of disease.

Disclosure: The authors have nothing to disclose.

[a] Neurology and Neurosurgery, Department of Veterinary Clinical Sciences, Purdue University College of Veterinary Medicine, Purdue University, Lynn Hall, 625 Harrison Street, West Lafayette, IN 47907, USA; [b] Neurology and Neurosurgery, Department of Clinical Sciences, Auburn University College of Veterinary Medicine, Auburn University, Greene Hall, 1130 Wire Road, Auburn, AL 36849, USA

* Corresponding author. Department of Veterinary Clinical Sciences, Purdue University, Lynn Hall, 625 Harrison Street, West Lafayette, IN 47907.

E-mail address: rbentley@purdue.edu

Vet Clin Small Anim 48 (2018) 63–83

http://dx.doi.org/10.1016/j.cvsm.2017.08.010 vetsmall.theclinics.com

Cases may present with multifocal meningoencephalomyelitis, intracranial lesions accompanying sinonasal lesions, ventriculitis, or a solitary CNS granuloma. Each of these presentations has its own features, incidence of multisystemic mycosis, differential diagnoses, pertinent diagnostic tests, and appropriate management, and is discussed separately in this article. Many organisms have been implicated in CNS mycosis and their predispositions vary. *Cryptococcus* spp have been associated with each of these clinical patterns but ventriculitis is atypical. *Blastomyces dermatitidis* often presents as an intracranial mass extending from the nasal cavity, but is also a chief cause of canine ventriculitis. *Cladophialophora bantiana* is neurotropic, often presenting as brain granulomas without extraneural lesions.

Much information is available regarding life cycles and microbiological features of the systemic mycoses.[1–5] Canine fungal discospondylitis has been studied, especially *Aspergillus* and *Paecilomyces*.[6–10] This article focuses on the clinical features, diagnosis, and management of fungal infections of the brain and spinal cord in dogs and cats.

SIGNALMENT, HISTORY, AND CLINICAL PRESENTATION

Fungal infections more often occur in younger animals, animals spending more time outdoors, and larger dogs.[1,2,11] Young German Shepherd dogs are overrepresented for aspergillosis.[10,12] However, indoor-only cats can develop mycoses.[3,5] Disease also occurs in older animals, including CNS cryptococcosis in cats[5,13] and many cases of solitary CNS granulomas (discussed later). Exposure to bird or bat feces sitting on soil (including house plants) is pertinent.[3,14]

Geographic location and travel history are critical. *Cryptococcus neoformans* is worldwide. *Cryptococcus gattii* is common around Vancouver Island and the northwestern United States, and is now recognized as a distinct species to *C neoformans*.[5] Most coccidioidomycosis cases are in animals that live in Arizona, in a neighboring state, or in animals that lived there up to 6 years previously.[1,15] Many blastomycosis cases are in the Midwest, the Ohio and Mississippi river valleys, or certain other clusters; proximity to bodies of water is a risk factor for dogs.[2,11,16] Most histoplasmosis cases are associated with the Mississippi, Ohio, or Missouri river valleys.[3]

Many CNS mycosis cases have progressive neurologic clinical signs over 0 to 14 days.[10,13,16–22] Transitory steroid responsiveness is common.[16,18] Longer neurologic histories occur, especially with cryptococcosis.[13] Neurologic clinical signs depend on localization. With multifocal meningoencephalomyelitis, forebrain and central vestibular deficits are common. In sinonasal mycosis with intracranial extension, seizures and other forebrain deficits are typical. With a solitary CNS granuloma, neurolocalization is often focal and forebrain or spinal. A cerebral mass with brain herniations may cause diffuse intracranial deficits. Cases with ventriculitis often have rapidly progressive brainstem disease.

When present, systemic signs precede the neurologic signs or occur concurrently. Systemic clinical signs are often present for days or a few weeks. However, cats with CNS cryptococcosis had extended extraneural histories (median 52 days, up to 4 years), which was significantly longer than in dogs (median 7 days).[13] There may be no clinical evidence of extraneural involvement. Specifics regarding extraneural disease are discussed later.

Multifocal Meningoencephalomyelitis Accompanying Systemic Disease

Multifocal meningoencephalomyelitis is especially common with hematogenous brain infection by *Cryptococcus* (**Box 1**). Usually, extraneural involvement is apparent

Box 1
Multifocal meningoencephalomyelitis accompanying systemic disease

Major pathogens of dogs and cats

- ***C neoformans*** **and** ***C gattii***
- ***Aspergillus terreus,*** *Aspergillus fumigatus*, and *Aspergillus deflectus*
- ***B dermatitidis***
- *Histoplasma capsulatum*

Individual canine case reports

- ***Cladophialophora bantiana***
- *Bipolaris* spp
- *Cladosporium cladosporioides*
- *Fusarium* spp
- *Paecilomyces* spp
- *Scopulariopsis chartarum*
- *Sporobolomyces roseus*

Individual feline case reports

- ***C bantiana***
- *Exophiala jeanselmei*
- *Ochroconis gallopavum*

(discussed later).[13,23,24] There may be no clinically detectable upper or lower respiratory tract involvement; percutaneous inoculation is possible.[23] Cases with concurrent sinonasal lesions are presented separately later.

Small animal CNS cryptococcosis is frequently forebrain or multifocal in character.[13,23–25] The pathogens are *C neoformans* (especially dogs) and *C gattii* (especially cats).[5,13] Cats develop cryptococcosis more frequently but dogs have more CNS involvement; the incidence of CNS mycosis is broadly similar.[5,13] Differences in the degree of CNS inflammation may depend on the host species (dog or cat) or fungal species (*C neoformans* or *C gattii*).[13]

In a sizable neurologic cryptococcosis case series, for dogs undergoing MRI, multifocal parenchymal T2-hyperintense lesions were most common, especially in the forebrain but also the cerebellum and cervical spinal cord.[13] There was ill-defined enhancement of parenchymal lesions. Meningeal enhancement was often diffuse and in some cases was the only finding. In cats, there were multifocal or solitary parenchymal brain lesions, especially in the cerebrum but also in the thalamus, cerebellum, midbrain, or optic chiasm.[13] Multifocal parenchymal lesions displayed T2 hyperintensity, T1 hypointensity, and peripheral contrast enhancement. One cat had normal imaging; MRI may be insensitive for feline meningitis. Concurrent sinonasal lesions were observed in a minority of these patients (discussed later). Cryptococcal organisms were identified in the cerebrospinal fluid (CSF) of 20 of 26 dogs and cats.[13]

Histopathologically, the forebrain and cerebellum were affected in most (dogs) or all (cats), with frequent brainstem lesions and less common spinal cord or ventricular lesions. All animals had meningeal involvement. Random, multifocal intraparenchymal pseudocysts were most common. In other cases, there was meningoencephalitis or exclusively meningitis.[13]

Other canine and feline cases of CNS cryptococcosis without sinonasal involvement confirm a tendency for seizures or central vestibular syndrome, concurrent ocular lesions and systemic disease, multifocal contrast-enhancing MRI lesions of the forebrain and cerebellum, cytologic identification of yeast in the CSF, and multifocal granulomatous lesions or cryptococcomas of the brain or meninges.[23–27]

Canine aspergillosis cases may involve combinations of azotemia, osteomyelitis, lymphadenopathy, and meningoencephalitis.[10,12] MRI has been reported for 10 dogs; *Aspergillus terreus* was most common.[10,12] Only 1 revealed a nasal mass invading the brain (discussed later).

In 5 canine aspergillosis cases there were multifocal brain lesions without sinonasal lesions (**Fig. 1**), in the forebrain (all cases) and brainstem (3 cases).[10,12] Most lesions were intra-axial, heterogeneous or hyperintense on T2 and fluid attenuation inversion recovery, T1-isointense to hypointense, and contrast enhancing. Mass effect was common. There was an extra-axial, strongly enhancing mass near the optic chiasm in 1 dog, an enhancing cerebral mass in another, and 1 hemorrhagic infarction. Concomitant meningeal enhancement was present in 3 dogs.

Interestingly, the other 4 dogs showed normal brain MRI (1.0–3.0 T).[10] One had a head tilt and diffuse paraspinal hyperesthesia. Cochlea and ocular changes were noted on MRI. Two other dogs had a head tilt, vestibular ataxia, and postural reaction deficits. It was thought that MRI may not have detected meningitis or ventriculitis. The other dog with normal brain imaging had a head tilt and myelopathy. Multifocal discospondylitis and a secondary intervertebral disk herniation were found on spinal MRI.

One variation of blastomycosis is multifocal brain disease without sinonasal lesions. In 2 dogs, there were multifocal intra-axial, and especially extra-axial lesions, predominantly in the forebrain but also the brainstem.[28] Lesions were generally T1 hypointense and T2 hyperintense with marked perilesional edema. The lesions and meninges enhanced strongly with contrast.

Histoplasma can cause diarrhea, multisystemic disease, and meningoencephalitis,[3,29] including seizures, vestibular syndrome, and organisms in the CSF.[30] Chronic granulomatous inflammation can involve the brain[29] but may be subclinical.[31] Reports of neurologic and advanced imaging features in the modern era are awaited.

Individual canine case reports describe multifocal meningoencephalitis, renal infection, and sometimes profound involvement of other organs with *Bipolaris*,[32] *Cladosporium cladosporioides*,[20] *Paecilomyces*,[33] or *Scopulariopsis chartarum*.[34] Note that *Bipolaris* and *Cladosporium* are members of the phaeohyphomycotic group. In single cases of *Fusarium*[19] or *Sporobolomyces roseus*,[17] systemic mycosis was not present. MRI or computed tomography (CT) may reveal multifocal, poorly defined contrast-enhancing lesions, especially in the forebrain.[17,19] Vasculitis, thrombosis, or hyphae within or around blood vessels support hematogenous brain infection.[17,19,20,32,34]

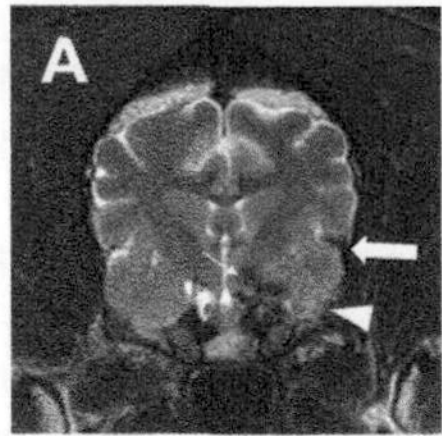

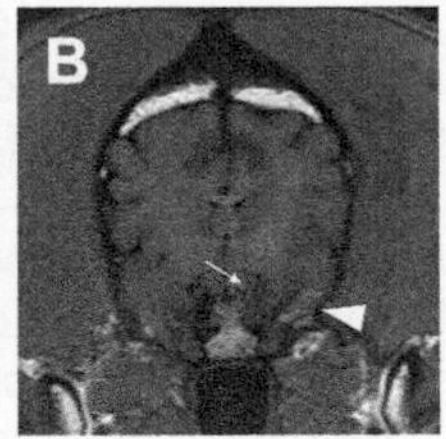

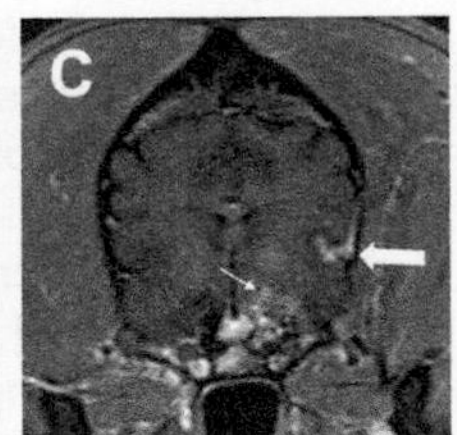

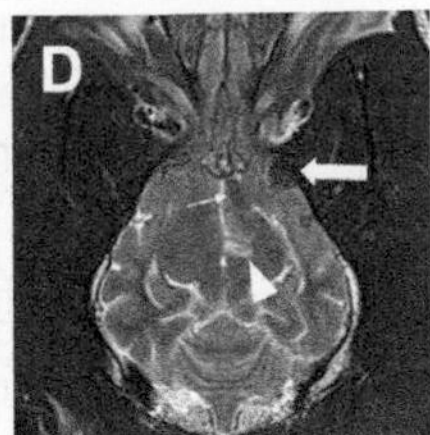

Fig. 1. Magnetic resonance images from a dog with multifocal aspergillosis meningoencephalitis. T2-weighted (*A*), precontrast T1-fluid-attenuated inversion recovery (FLAIR) (*B*), postcontrast fat-saturated T1-FLAIR (*C*) transverse images at the level of the cingulate gyrus, and dorsal T2-weighted image (*D*) at the level of the interthalamic adhesion. Intra-axial lesions are present within the basal nuclei (T2 hypointense; *arrows, A–D*), the pyriform lobe (T2 hyperintense; *arrowheads, A, B*), and the thalamus (T2 hyperintense; *arrowhead, D*). An extra-axial T2-hypointense strongly contrast-enhancing lesion (*large arrows*) is present in the meninges dorsal to the pyriform lobe (*A–D*) with another, smaller lesion just caudally (*D*). Note the normal cribriform plate (*D*).

Primarily discussed later, *C bantiana* has been associated with multifocal forebrain or disseminated lesions on necropsy of dogs and cats.[35–38] Other phaeohyphomycotic organisms causing multisystemic disease and rapid decline in cats include *Ochroconis gallopavum*[39] (frontal lobe gray discoloration) and *Exophiala jeanselmei*[40] (multifocal black cerebral and cerebellar granulomas).

The imaging and CSF analysis of animals with multifocal fungal meningoencephalomyelitis overlap with other infectious or inflammatory diseases, including granulomatous meningoencephalomyelitis in dogs. Mixed or neutrophilic pleocytosis is most common in mycosis and, except in cryptococcosis, the fungal organism is rarely identified in CSF (discussed later).[13,17,19] Imaging also overlaps with lymphoma, other round cell tumors, and metastatic tumors.[41] The detection of extraneural disease, if present, and the submission of serology are therefore particularly important.

Intracranial Lesions Accompanying Sinonasal Lesions

The major differential diagnoses for a nasal mass lesion and cribriform plate destruction are neoplasia and mycosis (**Box 2**).[42] The typical case is a dog or cat with a history of nasal discharge, epistaxis, or sneezing for 2 weeks to 1 year, without systemic mycosis.[42] Thoracic radiographs are often normal.[42–44] Lesions within the fronto-olfactory region and seizures are classic.[10,28,42,44] Cribriform plate penetration is also detected during rhinitis work-up in neurologically normal dogs.[42,45,46]

Sinonasal and intracranial canine blastomycosis is well reported (**Fig. 2**).[28,42,43,45] In a dog with seizures and forebrain deficits, MRI revealed a large mass spanning the nasal cavity, cribriform plate, and fronto-olfactory region and multiple intra-axial lesions. There was strong contrast enhancement of the mass, most brain lesions, 2 areas of ring enhancement, and meningeal enhancement.[28] In another MRI report, a retrobulbar contrast-enhancing mass extended into the calvarium without nasal involvement, causing behavior change and prechiasmatic blindness.[43] Given the marked osteolysis surrounding the optic canal and orbital fissure and extension along the floor of the vault, the preliminary diagnosis was neoplasia. Necropsy revealed blastomycosis.

CT is reported for 5 canine blastomycosis cases.[42,45] One dog displayed seizures with a normal interictal neurologic examination; the others were presented for nasal or ocular abnormalities. In 4 dogs, a contrast-enhancing nasal mass lesion traversed the cribriform plate; differential diagnoses were neoplasia or fungal rhinitis.[42] In the fifth, there was poorly enhancing material and osteolysis with only 1 small soft tissue density growth, more suggestive of mycosis.[45] In these cases, the frontal sinus, nasopharynx, and orbits were variably involved.[42,45] Note that fungal rhinitis is often bilateral but can be unilateral,[13,28,42,45] hampering discrimination from adenocarcinoma and other caudal nasal cavity neoplasms, which can also be unilateral or bilateral.[47,48]

Some cryptococcosis cases have lesions of the nasal cavity, fronto-olfactory region, and sporadic retrobulbar extension.[13] Sinonasal and intracranial lesions were revealed by MRI (2 cats and 2 dogs) or CT (1 dog).[13] Frank cribriform plate

Box 2
Intracranial lesions accompanying sinonasal (or retrobulbar) lesions

Major pathogens

- ***B dermatitidis*: mass lesions in dogs**
- ***C neoformans* and *C gattii*: rhinosinusitis in dogs and cats**
- *Aspergillus fumigatus*

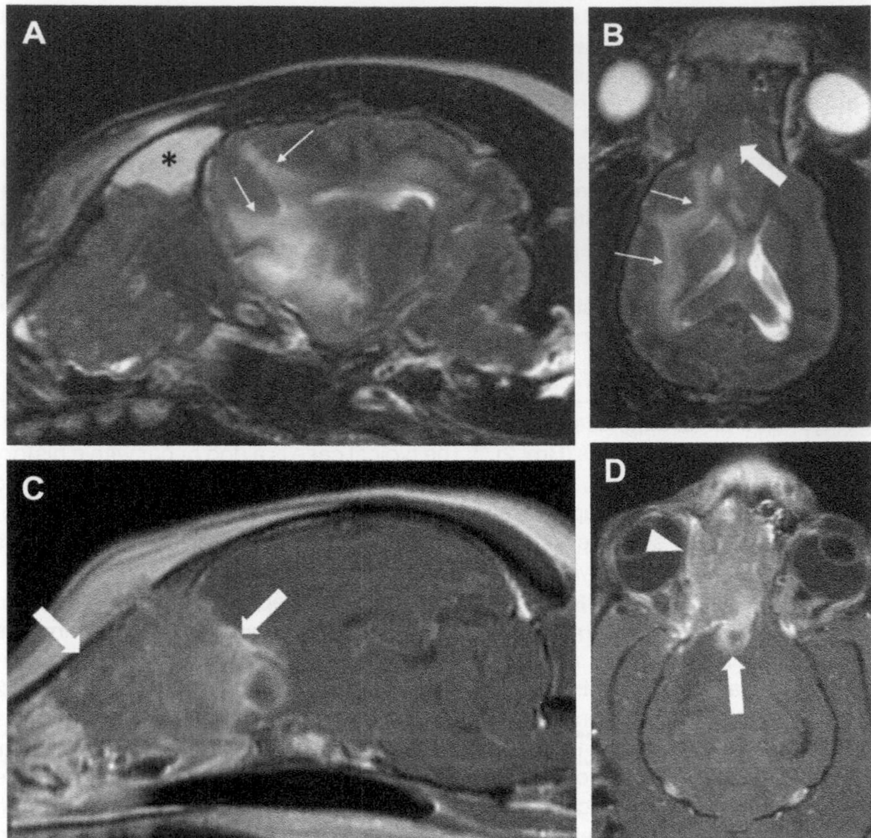

Fig. 2. A caudal nasal cavity, intracranial, and retrobulbar mass lesion with destruction of the cribriform plate in a dog with blastomycosis. T2-weighted right-parasagittal (*A*) and dorsal (*B*) images and T1-weighted postcontrast midsagittal (*C*) and dorsal (*D*) images. The mass (*large arrows*) is T2 hypointense to isointense compared with gray matter, strongly contrast enhancing, with a region of peripheral enhancement caudally. It completely obliterates the cribriform plate on the right side. There is extensive adjacent white matter tract edema (*arrows, A, B*). Mass effect is pronounced. The frontal nasal sinus is fluid filled (*asterisk* in *A*). Note the osteolysis of the maxillary bone between the nasal cavity and orbit, and extension into the right retrobulbar space (*arrowhead, D*). Differential diagnoses were nasal neoplasia or mycosis.

compromise was typical (4 of 5 animals), with frontal sinus fluid in cats, and individual dogs with a nasal cavity mass or frontal sinus nodules. In dogs with *C neoformans*, nasal and intracranial lesions occur without cribriform plate destruction.[5] Note that enhancement of the cribriform plate with loss of structural detail may be the only sinonasal lesion in CNS cryptococcosis.[44] In 1 dog with neurologic blindness and multiple cranial nerve deficits, cytology and culture of crusty nasal discharge confirmed *C neoformans*.[49] Even minor nasal clinical signs are important in neurologic patients.

Aspergillus fumigatus is a leading cause of fungal rhinitis in mesocephalic and dolichocephalic dogs.[4] Mucopurulent nasal discharge and nasal planum depigmentation may be followed by facial deformity, epiphora, or seizures[4] but reports are sparse. One dog with a seizure following 2 months of nasal clinical signs showed a contrast-enhancing nasal cavity and frontal lobe mass on MRI, with extensive adjacent brain edema.[10] A cat with nasal disease and unilateral exophthalmia developed sudden bilateral blindness.[50] MRI revealed optic chiasm enhancement. At necropsy, *A fumigatus* and optic chiasm meningitis and gliosis were identified.

For a nasal mass lesion with cribriform plate destruction, neoplasia and mycosis should be considered.[42] In some cryptococcosis cases, sinonasal and intracranial lesions are separated by an intact cribriform plate. Diagnosis may require demonstration of the fungal organism (eg, rhinoscopic biopsy and culture); however, extreme care must be taken during biopsy in cribriform plate compromise. Ventricular pneumocephalus and meningoencephalitis may occur postrhinotomy.[46]

Ventriculitis Accompanying Systemic Disease

Ventriculitis is well documented in canine blastomycosis (**Box 3**).[16,51,52] It may emerge in other mycoses. A hallmark is obstructive hydrocephalus and rapid neurologic decline. Fungal dissemination through the CSF probably follows hematogenous brain infection.[18]

Systemic disease is common. In 4 dogs with blastomyces ventriculitis, manifest extraneural clinical signs included ocular lesions, fungal arthritis, cutaneous lesions, or mandibular swelling, as well as abnormalities on laboratory work or thoracic radiographs.[16,51,52] However, in 1 dog, the only presenting clinical signs were neurologic, and in another a clinically silent pleuritic focus was the only extraneural necropsy finding.[16]

MRI, CT, and necropsy examinations have shown a periventricular distribution, with pyogranulomatous inflammation in and around ventricles, obstructive hydrocephalus, and meningitis (**Fig. 3**).[16,51,52] Lesions were most common in the lateral ventricles (bilaterally enlarged in all cases) and the third ventricle.[16,52] MRI revealed periventricular T2 hyperintensity; frequent involvement of the aqueduct, fourth ventricle, and cervical central canal; and meningeal contrast enhancement.[16] On CT and MRI, periventricular contrast enhancement was most prominent around the rostral horns.[16,51] The pituitary gland may be involved.[16,52]

In a rapidly deteriorating dog with *Trichosporon montevideense*, MRI was very similar.[18] Vomiting had been the only extraneural clinical sign. At necropsy, all fungal hyphae were periventricular, with no mycosis of other organs.

Advanced imaging features of human CNS cryptococcosis include ventriculomegaly and occasional frank ventriculitis.[53] Periventricular lesions, a dilated fourth ventricle, and ventriculomegaly have each occurred in individual small animals, typically accompanying multifocal parenchymal lesions.[13] Multifocal histologic ependymitis was reported, involving the ventricles, choroid plexus, or central canal.

One cat with ventriculitis caused by *Phoma eupyrena* phaeohyphomycosis died within 7 days.[54] MRI revealed lateral and third ventricle ventriculomegaly. There was loss of the ventricular lumen at the junction of the aqueduct and fourth ventricle junction, where ependymitis was found at necropsy. No extraneural involvement was detected.

Box 3
Ventriculitis accompanying systemic disease

Major pathogen	Individual cases
• ***B dermatitidis* (dogs)**	• *Trichosporon montevideense* (dogs) • *Cryptococcus* spp (dogs and cats) • *Phoma eupyrena* (cats)

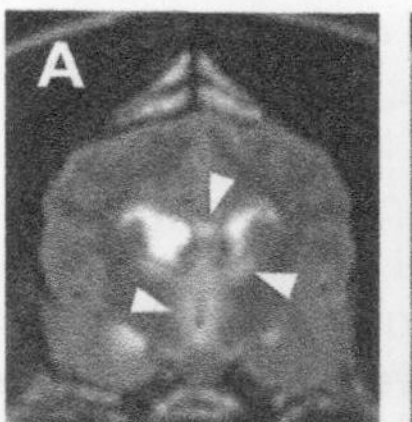

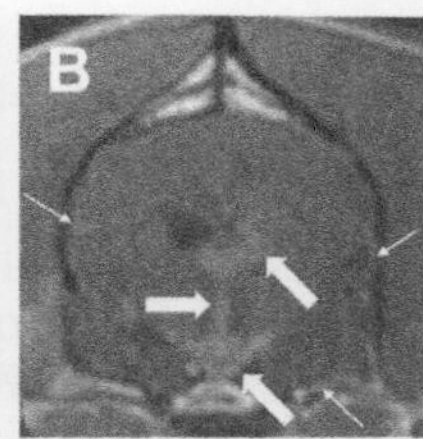

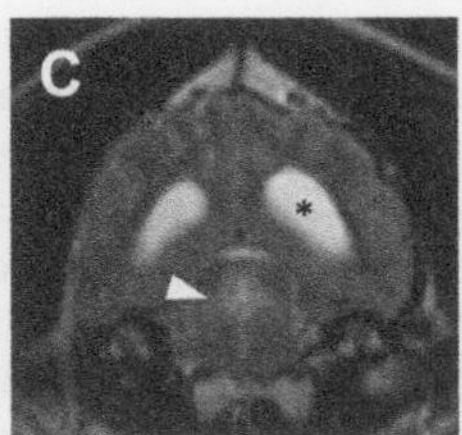

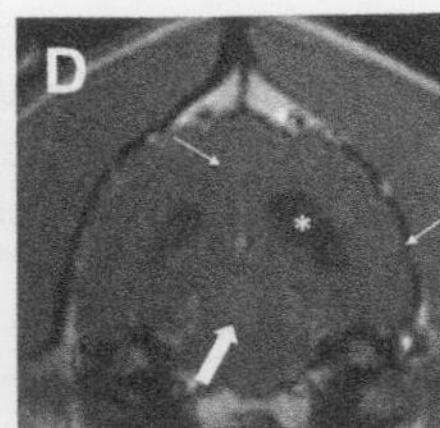

Fig. 3. Ventricular and periventricular magnetic resonance lesions in a dog with rapidly fatal blastomyces ventriculitis. T2-weighted (*A, C*) and T1-weighted postcontrast (*B, D*) transverse images at the level of the pituitary gland (*A, B*) or the mesencephalic aqueduct (*C, D*). There is periventricular T2 hyperintensity (*arrowheads*) within the corpus callosum, ventral to the lateral ventricles, and surrounding the third ventricle (*A*) and mesencephalic aqueduct (*C*). Contrast enhancement (*large arrows*) appears continuous through the left lateral ventricle ependyma and choroid plexus, third ventricle, pituitary gland, and surrounding leptomeninges (*B*) and encircles the mesencephalic aqueduct (*D*). There is segmental leptomeningeal contrast enhancement (*arrows*). Ventriculomegaly (*asterisks*) is asymmetric. Collapse of the subarachnoid space and gyral flattening (*A*) indicate mass effect.

This pattern of infection is distinct from other types of CNS mycosis because the rapidity of progression and especially the advanced imaging features are very different. Diagnostic evaluation must be prompt. Patients may need presumptive interventions before the results of diagnostic tests such as *Blastomyces* antigen are available.[52] Treatment of obstructive hydrocephalus and increased intracranial pressure is mandatory. Mortality is high. It has been suggested that surgical shunting of the lateral ventricles is indicated, including a temporary ventriculosubcutaneous shunt, which can be placed quickly and with inexpensive materials.[16]

Solitary Central Nervous System Granuloma with Varying Systemic Disease

A single granuloma on advanced imaging may occur in one of 2 settings, and in either situation can be mistaken for neoplasia (**Box 4**). The phaeohyphomycotic (pigmented hyphae) organism *Cladophialophora* is neurotropic and can form an intracranial granuloma without extracranial involvement. Systemic mycoses including *Coccidioides* can form a masslike granuloma with variable extraneural disease.

C bantiana (previously *Cladosporium bantianum*, *Cladosporium trichoides*, and *Xylohypha bantiana*) typically presents as brain granulomas without extraneural disease in dogs,[21,35,37] cats,[37,38,55–58] and humans.[59] Some dogs had concurrent abdominal and thoracic involvement[36,60,61] or an immunosuppressive comorbidity.[35–37] One cat

Box 4
Solitary central nervous system granulomas of dogs and cats

Major pathogens - extraneural disease often absent

- ***C bantiana***

Individual case report with no known extraneural disease

- *H capsulatum*

Major pathogens - extraneural disease variable

- ***Coccidioides* spp**
- *B dermatitidis*
- *Cryptococcus* spp

had severe lymphopenia of unclear cause and significance.[58] A single cerebral mass has been noted on MRI.[21,60] In 1 dog, a strongly T2-hyperintense and non–contrast-enhancing core had a mildly T2-hypointense and strongly enhancing rim, consistent with a well-defined spherical abscess.[21] At surgery, a cavity contained purulent discharge. In another dog, the granuloma was less well defined, with nonuniform enhancement and irregular shape.[60] Both displayed surrounding white matter tract edema, pronounced mass effect, and meningeal enhancement. Most animals have been diagnosed at necropsy, with findings that included a single unilateral cerebral or thalamic granuloma.[37,38,57,58] In 1 of these cases, the cerebral granuloma crossed the longitudinal fissure to the contralateral cortex. In another there were also smaller forebrain pyogranulomatous inflammatory foci. There was a single cerebellar granuloma in 1 dog.[61] Bilateral pigmented lesions of the rostral cerebrum[55] or multifocal gray or black pyogranulomas of the cerebrum or entire brain are possible.[35–38]

Serology is not available for *Cladophialophora*. Known for intracranial infection without systemic disease, antemortem diagnosis may only be possible through surgical excisional biopsy or minimally invasive biopsy.[21,60]

Coccidioidomycosis causes masslike CNS granulomas that can be mistaken for neoplasia in small animals.[62–66] Reports of a solitary mass on MRI with histologic confirmation of *Coccidioides*[15,67] indicate a median age around 7.5 years. Disease is often limited to a granuloma of the brain[15,65,66] or spinal cord.[15,67] Diagnosis has been challenging because MRI features overlap with neoplasia[15,67] and because of an incomplete relationship between seropositivity and clinical disease (discussed later). Definitive diagnosis requires cytologic, histologic, or microbiological identification of *Coccidioides*.[1,64] Some small animals with CNS granulomas had overt multisystemic disease, abnormalities on clinicopathology and thoracic radiography, or were diagnosed via aspiration of extraneural organs.[15,65] In others,[15,67] definitive diagnosis required excisional biopsy of the brain or spinal granuloma.

Coccidioides granulomas occur at various sites along the neuraxis, especially the frontal lobe or spinal cord. Some were T1 hyperintense and even T2 hypointense on MRI, possibly because of collagenous fibers and gliosis.[15] Most were T2 hyperintense and T1 isointense to hypointense. Intracranial extra-axial and intradural-extramedullary granulomas were strongly contrast enhancing, sometimes with a dural tail, but the suspicion of meningioma could be reduced by noting that the border with the parenchyma of the brain or spinal cord was indistinct or irregular.[15] One intradural-extramedullary granuloma was well defined.[67] Intracranial intra-axial and intramedullary granulomas showed varying but generally poor contrast enhancement and could not be discriminated from neoplasms such as glioma.[15] Some granulomas had a mixed intra-axial and extra-axial appearance, which is unusual for primary brain tumors but can occur with round cell neoplasms and infectious disease.[15] At surgery, when an intradural-extramedullary location is anticipated from MRI, an intramedullary lesion may be encountered.[15,67] Only 1 case had an extradural spinal mass with distinct demarcation from the neuroparenchyma on MRI.[15]

Other presentations of blastomycosis and cryptococcosis (discussed earlier) are more common but solitary CNS granulomas do occur (**Fig. 4**). Many small animals have been middle-aged or older. Although pulmonary involvement was identified radiographically in some cases,[28,42] in several no extraneural mycosis was identified,[68] despite exhaustive work-up[69] or complete necropsy.[14,22,70] A solitary intra-axial cerebral mass or intramedullary mass can occur with *Blastomyces*[22,28,42] or *Cryptococcus*[14,70,71] in dogs or cats. Common features on MRI[14,28,70] or CT[42,69] included a mass lesion with adjacent and often extensive edema. Contrast enhancement was strong and homogeneous with an irregular outline, or peripheral. One lesion

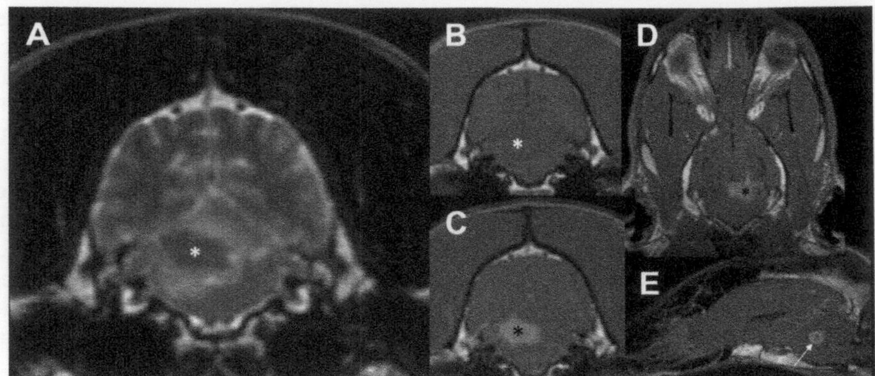

Fig. 4. Magnetic resonance images of a dog with a cerebellar blastomyces granuloma. Transverse images at the level of the vestibulocochlear nerves (*A–C*), dorsal image at the level of the flocculonodular lobe (*D*), and a right-parasagittal image (*E*) are T2 weighted (*A*), T1-weighted (*B*), or postcontrast T1 weighted (*C–E*). The mass (*asterisks*) is T2 hypointense compared with gray matter with surrounding hyperintensity (*A*). Slightly hypointense on T1 (*B*), it enhances strongly with irregular margins (*C, D*) and 1 region of peripheral enhancement (*arrow, E*). The mass appears most likely intra-axial but is continuous with contrast enhancement of the tentorium cerebelli. Note the lack of sinonasal involvement (*D, E*). The mass was considered most consistent with neoplasia and a granulomatous lesion was considered less likely.

was highly lobulated.[70] On MRI, lesions were T1 isointense to hypointense and heterogeneously T2 hyperintense; the center may be T2 hypointense.[14,28,70] The mass was hyperattenuating on CT.[42,69] In 1 feline with blastomyces cerebral granuloma, CT seemed most consistent with an extra-axial location but an intra-axial lesion was encountered surgically.[69] Based on MRI or CT, neoplasia was a major differential diagnosis or the presumptive diagnosis in all cases.[14,28,42,69,70] In 1 Doberman pinscher with no known extraneural disease, a ventral extradural myelographic compression at C6 to C7 was diagnosed as cervical spondylomyelopathy.[68] Surgery revealed a gelatinous white mass containing *Cryptococcus*.

Histoplasma caused spinal compression with no apparent systemic disease in 1 dog.[72] A strongly contrast-enhancing extradural lesion extended within 4 thoracic vertebrae on MRI, with irregular T2 hyperintensity of adjacent paravertebral muscles. The differential diagnoses included neoplasia and granuloma. Through excisional biopsy, a definitive diagnosis was achieved and ambulation was restored.

When present, meningeal enhancement on MRI or CT helps to decrease the suspicion of a primary brain tumor and increase the suspicion of an inflammatory process.[21,42] Adjacent edema is often extensive with fungal granulomas[21,28,42,64,69] but this can also occur with neoplastic lesions. CSF analysis is critical in differentiating from neoplasia and is usually inflammatory with fungal granulomas.[15,21,28,70] However, pleocytosis is not always present and normal CSF or mild changes are possible.[15,68] Mass effect may preclude safe CSF tap,[42] further hampering distinction from neoplasia.

These presentations are distinct because, based on age, advanced imaging features, and lack of findings on systemic work-up, granulomas may be confused with neoplasms. Serology may be imprecise (*Coccidioides*) or unavailable (*Cladophialophora*). Surgery may be required to achieve a definitive diagnosis and discrimination from neoplasia. Surgical excision improves the outcome of human patients with fungal granuloma.[73] There have been good outcomes with surgical resection and antifungal medications for a limited number of dogs and cats with solitary CNS granulomas[15,21,67–69,72] but outcomes have not been systematically compared with medical therapy. Medical-only therapy has been associated with good outcomes, persistent clinical signs,[15,28] or continued progression.[60] CNS phaeohyphomycosis is deadly. The only surviving small animal was also the only such animal treated surgically to date.[21] Similarly, in humans, medical-only fatality can be 100%, whereas with surgery some patients survive.[59,74]

Other Presentations

Not all cases present as multifocal meningoencephalomyelitis, sinonasal and intracranial lesions, ventriculitis, or a solitary CNS granuloma. Some cases show overlap, such as a masslike granuloma accompanying multifocal meningoencephalitis[10,12] or ventriculitis,[16] or a large pontine cryptococcoma with pinpoint cerebellar and renal lesions.[75] Without advanced imaging or necropsy, cases cannot be ascribed to one of the 4 groups. For example, in 1 young cat, intracranial *Paracoccidioides brasiliensis* progressed to uremic syndrome necessitating euthanasia.[76]

DIAGNOSIS

There is diagnostic utility to knowing the typical systemic presentations of fungal organisms.[77] In cats, cryptococcosis is associated with nasal (52% of 62 cats), cutaneous (45%), and ocular lesions (32%).[5] In dogs, neurologic clinical signs (61% of 31 dogs) predominated over ocular (45%) and nasal clinical signs (19%).[5] Canine blastomycosis involves the respiratory (88% of 115 dogs), lymphatic (67%), or ocular systems (52%).[11] In coccidioidomycosis in dogs, pneumonia classically occurs first, whereas osteomyelitis indicates dissemination. In cats, dermatologic and disseminated infections predominate.[1,63,78] *A fumigatus* is the foremost cause of canine mycotic rhinosinusitis, whereas *A terreus* causes discospondylitis or disseminated disease and rarely rhinitis.[4,79]

In CNS mycosis, nonspecific signs including anorexia, lethargy, weight loss, and (in dogs) vomiting are particularly common.[10,13,16–18,21,22] Importantly, fever is frequently absent.[10,15,16,21,22,28,43,51] Almost any organ can be affected. The respiratory tract and the eyes are leading extraneural sites.[10,11,13,33,44,80] Ocular lesions include fundic granulomas and uveitis.[10,28,33,44,51] The respiratory tract is the major route of entry but the organism may spread to hilar lymph nodes and hematogenously disseminate without clinical respiratory disease.[5,16,81] Thoracic radiographs can be normal.[16,17,19,25,28,33,42–44,50–52,69,72] Radiographs more often reveal interstitial, alveolar, or nodular pulmonary patterns or tracheobronchial lymphadenopathy.[16,28,42] Most[10,42,81] but not all[44] cases of sinonasal infection with intracranial extension have nasal clinical signs.

Findings on hematology, serum biochemistry, and urinalysis are exceedingly variable (**Box 5**). The results can be normal, mild and nonspecific, or suggest an infectious process or profound systemic disease. Feline immunodeficiency virus (FIV) antibody and feline leukemia virus antigen tests are highly recommended but usually negative in feline CNS mycosis.[1,13,40,50,69,76] Individual cases are positive, especially for FIV,[5,26] and retrovirus-associated immunosuppression could affect prognosis.[3]

It is imperative to image multiple body parts and take diagnostic samples as indicated. In CNS mycosis cases, demonstration of the causal organism may occur with nasal swab[81] or rhinoscopic biopsy,[42] scrapings of skin lesions,[44] FNA of myriad different sites,[15,23,28,33,44,51] or examination of urine sediment.[10,51,76]

Advanced imaging is reviewed for lesions of the nasal cavity, frontal sinus and cribriform plate,[10,28,42] eye,[10,28] temporalis muscle,[28] medial retropharyngeal and

Box 5
Clinicopathologic findings reported in small animal central nervous system fungal infections

Complete blood count, serum biochemistry, urinalysis	Normal Mild, nonspecific abnormalities Nonregenerative anemia Neutrophilia, monocytosis, increased alkaline phosphatase activity following recent steroidal therapy Inflammatory leukogram, often chronic Left-shifted neutrophilia Hyperglobulinemia Hypercalcemia (5% of canine blastomycosis) Azotemia, hyposthenuria Fungiuria
Fine-needle aspirate identification of fungal organisms	Anterior chamber, lymph node, pulmonary mass, mammary mass, bone marrow, arthrocentesis
CSF analysis	Normal Albuminocytologic dissociation Mixed pleocytosis (especially canine cryptococcosis) Neutrophilic pleocytosis (especially feline cryptococcosis) Mononuclear pleocytosis (especially blastomycosis) Eosinophilic pleocytosis
Identification of the organism in CSF	*Cryptococcus* spp Other fungal species sporadically identified Organisms identified with India ink

Data from Refs.[10,13–17,19–21,23–25,28,33,42–44,51,52,60,68–70,76,82,83]

mandibular lymph nodes,[13] mediastinum,[67] intervertebral discs,[10,79] and paravertebral muscle.[15,72]

The body temperature, physical examination, hematology, serum biochemistry, and thoracic radiographs should be evaluated for all cases, but each of these is often normal in individual patients. The absence of findings does not rule out brain or spinal cord mycosis.[28] The absence of extraneural disease can be particularly common in older animals with masslike brain or spinal granulomas.[14,21,68,69]

CSF nucleated cell count and protein levels are typically increased, often markedly (see **Box 5**). The type of pleocytosis varies. Mixed pleocytosis and neutrophilic pleocytosis are most common.[13] The eosinophil count is usually zero or low.[13–15] In canine cryptococcosis it ranges from 0% to 60%.[13,68,83] The nucleated cell count can be normal.[15,33,76] The presence of eosinophils, neutrophils, vacuolated macrophages, or albuminocytologic dissociation may still provide evidence of inflammation.[10,13,28,60,68]

Cryptococcal organism are identified in the CSF of most dogs and even more cats.[13] However, other organisms are observed only sporadically.[16,30,36] Fungal culture of the CSF is often negative[13,19] but can be positive.[10,13,25]

As discussed earlier, neurosurgery[15,21,68,69] or minimally invasive biopsy[60] achieves definitive diagnosis of CNS granulomas. In ventriculitis-induced hydrocephalus, *Blastomyces* may be detected in lateral ventricle CSF during shunting.[16]

Serology

Antigen tests are a mainstay in ruling in or ruling out small animal CNS mycosis (**Table 1**). *Blastomyces* galactomannan antigen detection is particularly sensitive in

Table 1
Sensitivity and specificity of diagnostic tests for small animal mycoses

Organism	Species	Test	Specimen	Sensitivity (%)	Specificity (%)	References
Blastomyces	Dogs	Ag (GMA)	Urine	94	High[a] (negative in 98% controls)	Spector et al,[84] 2008
			Serum	87	High[a] (negative in 100% controls)	
		Ab (AGID)	Serum	17	—	
		Ab (EIA for BAD-1)	Serum	95	Moderate–high[b]	Mourning et al,[94] 2015
Coccidioides	Dogs	Ag (GMA)	Serum	20	Uncertain[c]	Kirsch et al,[88] 2012
			Urine	3.5	Uncertain[c]	
		Ab (EIA)	Serum	95	96	Chow et al,[93] 2017
Cryptococcus	Cats	Ag (LCAT)	Serum	95–98[d]	100	Malik et al,[85] 1996
	Dogs	Ag (LCAT)	Serum	Moderate–high[e]	—	Trivedi et al,[5] 2011 Medleau et al,[86] 1990
Histoplasma	Dogs	Ag (EIA)	Urine	90	100	Cunningham,[87] 2015
Aspergillus	Dogs	Ab (AGID)	Serum	67–77	98–100	Sharman & Mansfield,[4] 2012
		Ab (ELISA)	Serum	88	97	Billen et al,[89] 2009
		Ag (GMA)	Serum	24 (sinonasal) 92 (systemic)	82 (sinonasal) 86 (systemic)	Garcia et al,[90] 2012
Beta-D-glucan assay	Any	Ag (beta-D-glucan)	Serum, CSF	Unknown[f] (77% in humans)	Unknown (85% in humans)	Falci et al,[91] 2017

Abbreviations: Ab, antibody; Ag, antigen; AGID, agar gel immunodiffusion (also known as agar gel double immunodiffusion); BAD-1, recombinant *Blastomyces* adhesin-1 repeat antigen; EIA, enzyme immunoassay; ELISA, enzyme-linked immunosorbent assay; GMA, galactomannan antigen (cell wall component of many fungi); LCAT, latex cryptococcal antigen test (also known as cryptococcal antigen latex agglutination serology [CALAS]).

[a] Unable to assess specificity (too few specimens from other mycoses; 96% false-positive in human histoplasmosis).

[b] Specificity 88% in histoplasmosis, 95% in healthy controls, 100% in nonfungal pulmonary diseases.

[c] False-positives were seen, especially in controls with histoplasmosis.

[d] False-negatives may be more common with localized or CNS disease.

[e] Positive in 9 of 9 dogs (Malik and colleagues,[85] 1996) or 15 of 18 dogs (Trivedi and colleagues,[5] 2011); positive in 9 of 11 dogs with neurologic cryptococcosis (Sykes and colleagues,[13] 2010). Median titer lower than in cats (Trivedi and colleagues,[5] 2011). Positive in CSF of dogs with negative sera (Sykes and colleagues,[13] 2010; Trivedi and colleagues,[5] 2011).

[f] Not thought to be positive in cases involving *Cryptococcus* or *Blastomyces*.

urine.[84] Although otherwise specific, false-positives occur in histoplasmosis cases. Cryptococcal antigen testing is routine and particularly sensitive in cats.[5,85,86] False-negatives may be more common with localized or CNS disease. If serum is negative, there is utility to submitting CSF.[5,13] Recently, *Histoplasma* antigen showed high sensitivity and excellent specificity.[87] *Coccidioides* antigen detection was disappointing.[88] Galactomannan antigen is usually negative in localized (eg, sinonasal or forebrain) aspergillosis.[4,89] However, sensitivity can be as high as 92% in dogs with disseminated disease,[79,90] in which it might be a useful screening test. False-positives occur with β-lactam antibiotic or Plasmalyte administration.[4,10,89] The beta-D-glucan antigen can be positive with any fungus except *Cryptococcus* or *Blastomyces*. The negative predictive value in humans is so high that antifungal therapy could be withheld based on a negative result.[91] It is offered for small animals but no published information is available.

Historically, antibody sensitivity has been poor. Fungal immunity is cell mediated more than humoral. In cats, *Coccidioides* agar gel immunodiffusion is fairly sensitive and specific; a clinically abnormal cat with any level of antibodies likely has coccidioidomycosis.[1,78] However, in Arizona, healthy dogs and coccidioidomycosis cases show similar results.[92] The breaking publication of canine antibody detection via enzyme immunoassay with high sensitivity and specificity is therefore exciting.[93] Detection of antibodies directed against an alternative *Blastomyces* antigen (recombinant *Blastomyces* adhesin-1 repeat antigen [BAD-1]) recently showed excellent

Table 2
The mechanism of action of antifungal agents

Antifungal Agent Class	Specific Agents	Mechanism of Action
Polyene antibiotic	Amphotericin B	Binds to ergosterol → disrupts fungal wall integrity → increased potassium permeability → fungal cell death
Azoles	Imidazoles (ketoconazole, miconazole), triazoles (fluconazole, itraconazole, voriconazole, posaconazole, ravuconazole)	Reduces ergosterol production via inhibition of the cytochrome p-450–dependent fungal enzyme lanosterol 14 a-desmethylase
Cytosine analogue	Flucytosine	Enters fungal cell via cytosine permease → converts to 5-fluorouracil → interferes with messenger RNA synthesis → inhibits fungal protein synthesis
Allylamines	Terbinafine	Inhibits squalene epoxidase in the ergosterol pathway → squalene accumulates within fungal cell → squalene is toxic to the fungal cell
Glucan synthesis inhibitors	Echinocandins (caspofungin, anidulafungin, micafungin)	Interferes with glucan synthesis → the fungal cell becomes osmotically unstable → cellular death

Data from Redmond A, Dancer C, Woods M. Fungal infections of the central nervous system: a review of fungal pathogens and treatment. Neurol India 2007;55:251–9.

Table 3
Antifungal agents commonly prescribed in veterinary medicine

Antifungal Medication	Dose	Success Against Selected Pathogens	Major Side Effects	Other
Fluconazole[13,95,98,99]	D: 2.5–15 mg/kg PO or IV q 12–24 h C: 25–50 mg/cat PO or IV q 12–24 h	*Coccidioides*, *Cryptococcus*, *Histoplasma*	Hepatotoxicity	Good CNS penetration
Itraconazole[13,72,95,98,99]	D, C: 5–10 mg/kg PO q 12–24 h	*Aspergillus*, *Blastomyces*, *Coccidioides*, *Cryptococcus*, *Histoplasma*	Hepatotoxicity	May be more effective in treatment of extradural masses (ie, those outside the BBB)
Ketoconazole[13,80,95,98,99]	D: 5–10 mg/kg PO q 12–24 h C: 50 mg/cat PO q 12–24 h	*Blastomyces*, *Coccidioides*, *Cryptococcus*, *Histoplasma*	Hepatotoxicity	Not an effective treatment of feline CNS *Cryptococcus*
Amphotericin B (liposomal)[13,95,98]	D: 2–3 mg/kg IV 3 times weekly (up to 9–12 treatments) C: 1 mg/kg IV 3 times weekly (up to 12 treatments)	*Cryptococcus*	Nephrotoxicity, hypokalemia	Liposomal and lipid complex formulations have better CNS penetration and less nephrotoxicity
Voriconazole[1,21,100]	D: 3.5–4 mg/kg PO q 12 h C: not recommended	*Aspergillus*, *Candida*, *Cryptococcus*	Neurologic effects (C) including visual changes, ataxia, paralysis	Expense
Flucytosine[98,99]	D: 50 mg/kg PO q 6–8 h C: 25–50 mg/kg PO q 6–12 h	—	Dermal eruptions	Never used as sole agent because of rapid development of resistance
Posaconazole[79,101]	D: 5 mg/kg PO q 12 h C: 5 mg/kg PO q 24 h	*Aspergillus*	Hepatotoxicity	Expense
Combination therapy[13,95,98,99]	See doses above	*Cryptococcus*	—	Combinations of amphotericin B, flucytosine, fluconazole, itraconazole

Abbreviations: C, cat; D, dog; IV, intravenous; PO, per os; q, every.

sensitivity, with 88% specificity even in coccidioidomycosis controls.[94] Serology for canine aspergillosis should be used in conjunction with other tests.[4,6,89]

MANAGEMENT

CNS involvement is a negative prognostic indicator for mycosis[95] and, in neurologic cryptococcosis, altered mental status further decreases the prognosis.[13] The CNS is a difficult location to treat effectively. This difficulty relates to the blood-brain barrier (BBB) and blood-CSF barrier. The presence of efflux pumps located within the BBB makes it impossible for some drugs to reach effective therapeutic levels within the CNS.[96,97] The efficacy of antifungal medications[98–101] depends on several factors: the fungal pathogen being treated, the susceptibility of the pathogen to therapeutics, the location of the pathogen within the CNS, and the ability for the drug to reach the pathogen.[102,103]

Table 2 shows the 5 main classes of antifungal medications: (1) polyene antibiotics, (2) azoles, (3) cytosine analogues, (4) allylamines, and (5) glucan synthesis inhibitors.[103] Some of these antifungal medications are more readily used in veterinary medicine than others. This difference in use is related to availability, safety, cost, and efficacy in veterinary species.

In general, an azole that penetrates the BBB is used, such as fluconazole,[104] voriconazole,[21] or posaconazole[79] (**Table 3**). Voriconazole is neurotoxic to cats.[100] Ketoconazole and itraconazole, mainstays in extraneural mycosis, are poor choices except perhaps with an extradural mass.[72,80] Combination therapy may be appropriate, using flucytosine or amphotericin B.[13,95] Liposomal (eg, AmBisome) or lipid complex (eg, Abelcet) amphotericin B formulations show improved CNS penetration and reduced nephrotoxicity.[63]

Prolonged duration of treatment is indicated. Ideally, the response to treatment is followed, for example by serial antigen quantification[105] or MRI and CSF,[21] which is highly beneficial when considering medication discontinuation. Microbiological cure may profoundly lag behind clinical cure.

Judicious short-term use of corticosteroids (eg, 0.5–1 mg/kg/d prednisone) may be beneficial when provided with meticulous supportive care; survival in the first 10 days was statistically significantly increased.[13] Patients may deteriorate when fungicidal therapy is started, then improve on coadministration of antiinflammatory corticosteroids.[28] It is thought that fungal die-off increases CNS inflammation. As discussed earlier, there is evidence in various species, especially humans, that surgery improves outcomes for fungal CNS granulomas.

REFERENCES

1. Graupmann-Kuzma A, Valentine BA, Shubitz LF, et al. Coccidioidomycosis in dogs and cats: a review. J Am Anim Hosp Assoc 2008;44:226–35.
2. Brömel C, Sykes JE. Epidemiology, diagnosis, and treatment of blastomycosis in dogs and cats. Clin Tech Small Anim Pract 2005;20:233–9.
3. Blache J, Ryan K, Arceneaux K. Histoplasmosis. Compend Contin Educ Vet 2011;33:E1–10.
4. Sharman MJ, Mansfield CS. Sinonasal aspergillosis in dogs: a review. J Small Anim Pract 2012;53:434–44.
5. Trivedi SR, Sykes JE, Cannon MS, et al. Clinical features and epidemiology of cryptococcosis in cats and dogs in California: 93 cases (1988–2010). J Am Vet Med Assoc 2011;239:357–69.

6. Garcia ME, Caballero J, Cruzado M, et al. The value of the determination of anti-aspergillus IgG in the serodiagnosis of canine aspergillosis: comparison with galactomannan detection. J Vet Med B Infect Dis Vet Public Health 2001;48:743–50.
7. Foley J, Norris C, Jang S. Paecilomycosis in dogs and horses and a review of the literature. J Vet Intern Med 2002;16:238–43.
8. Watt P, Robins G, Galloway A, et al. Disseminated opportunistic fungal disease in dogs: 10 cases (1982-1990). J Am Vet Med Assoc 1995;207:67–70.
9. Berry W, Leisewitz A. Multifocal *Aspergillus terreus* discospondylitis in two German shepherd dogs. J S Afr Vet Assoc 1996;67:222–8.
10. Taylor AR, Young BD, Levine GJ, et al. Clinical features and magnetic resonance imaging findings in 7 dogs with central nervous system aspergillosis. J Vet Intern Med 2015;29:1556–63.
11. Arceneaux K, Taboada J, Hosgood G. Blastomycosis in dogs: 115 cases (1980-1995). J Am Vet Med Assoc 1998;213:658–64.
12. Schultz RM, Johnson EG, Wisner ER, et al. Clinicopathologic and diagnostic imaging characteristics of systemic aspergillosis in 30 dogs. J Vet Intern Med 2008;22:851–9.
13. Sykes JE, Sturges BK, Cannon MS, et al. Clinical signs, imaging features, neuropathology, and outcome in cats and dogs with central nervous system cryptococcosis from California. J Vet Intern Med 2010;24:1427–38.
14. Belluco S, Thibaud JL, Guillot J, et al. Spinal cryptococcoma in an immunocompetent cat. J Comp Pathol 2008;139:246–51.
15. Bentley RT, Heng HG, Thompson C, et al. Magnetic resonance imaging features and outcome for solitary central nervous system *Coccidioides* granulomas in 11 dogs and cats. Vet Radiol Ultrasound 2015;56:520–30.
16. Bentley RT, Reese MJ, Heng HG, et al. Ependymal and periventricular magnetic resonance imaging changes in four dogs with central nervous system blastomycosis. Vet Radiol Ultrasound 2013;54:489–96.
17. Saey V, Vanhaesebrouck A, Maes S, et al. Granulomatous meningoencephalitis associated with *Sporobolomyces roseus* in a dog. Vet Pathol 2011;48:1158–60.
18. Bryan LK, Porter BF, Wickes BL, et al. Meningoencephalitis in a dog due to *Trichosporon montevideense*. J Comp Pathol 2014;151:157–61.
19. Evans J, Levesque D, de Lahunta A, et al. Intracranial fusariosis: a novel cause of fungal meningoencephalitis in a dog. Vet Pathol 2004;41:510–4.
20. Poutahidis T, Angelopoulou K, Karamanavi E, et al. Mycotic encephalitis and nephritis in a dog due to infection with *Cladosporium cladosporioides*. J Comp Pathol 2009;140:59–63.
21. Bentley R, Faissler D, Sutherland-Smith J. Successful management of an intracranial phaeohyphomycotic fungal granuloma in a dog. J Am Vet Med Assoc 2011;239:480–5.
22. McEwen SA, Hulland TJ. Cerebral blastomycosis in a cat. Can Vet J 1984;25:411–3.
23. Headley SA, Mota FCD, Lindsay S, et al. *Cryptococcus neoformans* var. grubii-induced arthritis with encephalitic dissemination in a dog and review of published literature. Mycopathologia 2016;181:595–601.
24. Newman SJ, Langston CE, Scase TJ. Cryptococcal pyelonephritis in a dog. J Am Vet Med Assoc 2003;222:180–3.
25. O'Toole T, Sato A, Rozanski E. Cryptococcosis of the central nervous system in a dog. J Am Vet Med Assoc 2003;222:1722–5.

26. Ramos-Vara J, Ferrer L, Visa J. Pathological findings in a cat with cryptococcosis and feline immunodeficiency virus infection. Histol Histopathol 1994;9:305–8.
27. Pal M. Feline meningitis due to *Cryptococcus neoformans* var. neoformans and review of feline cryptococcosis. Mycoses 1991;34:313–6.
28. Lipitz L, Rylander H, Forrest LJ, et al. Clinical and magnetic resonance imaging features of central nervous system blastomycosis in 4 dogs. J Vet Intern Med 2010;24:1509–14.
29. Brömel C, Sykes J. Histoplasmosis in dogs and cats. Clin Tech Small Anim Pract 2005;20:227–32.
30. Meadows RL, Macwilliams PS, Dzata G, et al. Diagnosis of histoplasmosis in a dog by cytologic examination of CSF. Vet Clin Pathol 1992;21:122–5.
31. Gilor C, Ridgway MD, Singh K. DIC and granulomatous vasculitis in a dog with disseminated histoplasmosis. J Am Anim Hosp Assoc 2011;47:e26–30.
32. Giri DK, Sims WP, Sura R, et al. Cerebral and renal phaeohyphomycosis in a dog infected with *Bipolaris* species. Vet Pathol 2011;48:754–7.
33. March P, Knowles K, Dillavou C, et al. Diagnosis, treatment, and temporary remission of disseminated paecilomycosis in a vizsla. J Am Anim Hosp Assoc 1996;32:509–14.
34. Welsh RD, Ely RAYW. *Scopulariopsis chartarum* systemic mycosis in a dog. J Clin Microbiol 1999;37:2102–3.
35. Migaki G, Casey H, Bayles W. Cerebral phaeohyphomycosis in a dog. J Am Vet Med Assoc 1987;191:997–8.
36. Schroeder H, Jardine J, Davis V. Systemic phaeohyphomycosis caused by *Xylohypha bantiana* in a dog. J S Afr Vet Assoc 1995;65:175–8.
37. Dillehay D, Ribas J, Newton J, et al. Cerebral phaeohyphomycosis in two dogs and a cat. Vet Pathol 1987;24:192–4.
38. Mariani CL, Platt SR, Scase TJ, et al. Cerebral phaeohyphomycosis caused by *Cladosporium* spp. in two domestic shorthair cats. J Am Anim Hosp Assoc 2002;38:225–30.
39. Padhye AA, Amster RL, Browning M, et al. Fatal encephalitis caused by *Ochroconis gallopavum* in a domestic cat (*Felis domesticus*). J Med Vet Mycol 1994;32:141–5.
40. Helms SR, McLeod CG. Systemic *Exophiala jeanselmei* infection in a cat. J Am Vet Med Assoc 2000;217:1858–61.
41. Bentley RT. Magnetic resonance imaging diagnosis of brain tumors in dogs. Vet J 2015;205:204–16.
42. Hecht S, Adams WH, Smith JR, et al. Clinical and imaging findings in five dogs with intracranial blastomycosis (*Blastomyces dermatiditis*). J Am Anim Hosp Assoc 2011;47:241–9.
43. Baron ML, Hecht S, Westermeyer HD, et al. Intracranial extension of retrobulbar blastomycosis (*Blastomyces dermatitidis*) in a dog. Vet Ophthalmol 2011;14:137–41.
44. Tiches D, Vite CH, Dayrell-Hart B, et al. A case of canine central nervous system cryptococcosis: management with fluconazole. J Am Anim Hosp Assoc 1998;34:145–51.
45. Wehner A, Crochik S, Howerth EW, et al. Diagnosis and treatment of blastomycosis affecting the nose and nasopharynx of a dog. J Am Vet Med Assoc 2008;233:1112–6.
46. Launcelott ZA, Palmisano MP, Stefanacci JD, et al. Ventricular pneumocephalus, cervical subarachnoid pneumorrhachis, and meningoencephalitis in a dog

following rhinotomy for chronic fungal rhinitis. J Am Vet Med Assoc 2016;248: 430–5.
47. Kraft SL, Gavin PR, DeHaan C, et al. Retrospective review of 50 canine intracranial tumors evaluated by magnetic resonance imaging. J Vet Intern Med 1997; 11:218–25.
48. Cramer S, Campbell G, Gray C, et al. Pathology in practice. Brain neoplasm. J Am Vet Med Assoc 2012;240:47–9.
49. Malik R, Craig A, Wigney D, et al. Combination chemotherapy of canine and feline cryptococcosis using subcutaneously administered amphotericin B. Aust Vet J 1996;73:124–8.
50. Barachetti L, Mortellaro CM, Di Giancamillo M, et al. Bilateral orbital and nasal aspergillosis in a cat. Vet Ophthalmol 2009;12:176–82.
51. Saito M, Sharp NJH, Munana K, et al. CT findings of intracranial blastomycosis in a dog. Vet Radiol Ultrasound 2002;43:16–21.
52. Gaunt MC, Taylor SM, Kerr ME. Central nervous system blastomycosis in a dog. Can Vet J 2009;50:959–62.
53. Cheng Y, Ling J, Chang F, et al. Radiological manifestations of cryptococcal infection in central nervous system. J Chin Med Assoc 2003;66:19–26.
54. Lapointe J, Higgins RJ, Sturges B. Phaeohyphomycotic ependymitis in a cat. J Vet Diagn Invest 1998;10:202–4.
55. Bouljihad M, Lindeman CJ, Hayden DW. Pyogranulomatous meningoencephalitis associated with dematiaceous fungal (*Cladophialophora bantiana*) infection in a domestic cat. J Vet Diagn Invest 2002;14:70–2.
56. Jang S, Biberstein E, Rinaldi M, et al. Feline brain abscesses due to *Cladosporium trichoides*. Sabouraudia 1997;15:115–23.
57. Shinwari M, Thomas A, Orr J. Feline cerebral phaeohyphomycosis associated with *Cladosporium bantianum*. Aust Vet J 1985;62:383–4.
58. Russell EB, Gunew MN, Dennis MM, et al. Cerebral pyogranulomatous encephalitis caused by *Cladophialophora bantiana* in a 15-week-old domestic shorthair kitten. J Feline Med Surg 2016;2:1–6.
59. Revankar SG, Sutton DA, Rinaldi MG. Primary central nervous system phaeohyphomycosis: a review of 101 cases. Clin Infect Dis 2004;38:206–16.
60. Añor S, Sturges BK, Lafranco L, et al. Systemic phaeohyphomycosis (*Cladophialophora bantiana*) in a dog-clinical diagnosis with stereotactic computed tomographic-guided brain biopsy. J Vet Intern Med 2001;15:257–61.
61. Newsholme S, Tyrer M. Cerebral mycosis in a dog caused by *Cladosporium trichoides*. Onderstepoort J Vet Res 1980;47:47–9.
62. Ramírez-Romero R, Silva-Pérez RA, Lara-Arias J, et al. Coccidioidomycosis in biopsies with presumptive diagnosis of malignancy in dogs: report of three cases and comparative discussion of published reports. Mycopathologia 2016;181:151–7.
63. Shubitz LF. Comparative aspects of coccidioidomycosis in animals and humans. Ann N Y Acad Sci 2007;1111:395–403.
64. Shubitz LF, Dial SM. Coccidioidomycosis: a diagnostic challenge. Clin Tech Small Anim Pract 2005;20:220–6.
65. Pryor WH, Huizenga CG, Splitter GA, et al. *Coccidioides immitis* encephalitis in two dogs. J Am Vet Med Assoc 1972;161:1108–12.
66. Burtch M. Granulomatous meningitis caused by *Coccidioides immitis* in a dog. J Am Vet Med Assoc 1998;212:827–9.
67. Foureman P, Longshore R, Plummer SB. Spinal cord granuloma due to *Coccidioides immitis* in a cat. J Vet Intern Med 2005;19:373–6.

68. Kerwin SC, McCarthy RJ, VanSteenhouse JL, et al. Cervical spinal cord compression caused by cryptococcosis in a dog: successful treatment with surgery and fluconazole. J Am Anim Hosp Assoc 1998;34:523–6.
69. Smith J, Legendre A, Thomas W, et al. Cerebral *Blastomyces dermatitidis* infection in a cat. J Am Vet Med Assoc 2007;231:1210–4.
70. Foster SF, Charles JA, Parker G, et al. Cerebral cryptococcal granuloma in a cat. J Feline Med Surg 2001;3:37–44.
71. Glass E, DeLahunta A, Kent M, et al. A cryptococcal granuloma in the brain of a cat causing focal signs. Prog Vet Neurol 1996;7:141–4.
72. Reginato A, Giannuzzi P, Ricciardi M, et al. Extradural spinal cord lesion in a dog: first case study of canine neurological histoplasmosis in Italy. Vet Microbiol 2014;170:451–5.
73. Dubey A, Patwardhan RV, Sampth S, et al. Intracranial fungal granuloma: analysis of 40 patients and review of the literature. Surg Neurol 2005;63:254–60.
74. Kantarcioglu A, de Hoog G. Infections of the central nervous system by melanized fungi: a review of cases presented between 1999 and 2004. Mycoses 2004;47:4–13.
75. Mandrioli L, Bettini G, Marcato PS, et al. Central nervous system cryptococcoma in a cat. J Vet Med A Physiol Pathol Clin Med 2002;49:526–30.
76. Gonzalez JF, Montiel NA, Maass RL. First report on the diagnosis and treatment of encephalic and urinary paracoccidioidomycosis in a cat. J Feline Med Surg 2010;12:659–62.
77. Dial SM. Fungal diagnostics: current techniques and future trends. Vet Clin North Am Small Anim Pract 2007;37:373–92.
78. Greene RT, Troy GC. Coccidioidomycosis in 48 cats: a retrospective study (1984-1993). J Vet Intern Med 1995;9:86–91.
79. Corrigan VK, Legendre AM, Wheat LJ, et al. Treatment of disseminated aspergillosis with posaconazole in 10 dogs. J Vet Intern Med 2016;30:167–73.
80. Gerds-Grogan S, Dayrell-Hart B. Feline cryptococcosis: a retrospective evaluation. J Am Anim Hosp Assoc 1997;33:118–22.
81. Krockenberger MB, Swinney G, Martin P, et al. Sequential opportunistic infections in two German shepherd dogs. Aust Vet J 2011;89:9–14.
82. Crews LJ, Sharkey LC, Feeney DA, et al. Evaluation of total and ionized calcium status in dogs with blastomycosis: 38 cases (1997-2006). J Am Vet Med Assoc 2007;231:1545–9.
83. Windsor RC, Sturges BK, Vernau KM, et al. Cerebrospinal fluid eosinophilia in dogs. J Vet Intern Med 2009;23:275–81.
84. Spector D, Legendre AM, Wheat J, et al. Antigen and antibody testing for the diagnosis of blastomycosis in dogs. J Vet Intern Med 2008;22:839–43.
85. Malik R, McPetrie R, Wigney DI, et al. A latex cryptococcal antigen agglutination test for diagnosis and monitoring of therapy for cryptococcosis. Aust Vet J 1996;74:358–64.
86. Medleau L, Marks M, Brown J, et al. Clinical evaluation of a cryptococcal antigen latex agglutination test for diagnosis of cryptococcosis in cats. J Am Vet Med Assoc 1990;196:1470–3.
87. Cunningham L. Sensitivity and specificity of *Histoplasma* antigen detection by enzyme immunoassay. J Am Anim Hosp Assoc 2015;51:306–10.
88. Kirsch EJ, Greene RT, Prahl A, et al. Evaluation of *Coccidioides* antigen detection in dogs with coccidioidomycosis. Clin Vaccine Immunol 2012;19:343–5.

89. Billen F, Peeters D, Peters IR, et al. Comparison of the value of measurement of serum galactomannan and *Aspergillus*-specific antibodies in the diagnosis of canine sino-nasal aspergillosis. Vet Microbiol 2009;133:358–65.
90. Garcia RS, Wheat LJ, Cook AK, et al. Sensitivity and specificity of a blood and urine galactomannan antigen assay for diagnosis of systemic aspergillosis in dogs. J Vet Intern Med 2012;26:911–9.
91. Falci DR, Stadnik CMB, Pasqualotto AC. A review of diagnostic methods for invasive fungal diseases: challenges and perspectives. Infect Dis Ther 2017; 6(2):213–23.
92. Shubitz LF, Butkiewicz CD, Dial SM, et al. Incidence of *Coccidioides* infection among dogs residing in a region in which the organism is endemic. J Am Vet Med Assoc 2005;226:1846–50.
93. Chow NA, Lindsley MD, McCotter OZ, et al. Development of an enzyme immunoassay for detection of antibodies against *Coccidioides* in dogs and other mammalian species. PLoS One 2017;12:e0175081.
94. Mourning AC, Patterson EE, Kirsch EJ, et al. Evaluation of an enzyme immunoassay for antibodies to a recombinant *Blastomyces* adhesin-1 repeat antigen as an aid in the diagnosis of blastomycosis in dogs. J Am Vet Med Assoc 2015; 247:1133–8.
95. O'Brien CR, Krockenberger MB, Martin P, et al. Long-term outcome of therapy for 59 cats and 11 dogs with cryptococcosis. Aust Vet J 2006;84:384–92.
96. Taylor E. Impact of efflux transporters in the brain on the development of drugs for CNS disorders. Clin Pharmacokinet 2002;41:81–92.
97. Sager G. Cyclic GMP transporters. Neurochem Int 2004;45:865–73.
98. Lavely J, Lipsitz D. Fungal infections of the central nervous system in the dog and cat. Clin Tech Small Anim Pract 2005;20:212–9.
99. Kerl M. Update on canine and feline fungal diseases. Vet Clin North Am 2003; 33:721–47.
100. Quimby JM, Hoffman SB, Duke J, et al. Adverse neurologic events associated with voriconazole use in 3 cats. J Vet Intern Med 2010;24:647–9.
101. McLellan GJ, Aquino SM, Mason DR, et al. Use of posaconazole in the management of invasive orbital aspergillosis in a cat. J Am Anim Hosp Assoc 2006;42: 302–7.
102. Balkis M, Leidich S, Mukherjee P, et al. Mechanisms of fungal resistance: an overview. Drugs 2002;62:1025–40.
103. Redmond A, Dancer C, Woods M. Fungal infections of the central nervous system: a review of fungal pathogens and treatment. Neurol India 2007;55:251–9.
104. Malik R, Wigney D, Muir D, et al. Cryptococcosis in cats: clinical and mycological assessment of 29 cases and evaluation of treatment using orally administered fluconazole. J Med Vet Mycol 1992;30:133–44.
105. Foy DS, Trepanier LA, Kirsch EJ, et al. Serum and urine *Blastomyces* antigen concentrations as markers of clinical remission in dogs treated for systemic blastomycosis. J Vet Intern Med 2014;28:305–10.

Diagnostic Imaging of Discospondylitis

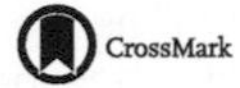

Catherine M. Ruoff, MS, DVM[a], Sharon C. Kerwin, DVM, MS[b,*], Amanda R. Taylor, DVM[c]

KEYWORDS

• Dog • Cat • Spine • MRI • CT • Radiography • Discospondylitis

KEY POINTS

- Radiography remains an important screening tool for diagnosis of discospondylitis; however, radiographic signs often lag behind clinical signs.
- Computed tomography (CT) is excellent for evaluating bone and may be useful both in diagnosis and follow-up imaging.
- MRI can identify sites of discospondylitis that are not yet radiographically visible and can reveal additional disease extension, such as spinal empyema.
- Fluoroscopic or CT-guided aspirates may be helpful in obtaining samples for culture, particularly as an alternative to open surgical biopsy.

Discospondylitis is a bacterial, or less commonly fungal or algal, spinal infection that is usually hematogenous in origin and begins as an infection of the cartilaginous end plates of the vertebral bodies with secondary involvement of the intervertebral disk.[1–3] Mixed bacterial infections are not uncommon, and combination bacterial and fungal infections have been reported.[4] Risk factors can include large breed, intact male status, recent corticosteroid treatment, or recent surgery (spinal surgery or surgery at a site remote to the spine).[5–9] In rare cases, a migrating foreign body (eg, grass awn) or epidural injection can cause discospondylitis.[10,11] In most cases, bacteria enter the vertebral bodies via the bloodstream from an infection at a distant site (eg, prostate infection). Bacteria colonize the highly vascular and slow-flowing metaphyseal and epiphyseal capillary beds with rapid extension into the disk as

Disclosure Statement: The authors have nothing to disclose.

[a] Department of Large Animal Clinical Sciences, College of Veterinary Medicine & Biomedical Sciences, Texas A&M University, College Station, TX 77843-4475, USA; [b] Department of Small Animal Clinical Sciences, College of Veterinary Medicine & Biomedical Sciences, Texas A&M University, College Station, TX 77843-4474, USA; [c] Department of Clinical Sciences, Auburn University College of Veterinary Medicine, Greene Hall, 1130 Wire Road, Auburn, AL 36849, USA
* Corresponding author.
E-mail address: skerwin@cvm.tamu.edu

Vet Clin Small Anim 48 (2018) 85–94
http://dx.doi.org/10.1016/j.cvsm.2017.08.007

well as the rest of the vertebral body. Although more common in dogs, discospondylitis has been reported in cats.[12,13] Although *Staphylococcus* spp are the most commonly reported etiologic agents, *Streptococcus*, *Brucella canis*, *Escherichia coli*, and *Enterobacter* are also common.[1,14–16] Clinicians should also keep in mind that less common etiologic agents, such as *Salmonella*, methicillin-resistant *Staphylococcus aureus*, *Erysipelothrix*, *Nocardia*, and many others, including a variety of fungi, may be diagnosed.[9,17–23] Some etiologic agents are sturdy and easy to grow in the laboratory, whereas others are fastidious and may be seen in tissue aspirates or histopathology but not grown in the microbiology laboratory.

Discospondylitis is notoriously difficult to diagnose: signs may include vague pain (usually localizing to the spine on direct palpation), lameness, fever, anorexia, weight loss, abdominal pain, and neurologic deficits ranging from mild ataxia to plegia, which can occur after pathologic spinal fracture or concurrent empyema.[14,24,25] Spinal pain is not always present and, therefore, may not be a reliable marker for disease resolution.[15] Although presentation can be peracute, clinical signs often wax and wane over a period of months to years. Imaging is critical to making the diagnosis yet can be challenging in individual patients. Clinicians may face the dilemma of when to stop antibiotics in patients with discospondylitis, because relapse is common with premature cessation of therapy.[16] In 1 large study, the duration of antimicrobial treatment in dogs followed until radiographic resolution of signs was 40 weeks to 80 weeks.[14] The role of imaging in confirming resolution of infection has yet to be determined.

A variety of imaging modalities have been used to identify sites of discospondylitis and include radiography, computed tomography (CT), MRI, myelography, epidurography, ultrasonography, and nuclear scintigraphy. In addition, fluoroscopy and CT can be used to aid in percutaneous image-guided aspirates of the affected disks.

RADIOGRAPHY

Radiography is a frequently used screening method for discospondylitis because it is readily available in most veterinary practices and is inexpensive and noninvasive. Common radiographic findings associated with discospondylitis include osteolysis of vertebral end plates and adjacent vertebral bodies with collapse of the intervertebral disk space (**Fig. 1**). There is also a variable amount of sclerosis adjacent to the osteolytic regions and osseous proliferation adjacent to the intervertebral disk spaces.[26–30] Because there is often a delay in development of radiographic signs, normal radiographs of the vertebral column do not rule out a diagnosis of discospondylitis, and additional imaging (MRI, CT, or repeat radiographs in several days to weeks) is often necessary to make a diagnosis.[1,31–33]

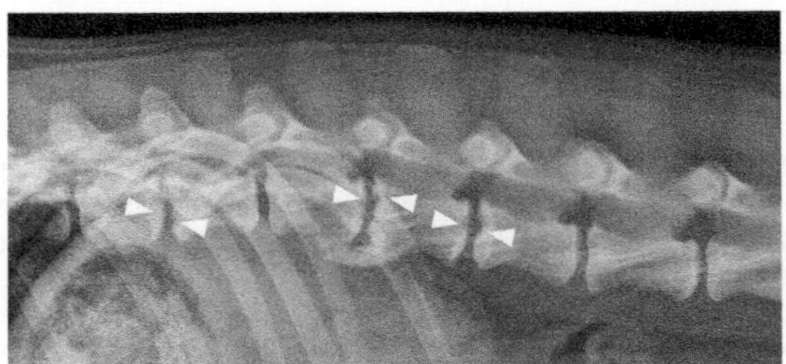

Fig. 1. Lateral radiograph of an adult pit bull with discospondylitis at T12-13, L1-2, and L2-3. There is osteolysis of the vertebral end plates (*arrowheads*), sclerosis of the adjacent bone, and narrowing of the intervertebral disk spaces at these sites.

One study found the radiographic appearance of discospondylitis can differ in juvenile dogs less than 6 months of age compared with adults. On initial radiographs, there was evidence of intervertebral disk space narrowing without evidence of vertebral end-plate osteolysis, which is typically seen in older dogs with discospondylitis. Subtle osteolysis of the adjacent vertebral end plates was seen at all of these sites on follow-up radiographs. Over time, a majority of these dogs developed osteolysis of the vertebral metaphyses with an appearance similar to discospondylitis in adult dogs; 8 of 10 dogs with discospondylitis lesions in the thoracolumbar vertebral column had a subluxation at the site of discospondylitis at the time of diagnosis or on follow-up radiographs.[34]

Physitis of the caudal vertebral physis has also been reported in young dogs and should be distinguished from discospondylitis. In vertebral physitis, osteolysis is initially restricted to the caudal vertebral physis. Eventually, collapse of the caudal vertebral body and spondylosis of the caudal aspect of the vertebral body occurs. In contrast, discospondylitis results in symmetric osteolysis of the vertebral end plates with sclerosis of the underlying bone and spondylosis deformans on the cranial and caudal aspects of the intervertebral disk space.[35]

COMPUTED TOMOGRAPHY

CT is useful in imaging discospondylitis because of its excellent depiction of bone. CT findings in dogs and cats with discospondylitis are similar to radiographic findings and include osteolysis of adjacent vertebral end plates with or without osteolysis of the underlying bone[13,28,36] (**Fig. 2**). CT has the potential to be more useful than radiography in the diagnosis of discospondylitis because CT can identify osseous lesions earlier in the disease process than radiography. Studies evaluating the sensitivity and specificity of CT for the diagnosis of discospondylitis, however, have not been performed.

MRI

MRI has become the imaging modality of choice for imaging discospondylitis and spinal infections in people,[37] and there are increasing reports of the use of MRI in the diagnosis of discospondylitis in small animals.[4,21,25,28,30,38,39] MRI has identified sites of discospondylitis that were not evident radiographically.[40] T2-weighted, precontrast and postcontrast T1-weighted, T2-weighted fat-saturated, and short-tau inversion recovery (STIR) MRI sequences are the most useful in the diagnosis of discospondylitis. The hydrated nucleus pulposus of the intervertebral disks,

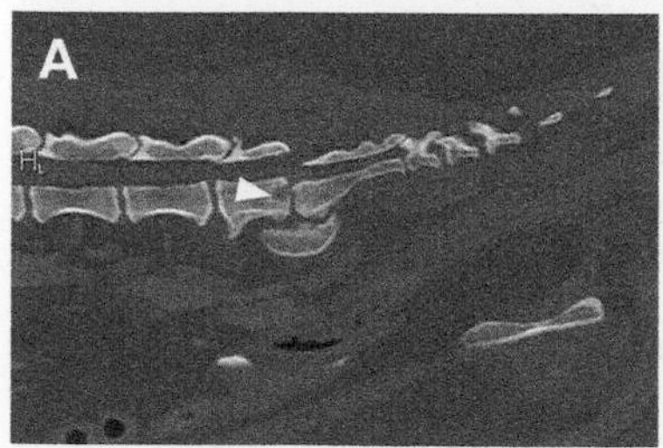

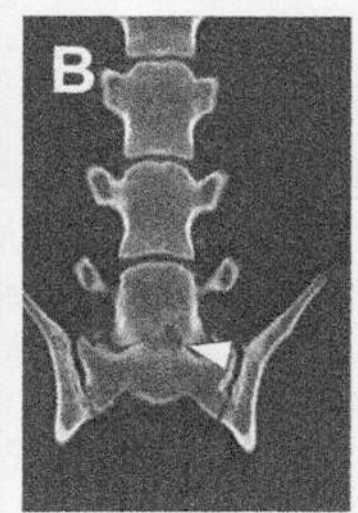

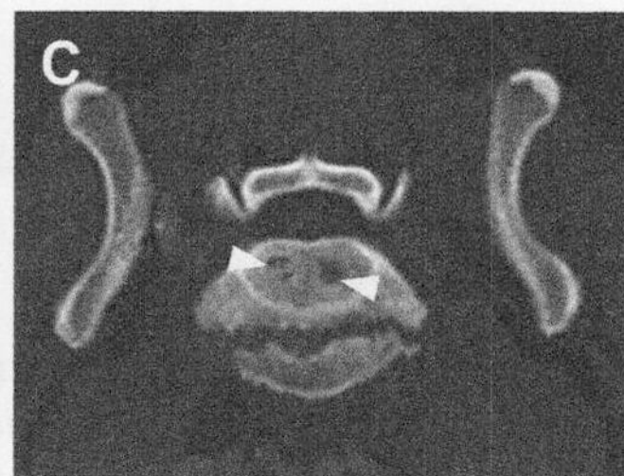

Fig. 2. Sagittal plane (*A*), dorsal plane (*B*), and transverse plane (*C*) bone window CT of an adult Australian cattle dog with discospondylitis at L7-S1. There is osteolysis of the vertebral end plates (*arrowheads*) with sclerosis of the adjacent vertebral bodies and narrowing of the L7-S1 intervertebral disk space.

cerebrospinal fluid, epidural fat, and most pathologic processes are hyperintense on T2-weighted images because of the high water content of these tissues. T1-weighted images depict bone better than T2-weighted images but have lower contrast than T2-weighted images. T1-weighted images made after intravenous administration of gadolinium depict lesions with increased blood supply. T2-weighted fat-saturated and STIR sequences are similar to T2-weighted images but with suppression of fat, which increases the conspicuity of many lesions.[41]

The MRI features of discospondylitis are fairly consistent. Affected vertebral end plates are usually T1 hypointense,[40] although 1 study reported mixed signal intensity on T1-weighted images in several dogs.[4] The vertebral end plates are usually T2 hypointense, although T2 hyperintensity has been reported in a few dogs[4,21,28,30,38,40] (**Fig. 3**). All of the vertebral end plates were reported to be STIR hyperintense in a study evaluating 17 sites of discospondylitis in 13 dogs,[40] whereas the vertebral end plates at 11 of 15 sites of discospondylitis were reported to be STIR hyperintense in another study.[4] There was contrast enhancement of the vertebral end plates at all 17 sites of discospondylitis in 1 study and at 11 of 19 sites in

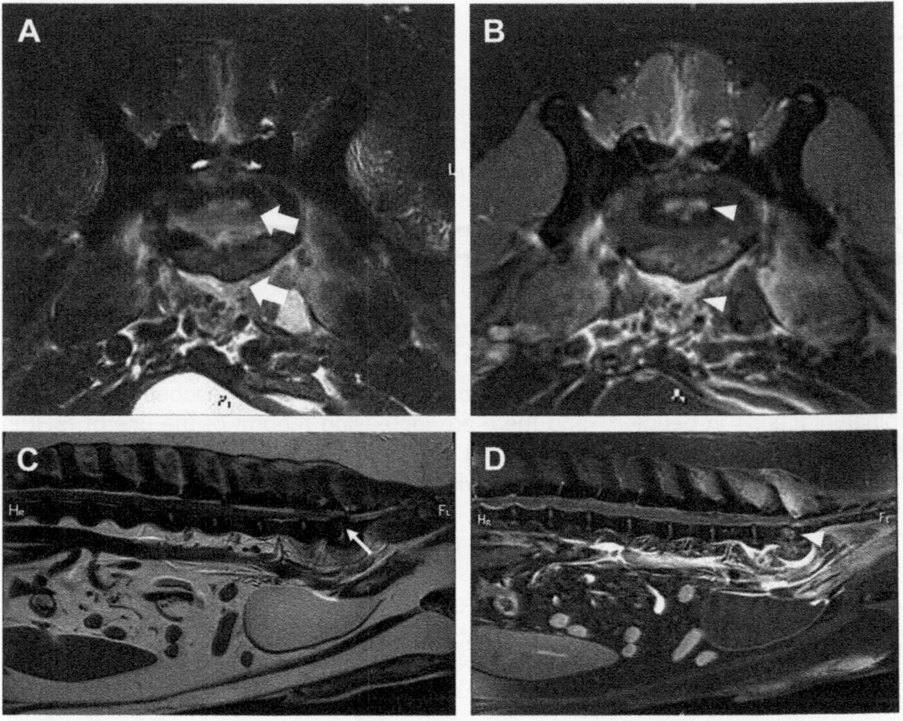

Fig. 3. MRI of the same dog as **Fig. 2**. (*A*) T2 fat-saturated transverse plane image through the L7-S1 intervertebral disk space. There is hyperintensity of the paraspinal soft tissues and ill-defined soft tissue within the vertebral canal (*block arrows*). (*B*) T1-weighted postcontrast image at the same level as in (*A*). There is contrast enhancement of the same tissues as well as the L7-S1 vertebral end plates (*arrowheads*). (*C*) T2-weighted sagittal plane image of the lumbar vertebral column. There is narrowing of the L7-S1 intervertebral disk space and T2 hypointensity of the vertebral end plates (*thin arrow*). (*D*) T1-weighted postcontrast image of the lumbar vertebral column. There is contrast enhancement of the paraspinal soft tissues and ill-defined tissue within the vertebral canal, as well as the L7-S1 vertebral end plates (*arrowheads*).

another study. Cortical lysis and irregularity of the vertebral end plates is a common feature identified on T1-weighted images, occurring in approximately 92.6% of sites in 1 study and 88.2% in another study.[4,40] Other processes can cause changes in the appearance of the vertebral end plates and include reactive end-plate changes, fatty infiltration of the body and end plates, end plate sclerosis, osteochondrosis, and Schmorl nodes. These processes, however, can usually be distinguished from discospondylitis by differences in signal intensity of the end plates and the appearance of the surrounding structures.[39]

The vertebral bodies adjacent to the affected vertebral end plates are usually abnormal. Affected vertebral bodies are usually T1 hypointense and T2 hypointense to isointense.[4,40] One-third to one-half of the vertebral body is most commonly affected, although the entire vertebral body can be affected. Signal intensity changes in the adjacent vertebrae are usually symmetric.[40] Contrast enhancement of the vertebral bodies is variable with all affected vertebral bodies contrast enhancing in 1 study, whereas only 4 of 18 affected vertebral bodies contrast enhanced in another study. Vertebral subluxation was a less common finding, occurring in 11.7% of dogs in 1 study and 14.8% of sites in another study.[4,40]

The soft tissues adjacent to the affected vertebrae are often abnormal. Affected intervertebral disks are usually hyperintense on STIR and T2-weighted images, whereas they are usually isointense on T1-weighted images and often contrast enhance.[4,28,30,40] There is variable T2 and STIR hyperintensity and contrast enhancement of the paraspinal soft tissues.[4,40] There is frequently extension of empyema into the epidural space resulting in compression of the spinal cord. Empyema is usually T1 hypointense to isointense and T2 and STIR hyperintense with contrast enhancement. This was seen in 17 of 23 dogs in 1 study and 15 of 17 sites in another study. Two patterns of contrast enhancement associated with epidural empyema have been reported: rim enhancement and diffuse enhancement. No correlation has been identified, however, associated with chronicity of discospondylitis and pattern of contrast enhancement.[21,25,40] T2 hyperintensity of the spinal cord has also been reported.[4,25] In a study of 23 discospondylitis sites, there was T2 hyperintensity of the spinal cord at 10 sites, 6 of which were focal at the level of extradural compression, whereas 4 were diffuse. There was no correlation, however, between the presence and type (focal or diffuse) of T2 hyperintensity of the spinal cord and severity of neurologic score.[4]

The thoracolumbar vertebral column and lumbosacral articulation has been reported to be the most commonly reported sites of discospondylitis. In 2 case series evaluating MRI findings associated with discospondylitis, the lumbosacral articulation was a frequent site of discospondylitis, accounting for 53% of lesions in 1 study and 16% of sites another study. Sites within the thoracic vertebral column were the next most common site followed by the lumbar vertebral column.[4,40] Not all these MRI studies, however, included the cervical spine, so it is possible there were additional sites of discospondylitis within the cervical region.

OTHER IMAGING MODALITIES

Myelography and epidurography have been used to evaluate discospondylitis, although these imaging modalities are used less frequently as the availability of MRI and CT has increased. In a study of 36 discospondylitis sites in 27 patients, there was compression of the spinal cord or cauda equine at 56% of the discospondylitis sites. Soft tissue was the cause of spinal cord compression at 73.7% of sites. Soft tissue and subluxation contributed to spinal cord compression in 13.3% of cases, whereas soft tissue and bone caused spinal cord compression in 6.6% of sites, and soft tissue, bone, and subluxation caused spinal cord compression in the remaining 6.6% of sites. In this study, no significant difference in degree of spinal cord compression and ambulatory status of the patient was identified. Additionally, no significant difference in the degree of spinal cord compression and outcome was identified.[42] The lack of correlation between degree of spinal cord compression and neurologic status of the patient is in contrast to studies using MRI to identify sites of discospondylitis that found that dogs with more severe spinal cord compression on MRI had worse neurologic scores. This could be due to the increased sensitivity of MRI in the identification of spinal cord compression.[4,40] Epidurography may be more useful than myelography in some cases of cauda equine compression secondary to discospondylitis.[30]

The use of ultrasonography and nuclear scintigraphy in the diagnosis of discospondylitis has occasionally been reported. In a case series of dogs less than 6 months old diagnosed with discospondylitis, ultrasound of the affected vertebrae and intervertebral disks was performed in 5 dogs. In these cases there was loss of reverberation artifact seen at normal intervertebral disk spaces and soft tissue bulging ventrally at the affected intervertebral disk spaces.[34] On bone phase nuclear scintigraphy images, there is focal marked increased radiopharmaceutical uptake centered on affected disk spaces.[30,43]

Fluoroscopy can be a useful modality to achieve image-guided percutaneous aspirates of potentially infected intervertebral disks.[33,35,44,45] Although blood and urine cultures can serve as surrogates for osteomyelitis, they may also grow different, unrelated bacteria or yield no growth at all.[14,46] One study described positive bacterial cultures in 9 of 10 dogs using fluoroscopically assisted disk aspirates, as opposed to growth on blood culture for only 1 of 6 dogs and positive urine cultures in 6 of 10 dogs.[33] Identification of the correct causative organism is critical to correct antimicrobial selection, so this technique, which has been reported for cervical and lumbar disks, is an attractive alternative to open surgical biopsy. The authors have also successfully used CT-guided aspirates to obtain diagnostic samples for culture in dogs with discospondylitis. Fluoroscopically guided percutaneous discectomy has also been reported, also with superior diagnostic results (causative bacteria identified in 9 of 10 dogs as opposed to 3 positive urine and 4 positive blood cultures). The authors also used the larger defect created by the trephine to allow for decompression and local injection of cefazolin. They reported complete resolution of clinical signs by 14 days in all dogs.[33] Long-term follow-up was not reported.

DIAGNOSTIC IMAGING AND FOLLOW-UP IN DISCOSPONDYLITIS

Radiographs are often used to monitor response to treatment of discospondylitis. Radiographic evidence of healing of discospondylitis includes replacement of lytic bone by osseous proliferation and ankylosis of the vertebrae, although radiographic improvement may lag significantly behind clinical improvement. In a study of 12 dogs who completely recovered from discospondylitis with antibiotic therapy alone, radiographs were made at 3-week intervals to monitor response to treatment. In dogs less than 1 year old, evidence of radiographic improvement was seen 3 weeks after initiation of treatment with increased osseous proliferation and sclerosis, although several dogs also had increased osteolysis compared with the initial radiographs. In dogs older than 1 year of age, there was increased osteolysis at 3 weeks after initiation of treatment without osseous proliferation or sclerosis evident radiographically, although dogs were improved clinically. In these dogs, increased osseous proliferation and sclerosis was not evident radiographically until 6 weeks to 12 weeks after beginning treatment.[31]

One study recommended continuing antimicrobial treatment until there is no radiographic evidence of disease, with markers of radiographic quiescence including absence of the lytic focus, smoothing and then loss of lytic focus, and replacement by bridging of the involved vertebrae.[14] As Shamir and coworkers[31] pointed out, however, differentiation of radiographic findings of chronic discospondylitis from the normal healing process, degenerative end-plate changes, or new superimposed infection in the presence of degenerative spine disease may be difficult and may not correlate with clinical signs. Although nuclear scintigraphy may be helpful in determining whether or not active infection is still present, it is not widely accessible and requires overnight hospitalization until a patient is cleared of radiation. In the authors' experience, clients are reluctant to allow this modality for follow-up in driving decision making. At the same time, many clients are anxious to stop administering expensive antibiotics to often very large dogs. Although MRI is arguably the most sensitive for soft tissue changes, the need for general anesthesia and expense often limits its use. The authors have used CT successfully in their hospital to help monitor the results of antibiotic therapy (**Fig. 4**). To date, however, there are no published data on what

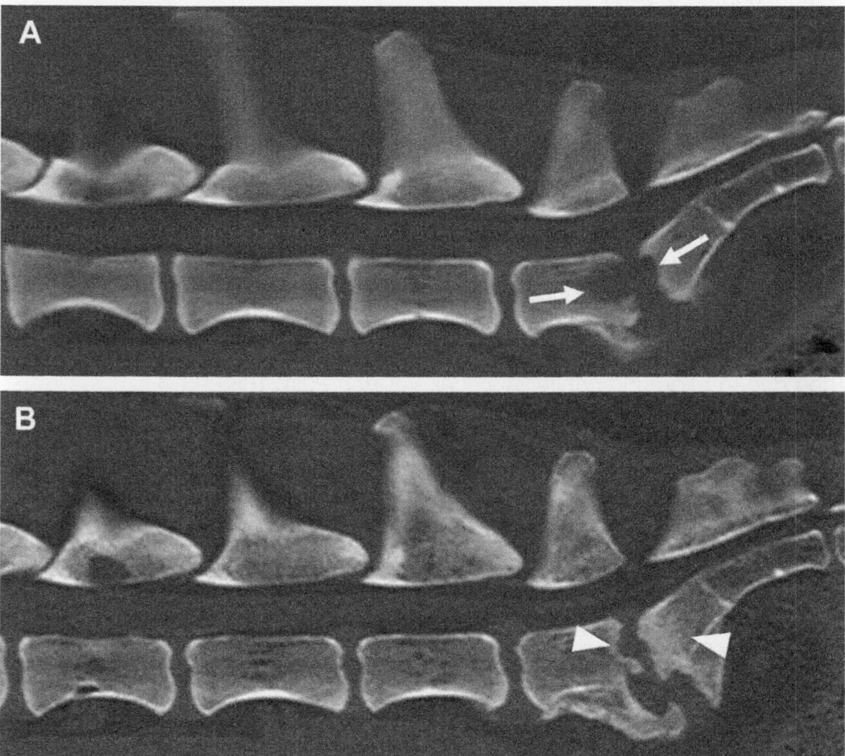

Fig. 4. Sagittal plane images of an adult Labrador retriever with discospondylitis at L7-S1 before (*A*) and after (*B*) 10 months of antibiotic administration. There is extensive osteolysis of the vertebral end plates and sclerosis of the adjacent bone prior to treatment (*arrows*). There is smoothly marginated osseous infilling of the sites of end-plate osteolysis with sclerosis of the underlying bone (*arrowheads*), although concave defects remain within the vertebral end plates. There is increased spondylosis deformans at L6-S1.

constitutes the best method for making the decision to stop treatment in cases of discospondylitis.

REFERENCES

1. Kornegay JN, Barber DL. Diskospondylitis in dogs. J Am Vet Med Assoc 1980; 177:337–41.
2. Dallman MJ, Dew TL, Tobias L, et al. Disseminated aspergillosis in a dog with diskospondylitis and neurologic deficits. J Am Vet Med Assoc 1992;200:511–3.
3. Manino PM, Oliveira F, Ficken M, et al. Disseminated protothecosis associated with diskospondylitis in a dog. J Am Anim Hosp Assoc 2014;50:429–35.
4. Harris JM, Chen AV, Tucker RL, et al. Clinical features and magnetic resonance imaging characteristics of diskospondylitis in dogs: 23 cases (1997-2010). J Am Vet Med Assoc 2013;242:359–65.
5. Bartels KE, Higbee RG, Bahr RJ, et al. Outcome of and complications associated with prophylactic percutaneous laser disk ablation in dogs with thoracolumbar disk disease: 277 cases (1992-2001). J Am Vet Med Assoc 2003;222:1733–9.
6. Kinzel S, Wolff M, Buecker A, et al. Partial percutaneous discectomy for treatment of thoracolumbar disc protrusion: retrospective study of 331 dogs. J Small Anim Pract 2005;46:479–84.
7. Canal S, Contiero B, Balducci F, et al. Risk factors for diskospondylitis in dogs after spinal decompression surgery for intervertebral disk herniation. J Am Vet Med Assoc 2016;248:1383–90.
8. Finnen A, Blond L, Parent J. Cervical discospondylitis in 2 Great Dane puppies following routine surgery. Can Vet J 2012;53:531–4.
9. Schwartz M, Boettcher IC, Kramer S, et al. Two dogs with iatrogenic discospondylitis caused by meticillin-resistant Staphylococcus aureus. J Small Anim Pract 2009;50:201–5.
10. Remedios AM, Wagner R, Caulkett NA, et al. Epidural abscess and discospondylitis in a dog after administration of a lumbosacral epidural analgesic. Can Vet J 1996;37:106–7.
11. Sutton A, May C, Coughlan A. Spinal osteomyelitis and epidural empyema in a dog due to migrating conifer material. Vet Rec 2010;166:693–4.
12. Hill MF, Warren-Smith C, Granger N. What is your diagnosis? Diskospondylitis. J Am Vet Med Assoc 2015;247:743–5.
13. Packer RA, Coates JR, Cook CR, et al. Sublumbar abscess and diskospondylitis in a cat. Vet Radiol Ultrasound 2005;46:396–9.
14. Burkert BA, Kerwin SC, Hosgood GL, et al. Signalment and clinical features of diskospondylitis in dogs: 513 cases (1980-2001). J Am Vet Med Assoc 2005; 227:268–75.
15. Hurov L, Troy G, Turnwald G. Diskospondylitis in the dog: 27 cases. J Am Vet Med Assoc 1978;173:275–81.
16. Kerwin SC, Lewis DD, Hribernik TN, et al. Diskospondylitis associated with Brucella canis infection in dogs: 14 cases (1980-1991). J Am Vet Med Assoc 1992;201:1253–7.
17. Mitten RW. Vertebral osteomyelitis in the dog due to Nocardia-like organisms. J Small Anim Pract 1974;15:563–70.
18. Bradney IW. Vertebral osteomyelitis due to *Nocardia* in a dog. Aust Vet J 1985;62: 315–6.
19. Houlton JEF, Jefferies AR. Infective polyarthritis and multiple discospondylitis in a dog due to Erysipelothrix rhusiopathiae. J Small Anim Pract 1989;30:35–8.

20. Golini L, Morgan JP, Glaus T, et al. Successful medical treatment of Erysipelothrix rhusiopathiae-induced lumbosacral diskospondylitis in a dog. Vet Rec 2012;170: 543.
21. Plessas IN, Jull P, Volk HA. A case of canine discospondylitis and epidural empyema due to Salmonella species. Can Vet J 2013;54:595–8.
22. Foster JD, Trepanier LA, Ginn JA. Use of linezolid to treat MRSP bacteremia and discospondylitis in a dog. J Am Anim Hosp Assoc 2014;50:53–8.
23. Hilligas J, Van Wie E, Barr J, et al. Vertebral osteomyelitis and multiple cutaneous lesions in a dog caused by Nocardia pseudobrasiliensis. J Vet Intern Med 2014; 28:1621–5.
24. Cabassu J, Moissonnier P. Surgical treatment of a vertebral fracture associated with a haematogenous osteomyelitis in a dog. Vet Comp Orthop Traumatol 2007;20:227–30.
25. De Stefani A, Garosi LS, McConnell FJ, et al. Magnetic resonance imaging features of spinal epidural empyema in five dogs. Vet Radiol Ultrasound 2008;49: 135–40.
26. Adamo PF, Cherubini GB. Discospondylitis associated with three unreported bacteria in the dog. J Small Anim Pract 2001;42:352–5.
27. Auger J, Dupuis J, Quesnel A, et al. Surgical treatment of lumbosacral instability caused by discospondylitis in four dogs. Vet Surg 2000;29:70–80.
28. Gonzalo-Orden JM, Altonaga JR, Orden MA, et al. Magnetic resonance, computed tomographic and radiologic findings in a dog with discospondylitis. Vet Radiol Ultrasound 2000;41:142–4.
29. Kinzel S, Koch J, Buecker A, et al. Treatment of 10 dogs with discospondylitis by fluoroscopy-guided percutaneous discectomy. Vet Rec 2005;156:78–81.
30. Kraft SL, Mussman JM, Smith T, et al. Magnetic resonance imaging of presumptive lumbosacral discospondylitis in a dog. Vet Radiol Ultrasound 1998;39:9–13.
31. Shamir MH, Tavor N, Aizenberg T. Radiographic findings during recovery from discospondylitis. Vet Radiol Ultrasound 2001;42:496–503.
32. Churcher RK. A dog with back pain. Aust Vet J 1996;74:17–8.
33. Fischer A, Mahaffey MB, Oliver JE. Fluoroscopically guided percutaneous disk aspiration in 10 dogs with diskospondylitis. J Vet Intern Med 1997;11:284–7.
34. Kirberger RM. Early diagnostic imaging findings in juvenile dogs with presumed diskospondylitis: 10 cases (2008-2014). J Am Vet Med Assoc 2016;249:539–46.
35. Jimenez MM, O'Callaghan MW. Vertebral physitis: a radiographic diagnosis to be separated from discospondylitis. Vet Radiol Ultrasound 1995;36:188–95.
36. De Risio L, Gnudi G, Bertoni G. What is your diagnosis? Sclerosis of the caudal vertebral body end plate of L7 and the cranial end plate of S1 and narrowing of the L7-S1 intervertebral disk space. J Am Vet Med Assoc 2003;222:1359–60.
37. Govender S. Spinal infections. J Bone Joint Surg Br 2005;87:1454–8.
38. Cherubini GB, Cappello R, Lu D, et al. MRI findings in a dog with discospondylitis caused by Bordetella species. J Small Anim Pract 2004;45:417–20.
39. Gendron K, Doherr MG, Gavin P, et al. Magnetic resonance imaging characterization of vertebral endplate changes in the dog. Vet Radiol Ultrasound 2012; 53(1):50–6.
40. Carrera I, Sullivan M, McConnell F, et al. Magnetic resonance imaging features of discospondylitis in dogs. Vet Radiol Ultrasound 2011;52:125–31.
41. Dennis R. Optimal magnetic resonance imaging of the spine. Vet Radiol Ultrasound 2011;52:S72–80.

42. Davis MJ, Dewey CW, Walker MA, et al. Contrast radiographic findings in canine bacterial discospondylitis: a multicenter, retrospective study of 27 cases. J Am Anim Hosp Assoc 2000;36:81–5.
43. Walker M, Platt SR, Graham JP, et al. Vertebral physitis with epiphyseal sequestration and a portosystemic shunt in a Pekingese dog. J Small Anim Pract 1999; 40:525–8.
44. Watt PR, Robins GM, Galloway AM, et al. Disseminated opportunistic fungal disease in dogs: 10 cases (1982-1990). J Am Vet Med Assoc 1995;207:67–70.
45. McKee WM, Mitten RW, Labuc RH. Surgical treatment of lumbosacral discospondylitis by a distraction-fusion technique. J Small Anim Pract 1990;31:15–20.
46. Lavely JA, Vernau KM, Vernau W, et al. Spinal epidural empyema in seven dogs. Vet Surg 2006;35:176–85.

Acute Herniation of Nondegenerate Nucleus Pulposus

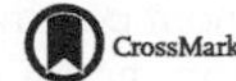

Acute Noncompressive Nucleus Pulposus Extrusion and Compressive Hydrated Nucleus Pulposus Extrusion

Steven De Decker, DVM, MVetMed, PhD*, Joe Fenn, BVetMed, MVetMed

KEYWORDS

- High-velocity low-volume disk extrusion • Traumatic disk extrusion • ANNPE
- HNPE • Spinal cord contusion

KEY POINTS

- Acute noncompressive nucleus pulposus extrusion is characterized by a sudden extrusion of nondegenerate nucleus pulposus without remaining spinal cord compression.
- Hydrated nucleus pulposus extrusion is characterized by a sudden extrusion of hydrated nucleus pulposus, which results in varying degrees of spinal cord compression.
- Dogs with acute noncompressive nucleus pulposus extrusion, and to a lesser extent dogs with hydrated nucleus pulposus extrusion, can present with characteristic clinical signs.
- MRI is the diagnostic modality of choice for both conditions. Specific MRI findings have been described for both conditions.
- Although there is consensus about the best treatment of acute noncompressive nucleus pulposus extrusion, the ideal treatment of hydrated nucleus pulposus extrusion is unknown.

INTRODUCTION

Acute intervertebral disk (IVD) herniation is the most common spinal emergency in dogs and can be defined as a localized displacement of IVD material beyond its normal anatomic boundaries.[1] Hansen type I IVD disease or IVD extrusion is the

---

The authors have nothing to disclose.
Department of Clinical Science and Services, Royal Veterinary College, University of London, Hatfield, Hertfordshire, UK
* Corresponding author. Department of Clinical Science and Services, Royal Veterinary College, University of London, Hawkshead Lane, North Mymms, Hatfield, Hertfordshire AL9 7TA, UK.
E-mail address: sdedecker@rvc.ac.uk

Vet Clin Small Anim 48 (2018) 95–109
http://dx.doi.org/10.1016/j.cvsm.2017.08.004 vetsmall.theclinics.com

most common and best characterized spinal cord condition in dogs.[2–4] In this condition, acute extrusion of dehydrated and calcified nucleus pulposus through a fully ruptured annulus fibrosus is preceded by advanced chondroid degeneration of the IVD and the nucleus pulposus in particular.[2] Acute spinal cord injury (SCI) in dogs with Hansen type I IVD disease is caused by a combination of spinal cord contusion and varying degrees of sustained spinal cord compression.[4–6] However, following continuous developments and increased availability of MRI in veterinary medicine, it is increasingly recognized that acute extrusions can also occur in nondegenerate or minimally degenerate nucleus pulposus. Although there is some discussion concerning the most appropriate terminology, 2 types of acute herniation of nondegenerate nucleus pulposus are currently recognized: acute noncompressive nucleus pulposus extrusion (ANNPE) and hydrated nucleus pulposus extrusion (HNPE). Differentiation and diagnosis is based on well-reported clinical characteristics and diagnostic imaging findings.[7,8] Several reports have now explored the typical clinical presentation, diagnostic findings, and management of ANNPE and HNPE, revealing some stark contrasts with traditional Hansen type I IVD extrusions and emphasizing the need for an accurate diagnosis in such cases.[7–14] Although both ANNPE and HNPE refer to an acute extrusion of nondegenerate nucleus pulposus and subsequent acute SCI, there are also important differences that might influence clinical decision-making regarding management and prognosis.

INTERVERTEBRAL DISK ANATOMY

Although a detailed description of canine IVD anatomy is beyond the scope of this article, an understanding of the basic anatomic concepts is desirable to understand the clinical characteristics and treatment recommendations for dogs with ANNPE and HNPE. All vertebral bodies, with the exception of the first and second vertebrae and the fused sacral vertebrae, are interconnected by an IVD.[15] The IVD is composed of a centrally located nucleus pulposus, an outer annulus fibrosus, the transitional zone, and adjacent vertebral endplates.[5] The healthy and nondegenerate nucleus pulposus is a mucoid, translucent, gelatinous structure (**Fig. 1**). It is well hydrated and is mainly composed of water.[16] The nucleus pulposus is surrounded by the annulus fibrosus, which consists of a network of concentrically organized collagen layers

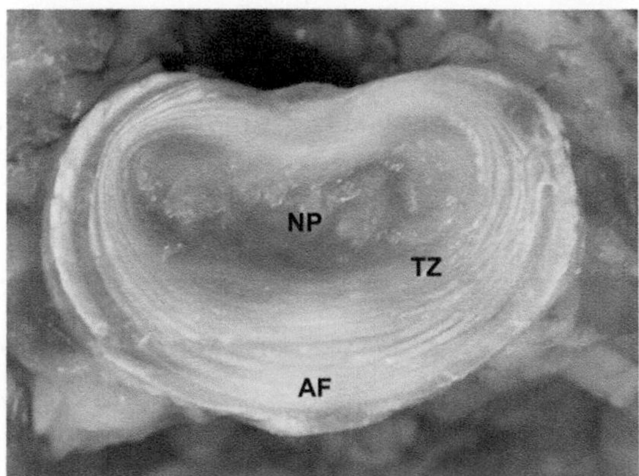

Fig. 1. Transverse section through a normally hydrated L1-L2 IVD illustrating the centrally located nucleus pulposus (NP), annulus fibrosus (AF), and transitional zone (TZ). Note the eccentric location of the NP and wider ventral AF.

forming fibrous lamellae. The annulus fibrosus is thicker ventrally than dorsally, which results in an eccentric localization of the nucleus pulposus in the IVD.[15] The thinner dorsal annulus fibrosus in combination with the eccentric location of the nucleus pulposus are thought to predispose the nucleus pulposus to extrude in a dorsal direction toward the vertebral canal and spinal cord.[15] The most central part of the annulus fibrosus is more cartilaginous and forms the interconnection between the nucleus pulposus and annulus fibrosus. This well-demarcated region is called the transitional zone.[2,5] The dorsal and ventral borders of the IVD are formed by, respectively, the dorsal and ventral longitudinal ligament, whereas the cranial and caudal borders are formed by the cartilaginous vertebral endplates.[15] These vertebral endplates have an important role in supplying the IVD with nutrients. Small molecules can reach the different components of the IVD through diffusion and osmosis from the capillary buds through the vertebral endplates.[17] The nucleus pulposus is a remnant of the embryologic notochord; the predominant cell type of the nondegenerate nucleus pulposus is, therefore, the notochordal cell. The transitional zone contains chondrocytelike cells, the outer layer of the annulus fibrosus contains fibrocytelike cells, and the more central layers of the annulus contain a mixed population of fibrocytes and chondrocytelike cells.[18] IVD degeneration is a complex and multifactorial process and is associated with changes in the composition of these cells and their associated extracellular matrix. Early IVD degeneration is characterized by histologic changes in the nucleus pulposus, which can be summarized as a gradual replacement of notochordal cells by chondrocytelike cells.[5,18] Clinically irrelevant degenerative changes of the IVD, however, also occur during the physiologic process of aging[19]; changes seen in early pathologic IVD degeneration can be indistinguishable from age-related changes.[5]

ACUTE NONCOMPRESSIVE NUCLEUS PULPOSUS EXTRUSION

There have been several terms used historically to describe this condition, with the current consensus of ANNPE used as it describes the key features of a sudden extrusion of nondegenerate nucleus pulposus, causing spinal cord contusion without significant compression.[7,13] Previous terms used have included traumatic disk extrusion, high-velocity low-volume disk extrusion, traumatic disk prolapse, and Hansen type III IVD disease.[2,20–22] ANNPEs have been diagnosed in dogs and less frequently in cats[23,24] and typically present with a very characteristic peracute onset of clinical signs during exercise or following trauma.[7,13,24] Clinical signs are distributed according to the neuroanatomical location and extent of the lesion and typically stabilize within 24 hours before improving or remaining static depending on the SCI severity.[7,13]

Pathophysiology

Understanding the pathogenesis of ANNPE requires an appreciation of the normal canine IVD anatomy outlined earlier. The strong osmotic gradient within the normal, nondegenerate nucleus pulposus acts to draw water into the nucleus pulposus and therefore create a naturally high intradiscal pressure.[5] The combination of this healthy hydrated nucleus pulposus surrounded by a dense and fibrous annulus fibrosus allows mobility as well as great stability.[5] The normal IVD is, therefore, able to withstand marked variations of physiologic loading and biomechanical stress without suffering structural compromise. However, in circumstances whereby the vertebral segment and IVD are subjected to supraphysiologic forces, such as during intense exercise or trauma, structural integrity may fail.[22] In such a scenario, a small tear may occur in the complex lamellar structure of the annulus fibrosus, leading to a sudden extrusion of nondegenerate nucleus pulposus material dorsally into the vertebral canal (an ANNPE). It has been suggested that the annular lamellae in dogs are more vulnerable to such tears with increasing age.[25] In ANNPE the nuclear material is hypothesized to extrude with great force, causing a focal contusive injury to the adjacent spinal cord.[7] As the extradural material is nondegenerate and, therefore, highly hydrated, it typically rapidly dissipates or is resorbed, leaving minimal to no spinal cord compression.[7,22]

This hypothesis is supported by postmortem findings in affected dogs of small tears in the dorsal annulus as well as extradural nondegenerate nucleus pulposus material in the vertebral canal.[26] The adjacent region of the spinal cord may demonstrate evidence of focal contusive injury, hemorrhage, and necrosis.[26]

Clinical Presentation and Differential Diagnosis

Dogs with ANNPE often have a characteristic clinical presentation and present with a peracute onset of often severe neurologic deficits; clinical signs are lateralized in up to 90% of affected cases[13] and are nonprogressive after the initial 24 hours.[7,10,13] Although dogs often vocalize at the onset of clinical signs and a moderate degree of spinal hyperesthesia can be noted on initial clinical examination, this condition is typically not associated with severe or sustained spinal pain.[7,13] A study has indicated that these specific clinical characteristics are indeed significantly associated with a diagnosis of ANNPE and that they can be used to raise a high clinical index of suspicion for this particular disorder.[1] Clinical signs are associated with intense exercise, such as running, in approximately 60% of cases and external trauma in up to 40% of affected animals.[7] Although any breed can be affected, older large-breed dogs, and especially Border Collies, seem vulnerable for this condition.[13]

This clinical presentation is very similar and almost indistinguishable from dogs with ischemic myelopathy or fibrocartilaginous embolic myelopathy.[22] Ischemic myelopathy should, therefore, be considered the most important differential diagnosis for ANNPE. Although both conditions can be differentiated by MRI,[27,28] a recent study identified differences in clinical presentation between dogs with ANNPE and ischemic myelopathy.[13] Dogs with ANNPE were significantly older (mean age of 7.0 years for dogs with ANNPE), were more likely to have a history of vocalization at the onset of clinical signs (in 62% of dogs with ANNPE), had spinal hyperesthesia more often (48% of dogs with ANNPE) during initial examination, and had a lesion affecting the C1-C5 spinal cord segments more often compared with dogs with ischemic myelopathy.[13] Dogs with ischemic myelopathy more likely had a lesion affecting the L4-S3 spinal cord segments compared with dogs with ANNPE.[13] Compared with the general hospital population, Border Collies were overrepresented for ANNPE, whereas English Staffordshire bull terriers were overrepresented for ischemic myelopathy.[13] As outlined earlier, the onset of clinical signs is associated with external trauma in up to 40% of dogs with ANNPE.[7] This association is also reflected in earlier reports referring to this condition as "traumatic disk extrusion."[21] This finding highlights that ANNPE should be considered in animals with spinal cord dysfunction immediately after external trauma and that ANNPE should be considered an important differential diagnosis for vertebral fracture and luxation.

Although Hansen type I IVD disease is the most common canine spinal emergency, affected animals often present with a different clinical presentation compared with dogs with ANNPE.[1] Dogs with Hansen type I IVD disease most commonly present with an acute instead of peracute onset of clinical signs. Clinical signs are often progressive beyond the first 24 hours after their onset. Affected animals more commonly display spinal hyperesthesia, and clinical signs are not often obviously lateralized.[3]

Diagnosis

It is often possible to reach a high clinical index of suspicion for ANNPE before diagnostic tests being performed because of the highly characteristic clinical presentation.[1] When making a presumptive diagnosis based on clinical presentation, it should be emphasized to the owner that any deterioration or failure to improve as expected should lead to a reevaluation of the diagnosis. A definitive diagnosis of ANNPE can only be achieved through visualization and histologic examination of extruded nondegenerate nucleus pulposus material in the vertebral canal.[26] However, as this can only be confirmed on postmortem examination, in clinical cases a presumptive antemortem diagnosis is based on combining the typical clinical presentation with supportive diagnostic imaging findings.[7,27,28] The potential uses and limitations of individual diagnostic tests are outlined later.

Radiography and myelography

The main use for survey radiographs is to rule out vertebral fractures and subluxations in cases with a history of external trauma immediately preceding the onset of clinical signs. However, the sensitivity for detecting vertebral fractures and subluxations using survey radiographs is only 72.0% and 77.5%, respectively.[29] In ANNPE it can be possible to identify a narrowed IVD space on survey radiographs. This radiographic finding is, however, not specific for animals with ANNPE.

Although myelography has now largely been superseded by advanced cross-sectional imaging modalities, it can be used to exclude compressive spinal conditions, such as Hansen type I IVD extrusion.[30] In ANNPE, myelography may reveal a small, focal extradural lesion overlying an IVD, with an adjacent intramedullary pattern due to focal spinal cord swelling.[9] However, it will not allow accurate differentiation between ANNPE and other causes of an intramedullary lesion, such as ischemic myelopathy.

Computed tomography

As with myelography, computed tomography (CT) can be used to exclude selected compressive conditions, such as Hansen type I IVD extrusion,[30,31] as well as being the diagnostic imaging modality of choice for excluding vertebral fractures and subluxations.[29] However, CT will also not allow differentiation between other intramedullary spinal cord lesions. The use of CT or myelography does, however, allow the exclusion of differential diagnoses that require urgent surgical intervention. It can, therefore, guide an appropriate management plan if no MRI is available.

MRI

MRI is the diagnostic imaging modality of choice for diagnosing ANNPE (**Fig. 2**).[7,27] The following criteria can be used to make a presumptive diagnosis of ANNPE using MRI[7]:

- Focal intramedullary spinal cord T2-weighted hyperintensity (typically isointense on T1-weighted sequences)
- Lesion located overlying an IVD space, often lateralized
- Reduction in volume of the T2-weighted hyperintense nucleus pulposus
- Mild narrowing of the affected IVD space
- Small volume of extradural material or signal intensity change dorsal to the affected IVD, with minimal to no spinal cord compression

The intramedullary lesion, representing an area of spinal cord edema secondary to contusive injury, is typically well demarcated and may affect gray matter preferentially.

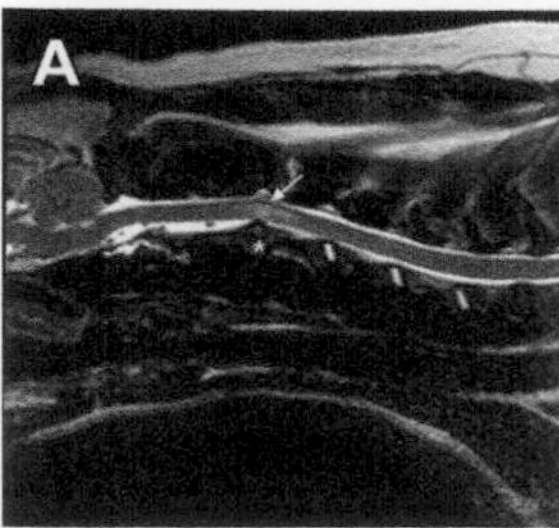

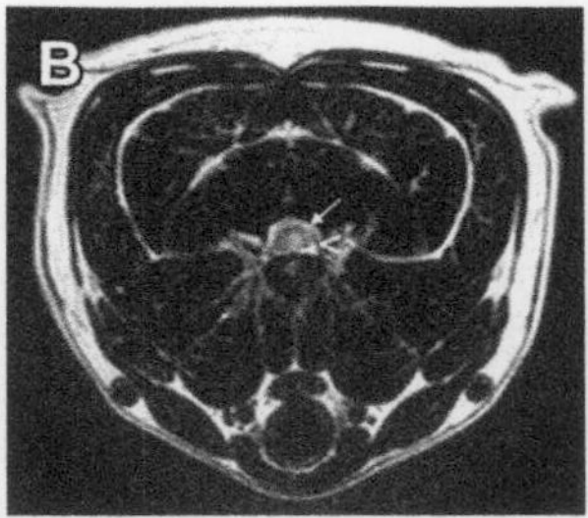

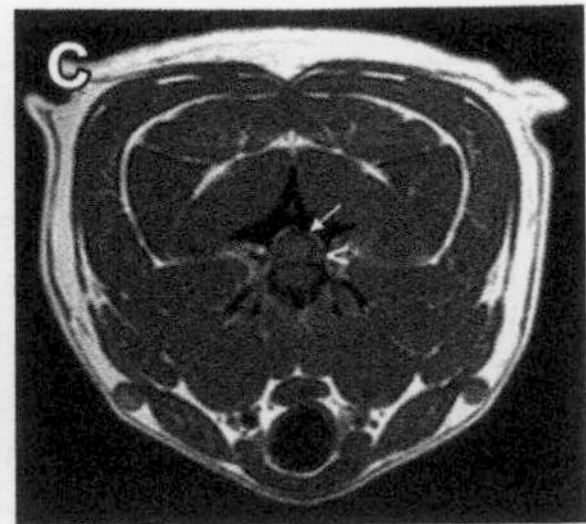

Fig. 2. (*A*) Midsagittal T2-weighted MRI of the cervical vertebral column of a dog with a C2-C3 ANNPE. There is a focal, intramedullary hyperintensity of the spinal cord immediately dorsal to the C2-C3 IVD space (*arrow*). The C2-C3 IVD nucleus pulposus has a markedly reduced volume and signal intensity (*asterisk*). (*B*) Transverse T2-weighted image at the level of the C2-C3 IVD space. There is a focal, lateralized intramedullary hyperintensity of the spinal cord predominantly affecting the gray matter (*arrow*). There is also a small volume of markedly hyperintense extradural material ventrolateral to the spinal cord (*open arrowhead*), causing minimal compression. (*C*) Transverse T1-weighted MRI at the same level as (*B*). The intramedullary lesion is isointense to spinal cord gray matter (*arrow*), and the extradural material is hypointense to adjacent epidural fat (*open arrow*).

Although mild postcontrast enhancement of the lesion on T1-weighted sequences has been reported,[21] usually this is not present.[7] In dogs with this typical clinical presentation, a common differential diagnosis for such a focal intramedullary spinal cord T2-weighted hyperintensity is ischemic myelopathy.[7,27] A recent study has shown moderate interobserver and moderate to good intraobserver agreement for differentiating between ANNPE and ischemic myelopathy using the criteria outlined earlier.[27] The findings of this study also suggested that a smaller, focal intramedullary lesion length is more often associated with a diagnosis of ANNPE compared with longer lesions in ischemic myelopathy as well as lesions diagnosed as ANNPE being more often lateralized.[27]

Treatment

There are currently no neuroprotective treatments available with proven efficacy in directly treating the contusive primary SCI. Treatment of ANNPE, therefore, involves supportive medical management, consisting of restricted activity, supportive nursing care, and physical rehabilitation.[7] As 48% to 57% of dogs with ANNPE present with evidence of spinal hyperesthesia,[7,13] appropriate analgesia may be indicated for the first few days. Restricted activity with short lead walks has been recommended in the management of ANNPE for a period of 4 to 6 weeks, to minimize the risk of further extrusion of nuclear material.[7,22] Nursing care requirements essential to prevent complications and aid recovery vary between cases depending on the severity of neurologic dysfunction, and may involve

- Manual bladder expression or urinary catheter maintenance in cases of urinary incontinence
- Monitoring for and management of respiratory dysfunction in severe cervical myelopathies, which includes turning recumbent patients every 4 hours to avoid lung atelectasis or accumulations of secretions
- Prevention of dermatologic consequences of prolonged recumbency, such as urine scald, pressure sores, and decubital ulcers
- Nutritional support to maintain body condition and support physical rehabilitation

Physical rehabilitation is increasingly recognized as important in supporting the recovery of patients with SCIs in both human and veterinary medicine.[32,33] The aims and requirements of physical therapy will be dictated by the severity of neurologic dysfunction but typically aim to maintain joint range of motion, minimize muscle atrophy, and prevent patient discomfort during the recovery period.[34]

Outcome

Overall recovery rates are variable with successful outcomes ranging from 66.7% to 100%.[7,9,13,21] It is, however, difficult to compare findings between studies due partly to differences in definitions of successful outcome, inclusion criteria, and management protocols, as well as the limited number of animals with the most severe injuries.[7,9,13,21] **Table 1** shows a summary of outcome data in studies including at least 10 dogs. Factors reported to be associated with a poor prognosis include severity of neurologic dysfunction and the extent of intramedullary lesions on MRI.[7] Severity of neurologic dysfunction has been shown to be associated with an unsuccessful outcome, with 0 out of 8 cases with paraplegia and absent nociception and only 7 out of 13 tetra/paraplegic dogs with intact nociception having successful outcomes in one study.[7] In the same study, all 21 dogs with less severe neurologic grades had successful outcomes.[7] Although the long-term outcome has only been reported for a limited number of cases with paraplegia and loss of nociception, only 2 of a total of 14 reported dogs were reported to have a successful outcome (see **Table 1**).[7,13,21]

Using MRI, the outcome has been shown to be associated with the length of the intramedullary T2-weighted hyperintensity on sagittal images and lesion cross-sectional area as a percentage of total spinal cord area on transverse images.[7] The maximal cross-sectional lesion area has been suggested to represent the best predictor of outcome in dogs with ANNPE, with a cutoff value of greater than 90% to predict an unsuccessful outcome with a sensitivity of 86% and specificity of 96%.[7] Several studies have found urinary or fecal incontinence to be a possible long-term complaint following ANNPE, with 10 out of 42,[7] 7 out of 46,[9] and 7 out of 26[13] dogs experiencing long-term reduced urinary or fecal continence (see **Table 1**). The ability to manage the consequences of urinary or fecal incontinence may, therefore, be an important factor in determining long-term outcome as well as an important consideration in the care of affected animals.[7,13]

Overall recovery times following ANNPE are variable and are likely influenced by the severity of SCI.[7] Reported recovery times in dogs diagnosed with ANNPE include median durations of hospitalization from 3.0 (range 0–58)[13] to 4.5 (range 0–29)[7] days, with time to independent ambulation varying from a median of 2.0[13] (range 0–84) to 16.5[7] days (range 2–93). It may take several months before maximum improvement is reached, with a median time to maximum clinical improvement of 2 months (range 0–48) reported in one study.[13]

Acute Noncompressive Nucleus Pulposus Extrusion in Cats

Although ANNPE has also been reported in cats, the current literature is limited to case reports and small case series.[20,23,24] Affected cats also present with a peracute onset of nonprogressive and variably painful clinical signs.[23,24] In contrast to dogs, cats most often present with symmetric instead of lateralized clinical signs and up to three-quarters of affected cats present after external trauma, such as a road-traffic accident or a fall from a height.[24] This finding highlights that also in cats ANNPE should be considered an important differential diagnosis for vertebral fracture and luxation. The cervical spinal cord segments are not often affected in cats.[24] Although prognosis for neurologic improvement is good, it seems unlikely for affected cats to experience a

Table 1
Long-term follow-up of studies including more than 10 dogs diagnosed with acute noncompressive nucleus pulposus extrusion

Reference	Number of Dogs	Dogs Reported to Demonstrate Functional Recovery (%)	Dogs with Long-term Continence Data Available	Dogs with Long-term Reduced Continence	Comment
Chang et al,[21] 2007	11	10 (90.0)	0	Data not available	10 out of 11 dogs recovered partially or completely, including 2 of 3 with loss of nociception
De Risio et al,[7] 2009	42	28 (66.7)	42	10 (23.8)	Success defined as able to perform daily activities and complete urinary and fecal continence; unsuccessful outcome in all 8 cases with loss of nociception
McKee et al,[9] 2010	46	46 (100)	46	7 (15.2)	Outcome reported as ability to urinate; 2 dogs with loss of nociception euthanized shortly after diagnosis and not included in follow-up
Fenn et al,[13] 2016	37	30 (81.1)	26	7 (26.9)	Success defined as able to perform daily activities and complete urinary and fecal continence; unsuccessful outcome in all 3 cases with loss of nociception

full neurologic recovery. A recent case series indicated that all cats for which long-term outcome was available had regained an ambulatory status, but none of them had become neurologically normal.[24]

HYDRATED NUCLEUS PULPOSUS EXTRUSION

More recently, another type of minimally to nondegenerate nucleus pulposus extrusion has been reported in dogs.[8,35] In contrast to animals with ANNPE, an amount of well-hydrated, gelatinous, extradural material can be identified in the vertebral canal, which is associated with varying degrees of spinal cord compression.[8] Although there is some controversy about the most appropriate terminology,[8,14,36] acute compressive HNPE is currently considered most appropriate.[36] Because of similarities between MRI findings in dogs and discal cysts in humans, this condition was initially referred to as "canine intraspinal discal cysts."[35] Human discal cysts are extradural lesions that communicate with the IVD. Affected people present most often with a chronic progressive history of a painful lumbar radiculopathy. Surgery in people confirms an obvious cyst wall, consisting of dense fibrous connective tissue; the serous or serosanguinous content of these cysts lack IVD material.[37] Dogs, however, present with an acute onset of clinical signs; surgery has not been able to demonstrate an obvious capsule or cyst wall delineating the extradural material and cytologic or histopathologic evaluation of the liquid extradural material has consistently revealed findings compatible with minimally degenerate nucleus pulposus.[8,11,12,14,35] It has, therefore, been suggested that these lesions should not be referred to as canine intraspinal discal cysts and that acute compressive HNPE might seem more appropriate.[36] Because cytologic and histologic examination of collected extradural material consistently reveals a degree of partial nucleus pulposus degeneration, it has more recently been suggested to refer to this condition as partially degenerated disk extrusions.[14] As outlined earlier, it can, however, be impossible to distinguish changes seen in early pathologic IVD degeneration from age-related changes.[5] Although the pathophysiology of HNPE is currently unknown, there are possible similarities with ANNPE with extrusion of hydrated nucleus pulposus through a single fissure in the dorsal annulus fibrosus secondary to sudden changes in IVD pressure and biomechanics.[12]

Clinical Presentation and Differential Diagnosis

HNPE has a predilection for the cervical region; clinical signs are, therefore, reflected by acute cervical spinal cord dysfunction. Clinical signs are often severe and symmetric (ie, not lateralized) with nonambulatory tetraparesis and tetraplegia being the most common clinical presentations. Cervical spinal hyperesthesia is only noted in a minority of cases.[8,11,12,38,39] Although so far only one case has been reported with possible HNPE affecting the thoracolumbar vertebral column,[35] the authors of this article have seen several dogs with clinical and imaging findings compatible with thoracolumbar HNPE (**Fig. 3**). Cervical HNPE can affect small and large chondrodystrophic and nonchondrodystrophic dogs.[8,11,38,39] Affected animals are generally older, with a median age around 9 years.[8,39] Onset of clinical signs is spontaneous and only rarely associated with intense physical exercise.[8,12,39]

Differential diagnoses for cervical compressive HNPE include other causes of acute cervical myelopathies, such as cervical ANNPE, ischemic myelopathy, and compressive Hansen type I IVD extrusion. In contrast to dogs with ANNPE or ischemic myelopathy, the onset of clinical signs is only rarely associated with intense physical exercise and neurologic deficits are typically symmetric.[8,11,12] Dogs with cervical HNPE have more severe neurologic deficits and less severe cervical hyperesthesia compared

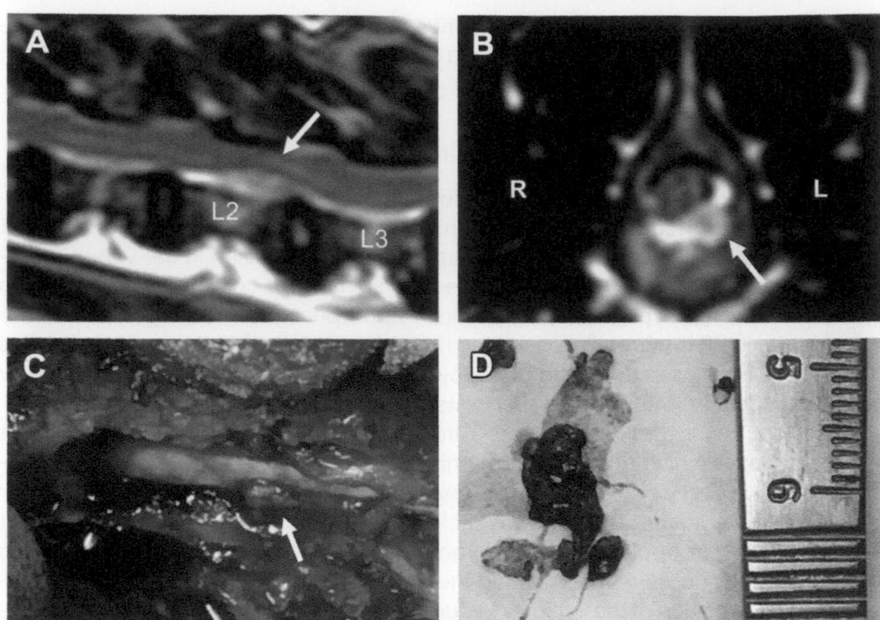

Fig. 3. (*A*) Midsagittal T2-weighted MRI of a dog with an L2-L3 compressive HNPE. Note the hyperintense nature of the extruded material (*arrow*) and decreased volume of hydrated nucleus pulposus in the L2-L3 IVD. (*B*) Transverse T2-weighted image at the level of the L2-L3 IVD space. There is left lateralized ventral extradural compression of hyperintense material (*arrow*). (*C*) Intraoperative image of the same dog illustrating focal spinal cord compression (*arrow*). (*D*) The gelatinous nature of the compressive material can be appreciated after surgical removal.

with dogs with other compressive cervical myelopathies, such as acute Hansen type I cervical IVD extrusions.[38]

Diagnosis

MRI is the diagnostic modality of choice to diagnose HNPE; several studies have reported consistent, almost pathognomonic MRI findings.[8,11,12,14] MRI abnormalities in dogs with cervical HNPE include (**Fig. 4**)

- Ventral, midline, extradural compressive material homogenous hyperintense on T2-weighted sequences and isointense in all sequences to normal, nondegenerate, nucleus pulposus lying immediately dorsal to the affected IVD.
- The compressive material can have a characteristic bilobed or seagull appearance, which can possibly be explained by the location of the compressive material ventral to the apparent intact dorsal longitudinal ligament.[12]
- The affected IVD space is narrowed and has a reduced volume of nucleus pulposus and an ill-defined dorsal annulus fibrosus.[8]
- The overlying spinal cord can demonstrate focal intraparenchymal hyperintensity suggestive of spinal cord contusion, and the extruded material can demonstrate variable degrees of contrast enhancement.[8,12,14]

A recent study has evaluated the usefulness of CT to evaluate cervical HNPE. Although unenhanced CT was not useful in detecting a lesion, IV contrast-enhanced

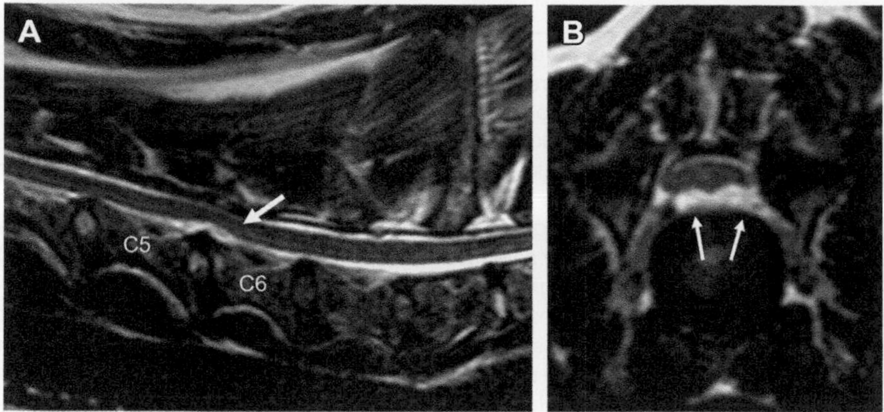

Fig. 4. (*A*) T2-weighted sagittal MRI of a dog with a C5-C6 acute compressive HNPE. A ventral extradural compression overlying the C5-C6 IVD is visible (*arrow*). The compressive material has the same intensity as normally hydrated nucleus pulposus. The IVD space is mildly narrowed and contains a reduced volume of normally hydrated nucleus pulposus. (*B*) T2-weighted transverse MRI at the C5-C6 IVD space. The extruded material has the typical bilobed or seagull appearance (*arrows*).

CT revealed a lesion in all but one case. The observed lesion was a well-demarcated hypodense lesion dorsal from the IVD space showing rim enhancement.[39] Contrast-enhanced CT had a sensitivity of 91% and specificity of 100% to differentiate between HNPE and Hansen type I IVD extrusion.[39]

Extruded material removed during surgery can have a white, waterlike, opaque, and liquid to gelatinous appearance.[8,12,14] Cytology and histology of compressive material reveals findings compatible with nucleus pulposus with evidence of early degeneration (**Fig. 5**).[11,12,14,39]

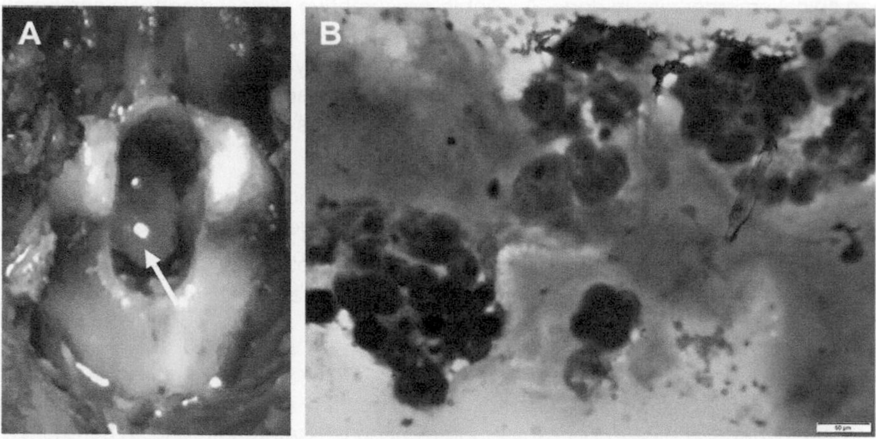

Fig. 5. (*A*) Intraoperative image of the same dog as in **Fig. 4**. The transparent waterlike extruded material is visible (*arrow*) after completion of the ventral slot. (*B*) Impression smear cytology of the extruded material reveals basophilic cells with characteristics of notochordal cell and chondrocytes, consistent with extruded nucleus pulposus with signs of early degeneration (hematoxylin-eosin, bar is 50 μm).

Treatment and Outcome

Outcomes seem to depend on the severity of clinical signs, with unsuccessful cases demonstrating tetraplegia with respiratory compromise at initial presentation.[8,39] Despite these often severe neurologic deficits, good outcomes, characterized by rapid and complete neurologic recoveries, have been reported after both medical and surgical treatment.[8,11,12,35,39,40] Medical management can consist of restricted exercise in combination with appropriate nursing care, physiotherapy, hydrotherapy, and appropriate antiinflammatory drugs and analgesia. Surgical treatment typically consists of decompressive surgery by a ventral slot procedure. The ideal type of treatment is currently uncertain.[36,39] Although it is unclear which dogs would benefit from surgical therapy instead of medical management, the combination of severe neurologic signs and obvious spinal compression on MRI have been considered indications for surgical treatment.[1,8,12] The acute onset of severe clinical signs and reported rapid improvements after initiation of medical treatment could suggest that spinal cord contusion plays a major role in the pathophysiology of HNPE, questioning the value of surgical decompression in this condition.[11] Furthermore, several reports have indicated spontaneous regression of extradural compressive material in animals that underwent medical management.[11,40] Further research is, therefore, necessary to compare the clinical presentation and outcome of dogs treated medically or surgically for cervical acute compressive HNPE. A recent study has compared the clinical presentation and outcome of 18 dogs treated medically and 16 dogs treated surgically for cervical HNPE. Although more dogs in the surgical group demonstrated cervical hyperesthesia, no other significant differences were seen for signalment, clinical presentation, or imaging findings. All dogs for which a long-term outcome was available had experienced an excellent neurologic recovery, and no significant differences in short- and long-term outcome variables were seen between dogs treated surgically or medically for cervical HNPE.[41]

SUMMARY

ANNPE and acute compressive cervical HNPE are increasingly recognized as common spinal emergencies in dogs. A reliable presumptive clinical diagnosis can be obtained by combining typical clinical characteristics and well-described MRI findings. Although the pathophysiology of both conditions is not yet fully elucidated, good outcomes can be obtained if appropriate treatment is initiated. Further research is needed to evaluate the best type of treatment in dogs with acute compressive cervical HNPE.

ACKNOWLEDGMENTS

The authors wish to thank Dr Laureen Peters and Dr Thomas Eley from the Department of Pathobiology and Population Sciences, Royal Veterinary College, University of London for their help with the preparation and interpretation of **Figs. 1** and **4**.

REFERENCES

1. Cardy TJ, De Decker S, Kenny PJ, et al. Clinical reasoning in canine spinal disease: what combination of clinical information is useful? Vet Rec 2015;177:171.
2. Hansen HJ. A pathologic-anatomical study on disc degeneration in dog. Acta Orthop Scand 1952;11:4–119.
3. Brisson BA. Intervertebral disc disease in dogs. Vet Clin North Am Small Anim Pract 2010;40:829–58.

4. Jeffery ND, Levine JM, Olby NJ, et al. Intervertebral disk degeneration in dogs: consequences, diagnosis, treatment and future directions. J Vet Intern Med 2013;27:1318–33.
5. Bergknut N, Smolders LA, Grinwis GC, et al. Intervertebral disc degeneration in the dog. Part 1: anatomy and physiology of the intervertebral disc and characteristics of intervertebral disc degeneration. Vet J 2013;195(3):282–91.
6. Granger N, Carwardine D. Acute spinal cord injury: tetraplegia and paraplegia in small animals. Vet Clin North Am Small Anim Pract 2014;44(6):1131–56.
7. De Risio L, Adams V, Dennis R, et al. Association of clinical and magnetic resonance imaging findings with outcome in dogs with presumptive acute noncompressive nucleus pulposus extrusion: 42 cases (2000–2007). J Am Vet Med Assoc 2009;234(4):495–504.
8. Beltran E, Dennis R, Doyle V, et al. Clinical and magnetic resonance imaging features of canine compressive cervical myelopathy with suspected hydrated nucleus pulposus extrusion. J Small Anim Pract 2012;53(2):101–7.
9. McKee WM, Downes CJ, Pink JJ, et al. Presumptive exercise-associated peracute thoracolumbar disc extrusion in 48 dogs. Vet Rec 2010;166(17):523.
10. Henke D, Gorgas D, Flegel T, et al. Magnetic resonance imaging findings in dogs with traumatic intervertebral disk extrusion with or without spinal cord compression: 31 cases (2006–2010). J Am Vet Med Assoc 2013;242(2):217–22.
11. Manunta ML, Evangelisti MA, Bergknut N, et al. Hydrated nucleus pulposus herniation in seven dogs. Vet J 2015;203(3):342–4.
12. Dolera M, Malfassi L, Marcarini S, et al. Hydrated nucleus pulposus extrusion in dogs: correlation of magnetic resonance imaging and microsurgical findings. Acta Vet Scand 2015;57(1):58.
13. Fenn J, Drees R, Volk HA, et al. Comparison of clinical signs and outcomes between dogs with presumptive ischemic myelopathy and dogs with acute noncompressive nucleus pulposus extrusion. J Am Vet Med Assoc 2016;249(7):767–75.
14. Falzone C. Canine acute cervical myelopathy: Hydrated nucleus pulposus extrusion or intraspinal discal cysts? Vet Surg 2017;46(3):376–80.
15. King AS, Smith RN. A comparison of the anatomy of the intervertebral disc in dog and man: with reference to herniation of the nucleus pulposus. Br Vet J 1955;3:135–49.
16. Ghosh P, Taylor TK, Braund KG. The variation of the glycosaminoglycans of the canine intervertebral disc with ageing. I. chondrodystrophoid breed. Gerontology 1977;23:87–98.
17. Urban JP, Smith S, Fairbank JC. Nutrition of the intervertebral disc. Spine 2014;29:2700–9.
18. Bergknut N, Meij BP, Hagman R, et al. Intervertebral disc disease in dogs – part 1: a new histological grading scheme for classification of intervertebral disc degeneration in dogs. Vet J 2013;195:156–63.
19. De Decker S, Gielen IM, Duchateau L, et al. Low-field magnetic resonance imaging findings of the caudal portion of the cervical region in clinically normal Doberman pinschers and foxhounds. Am J Vet Res 2010;71:428–34.
20. Lu D, Lamb CR, Wesselingh K, et al. Acute intervertebral disc extrusion in a cat: clinical and MRI findings. J Feline Med Surg 2002;4:65–8.
21. Chang Y, Dennis R, Platt SR, et al. Magnetic resonance imaging of traumatic intervertebral disc extrusion in dogs. Vet Rec 2007;160(23):795–9.

22. De Risio L. A review of fibrocartilaginous embolic myelopathy and different types of peracute non-compressive intervertebral disk extrusions in dogs and cats. Front Vet Sci 2015;18:24.
23. Chow K, Beatty JA, Voss K, et al. Probable lumbar acute non-compressive nucleus pulposus extrusion in a cat with acute onset paraparesis. J Feline Med Surg 2012;14(10):764–7.
24. Taylor-Brown FE, De Decker S. Presumptive acute non-compressive nucleus pulposus extrusion in 11 cats: clinical features, diagnostic imaging findings, treatment and outcome. J Feline Med Surg 2015;19(1):21–6.
25. Schollum ML, Robertson PA, Broom ND. How age influences unravelling morphology of annular lamellae–a study of interfibre cohesivity in the lumbar disc. J Anat 2010;216(3):310–9.
26. Griffiths IR. A syndrome produced by dorso-lateral" explosions" of the cervical inter-vertebral discs. Vet Rec 1970;87:737–41.
27. Fenn J, Drees R, Volk HA, et al. Inter- and intraobserver agreement for diagnosing presumptive ischemic myelopathy and acute noncompressive nucleus pulposus extrusion in dogs using magnetic resonance imaging. Vet Radiol Ultrasound 2016;57(1):33–40.
28. Specchi S, Johnson P, Beauchamp G, et al. Assessment of interobserver agreement and use of selected magnetic resonance imaging variables for differentiation of acute noncompressive nucleus pulposus extrusion and ischemic myelopathy in dogs. J Am Vet Med Assoc 2016;248:1013–21.
29. Kinns J, Mai W, Seiler G, et al. Radiographic sensitivity and negative predictive value for acute canine spinal trauma. Vet Radiol Ultrasound 2006;47(6):563–70.
30. Israel SK, Levine JM, Kerwin SC, et al. The relative sensitivity of computed tomography and myelography for identification of thoracolumbar intervertebral disk herniations in dogs. Vet Radiol Ultrasound 2009;50(3):247–52.
31. Schroeder R, Pelsue DH, Park RD, et al. Contrast-enhanced CT for localizing compressive thoracolumbar intervertebral disc extrusion. J Am Anim Hosp Assoc 2011;47(3):203–9.
32. Morawietz C, Moffat F. Effects of locomotor training after incomplete spinal cord injury: a systematic review. Arch Phys Med Rehabil 2013;94(11):2297–308.
33. Bennaim M, Porato M, Jarleton A, et al. Preliminary evaluation of the effects of photobiomodulation therapy and physical rehabilitation on early postoperative recovery of dogs undergoing hemilaminectomy for treatment of thoracolumbar intervertebral disk disease. Am J Vet Res 2017;78(2):195–206.
34. Campbell MT, Huntingford JL. Nursing care and rehabilitation therapy for patients with neurologic disease. In: Dewey CW, da Costa RC, editors. Practical guide to canine and feline neurology. 3rd edition. New York: Wiley Blackwell; 2015. p. 559–84.
35. Konar M, Lang J, Flühmann G, et al. Ventral intraspinal cysts associated with the intervertebral disc: magnetic resonance observations in seven dogs. Vet Surg 2008;37:94–101.
36. Lowrie ML, Platt SR, Garosi LS. Extramedullary spinal cysts in dogs. Vet Surg 2014;43:650–62.
37. Chiba K, Toyama Y, Matsumoto M, et al. Intraspinal cyst communication with the intervertebral disc in the lumbar spine: discal cyst. Spine 2001;26:2112–8.
38. Hamilton T, Glass E, Drobatz K, et al. Severity of spinal cord dysfunction and pain associated with hydrated nucleus pulposus extrusion in dogs. Vet Comp Orthop Traumatol 2014;27:313–8.

39. Royaux E, Martlé V, Kromhout K, et al. Detection of compressive hydrated nucleus pulposus extrusion in dogs with multislice computed tomography. Vet J 2016;216:202–6.
40. Kamishina H, Ogawa H, Katayama M, et al. Spontaneous regression of a cervical intraspinal cyst in a dog. J Vet Med Sci 2010;72:349–52.
41. Borlace T, Gutierrez-Quintana R, Taylor-Brown FE, et al. Comparison of medical and surgical treatment for acute cervical compressive hydrated nucleus pulposus extrusion in dogs. Vet Rec 2017. http://dx.doi.org/10.1136/vr.104528.

Head Trauma

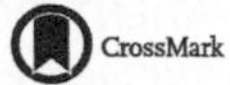

Kendon W. Kuo, DVM, MS[a,*], Lenore M. Bacek, DVM, MS[a],
Amanda R. Taylor, DVM[b]

KEYWORDS

- Head trauma • Traumatic brain injury • Intracranial pressure • Dog • Cat

KEY POINTS

- The goal of managing head trauma is the prevention and treatment of secondary injury.
- Systemic assessment and stabilization should occur before neurologic assessment.
- Validated assessment methods, such as the Modified Glasgow Coma Score and Animal Trauma Triage Score, may serve as guidelines for predicting outcome.
- Treatment is guided toward minimizing secondary injury and considering respiratory and cardiovascular systems, analgesia, anxiety, nutrition, and recumbency care.
- Assessments should be performed frequently to determine if a change in patient status has occurred.

INTRODUCTION

Head trauma is a common cause of morbidity and mortality in small animals. In dogs with severe blunt trauma, head trauma occurs in approximately 25% and is associated with increased mortality.[1] Reported mortality rates in dogs with head trauma range from 18% to 24%.[1,2] Approximately 50% of dogs and cats present with head trauma owing to motor vehicle accidents and crush injuries, respectively. Other causes include falls from height, bite wounds, gunshots, and other accidental or intentional human-inflicted trauma. Head trauma may lead to traumatic brain injury (TBI), defined as a structural or physiologic disruption of the brain by an external force. Rapid recognition and response is required to ensure the best outcome. Dogs and cats compensate remarkably well to losses in cerebral tissue.[3] Although the initial appearance of a head traumatized patient may be discouraging, even patients with severe neurologic deficits can recover with appropriate care. This article reviews the pathophysiology of head trauma, patient assessment and diagnostics, and treatment recommendations.

Disclosure Statement: None.
[a] Emergency and Critical Care, Department of Clinical Sciences, College of Veterinary Medicine, Auburn University, 1220 Wire Road, Auburn, AL 36849- 5540, USA; [b] Neurology/Neurosurgery, Department of Clinical Sciences, College of Veterinary Medicine, Auburn University, 1220 Wire Road, Auburn, AL 36849- 5540, USA
* Corresponding author.
E-mail address: kwk0003@auburn.edu

Vet Clin Small Anim 48 (2018) 111–128
http://dx.doi.org/10.1016/j.cvsm.2017.08.005 vetsmall.theclinics.com

PATIENT EVALUATION OVERVIEW

Normal Brain Physiology and Compensatory Mechanisms

Cerebral perfusion pressure (CPP) is the pressure gradient driving cerebral blood flow (CBF), including delivery of oxygen and metabolites. CPP is defined as the mean arterial pressure (MAP) minus the intracranial pressure (ICP): CPP = MAP − ICP. CBF is a function of CPP and cerebral vascular resistance (CVR): CBF = CPP/CVR. CVR is dependent on blood viscosity and vessel diameter: CVR = $L\eta/\pi r^4$, where L is vessel length, η is viscosity, and r is vessel radius.[4] A major mechanism controlling CVR is pressure autoregulation, the intrinsic ability of the vasculature to maintain a constant CBF and ICP over a wide range of pressure (MAP of 50–150 mm Hg). Chemical autoregulation with $Paco_2$ also influences CVR via vessel diameter.[4]

ICP is the pressure inside the skull exerted by the intracranial contents. The Monro-Kellie hypothesis states that the sum of the volumes of brain parenchyma, intracranial blood, and cerebrospinal fluid is constant. Any change in volume without a compensatory decrease in another component will cause an increase in pressure. With head trauma, hemorrhage or edema add to the volume. Increases in volume are buffered by fluid shifts in the brain vasculature and cerebrospinal fluid. This accommodation is known as intracranial compliance, or the change in volume per unit change in pressure.

In normal conditions, intracranial compliance is high and changes in intracranial volume minimally affect ICP. However, when the volume buffering capacity is exceeded, increases in volume directly increase ICP. High ICP decreases CPP, leading to ischemia and neuronal death.[4]

Brain injury is divided into primary and secondary injury. This distinction is valuable in understanding pathophysiology and highlights the goal in managing head trauma: prevention and treatment of secondary injury.

Primary Injury

The physical disruption of intracranial structures at the time of impact. Concussion is the mildest injury characterized by a loss of consciousness with no associated histopathologic lesions. Contusion is bruising of the brain parenchyma. Laceration is disruption of the brain parenchyma and is the most severe form of primary injury. Hemorrhage, hematoma formation, and subsequent compression of the brain parenchyma may also occur. Locations of hematoma formation include within brain parenchyma (intraaxial) and in the subarachnoid, subdural, and epidural spaces (extraaxial). In a study of dogs with mild head injury, 89% had skull fractures and 11% had intracranial hemorrhage.[5] In dogs and cats with severe head injury, nearly all (96%) had evidence of intracranial hemorrhage.[6] Primary injury is beyond the clinician's control and sets the stage for secondary injury.

Secondary Injury

Occurs minutes to days after the initial insult and involves a complex cascade of local and systemic derangements. Brain trauma results in excessive excitatory neurotransmitter release leading to further neuronal damage or death in a vicious cycle of *excitotoxicity*. The accumulation of neurotransmitters such as glutamate cause an influx of sodium and calcium resulting in depolarization and further release of neurotransmitters. Excessive sodium causes cytotoxic edema, whereas calcium activates destructive proteases, lipases, and endonucleases.

Other local contributors of secondary injury include depletion of adenosine triphosphate, production of reactive oxygen species, nitric oxide accumulation, and lactic acidosis.[7]Systemic derangements worsen brain injury by compromising cerebral perfusion. Hypotension, hypoxia, systemic inflammation, hyperglycemia or hypoglycemia, hypercapnia or hypocapnia, hyperthermia, and abnormalities in electrolytes or acid–base balance all contribute.[8]

Increased intracranial pressure

Intracranial hypertension perpetuates secondary injury. If severe, it may lead to brainstem compression, resulting in a depressed mental, cardiac, and respiratory function. Brain herniation and death are possible. This triggers the Cushing's reflex or cerebral ischemic response. With severely increased ICP, CBF decreases allowing CO_2 to accumulate locally. The vasomotor center of the brain detects the increase in CO_2 and triggers sympathetic discharge causing peripheral vasoconstriction to increase MAP and maintain CPP. Baroreceptors sense the hypertension, triggering a reflex bradycardia. In a patient with decreased mentation, a combination of hypertension and bradycardia indicates a potentially life-threatening increase in ICP requiring prompt treatment.[4]

Other findings with increased ICP include sudden decrease in mentation, pupillary light reflex, decerebrate posture (opisthotonus with hyperextension of all 4 limbs), and loss of physiologic nystagmus.[9] With severe head trauma, blood pressure autoregulation can be lost focally or globally, partially or completely. A partial loss resets the lower MAP extreme to a higher value (eg, from 50 mm Hg to 80 mm Hg). Without pressure autoregulation, CBF becomes directly proportional to systemic blood pressure, highlighting the importance of maintaining optimal blood pressure when treating head trauma cases.

SYSTEMIC ASSESSMENT

Head trauma patients are triaged and assessed for life-threatening injuries and systemic derangements, which contribute to secondary injury. Approximately 60% of human TBI patients have concurrent injuries.[9] See **Fig. 1** for overview of patient assessment.

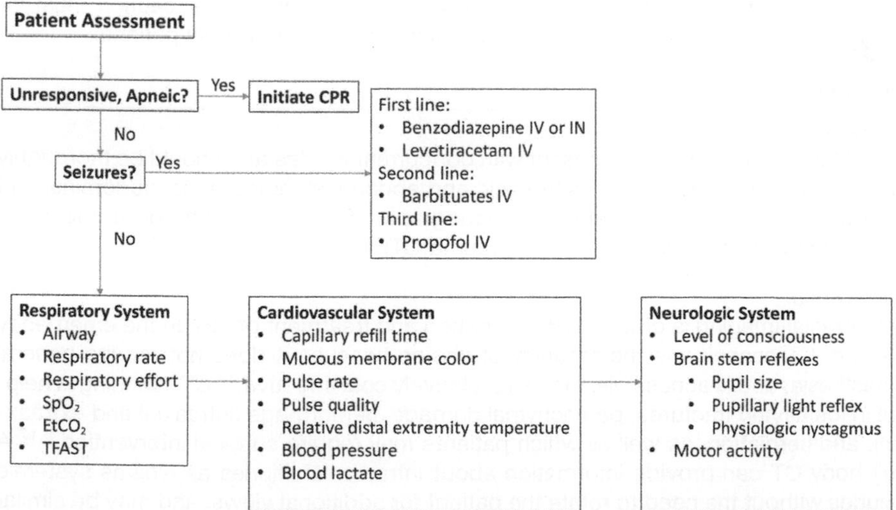

Fig. 1. Overview of patient assessment after head trauma. CPR, cardiopulmonary resuscitation; $EtCO_2$, end-tidal carbon dioxide; SpO_2, saturation of peripheral oxygen; TFAST, thoracic focused assessment with sonography for trauma.

Trauma patients may present in shock, and a full neurologic assessment should occur after patients are resuscitated and stabilized. The main goal is to establish normovolemia and appropriate oxygenation and ventilation. Assessment of the cardiovascular system should focus on the perfusion parameters (mentation, mucous membrane color, capillary refill time, pulse rate, pulse quality, and relative distal extremity temperature). Respiratory rate, respiratory effort, and thoracic auscultation may indicate respiratory compromise. Point-of-care thoracic ultrasound imaging may detect pneumothorax, pleural effusion, and parenchymal disease (contusion).[10]

Neurologic Assessment

Neurologic examination is performed without the influence of analgesia and interpreted based on the patient's stability and condition. For example, miosis may be due to traumatic uveitis or Horner's syndrome; segmental reflexes may be diminished by limb pathology such as fractures. Initial examination is focused on mentation, brain stem reflexes, and motor activity/posture to assign a score using the Modified Glasgow Coma Scale (MGCS), which has been validated in dogs (**Box 1**). The MGCS assesses 3 categories: motor activity, brainstem reflexes, and level of consciousness, with a total score of 18 (each category with a maximum score of 6) being normal. The MGCS is useful for serial monitoring and can be performed as frequently as every 30 minutes in critical patients. MGCS is a useful prognostic tool. Studies have shown that an MGCS of 8 within the first 48 hours of hospitalization approximates a 50% probability of survival.[2,11]

The animal trauma triage (ATT) score is another severity scoring system with several studies confirming its strong prognostic value.[1,11–14] The ATT score is based on 6 categories (body systems) scored on a scale of 0 to 3 with 0 being normal. In dogs with head trauma, a score of 9 approximated a 50% probability of survival.[11] A recent retrospective study determined the strongest predictor for non-survival was a decreased MGCS. This study also found that poor perfusion, higher ATT score, intubation or the need for hypertonic saline (HTS) were all associated with a worse outcome.[11] While scoring systems may help guide owners and veterinarians, caution must be exercised, as they are not designed to predict survival in individual patients.

Imaging

Extracranial

Head trauma patients often present with concurrent injuries and should be thoroughly evaluated with imaging such as thoracic and abdominal radiographs, abdominal and thoracic focused assessment with sonography for trauma, and/or a full body computed tomography (CT) scan (ie, trauma CT).[15,16]

Intracranial

Intracranial imaging is crucial to identification and treatment of TBI. In the emergency setting, CT scanning is the modality of choice because it does not require general anesthesia, and is accessible, fast, and relatively cost effective.[17] CT scanning is helpful in identifying fractures, parenchymal damage, hemorrhage (intraaxial and extraaxial), and herniation, as well as which patients may require surgical intervention.[5,17] A full body CT can provide information about intracranial injuries as well as systemic injuries without the need to rotate the patient for additional views, and may be similar in cost to multiple radiographic projections.[18]

Although CT is the primary imaging modality for TBI, MRI is more sensitive for smaller lesions. Because MRI requires general anesthesia, takes longer, and is less

Box 1
Modified Glasgow Coma Scale monitoring sheet

Date	Time	MA	BSR	LOC	Total Score	Initials

Motor Activity (MA)

6 = Normal gait/spinal reflexes
5 = Hemiparesis/tetraparesis
4 = Recumbent, intermittent extensor rigidity
3 = Recumbent, constant extensor rigidity
2 = Recumbent, constant extensor rigidity, opisthotonus
1 = Recumbent, depressed or absent spinal reflexes and muscle tone

Brain stem reflexes (BSR)

6 = Normal pupillary light response (PLR), normal oculocephalic reflexes
5 = Slow PLR, normal to depressed oculocephalic reflexes
4 = Bilateral miosis, normal to depressed oculocephalic reflexes
3 = Pinpoint pupils, depressed to absent oculocephalic reflexes
2 = Unilateral, unresponsive mydriasis, depressed to absent oculocephalic reflexes
1 = Bilateral, unresponsive mydriasis, depressed to absent oculocephalic reflexes

Level of consciousness (LOC)

6 = Occasional periods of alertness and responsive to environment
5 = Depression or delirium, capable of responding, but response may be inappropriate
4 = Semicomatose, responsive to visual stimuli
3 = Semicomatose, responsive to auditory stimuli
2 = Semicomatose, responsive only to repeated noxious stimuli
1 = Comatose, unresponsive to repeated noxious stimuli

readily available, it may not be appropriate for unstable patients.[19] A recent study in dogs demonstrated the prognostic value of early MRI in dogs with TBI, including prediction of posttraumatic epilepsy.[20]

PHARMACOLOGIC TREATMENT OPTIONS

Fluid Therapy

Although the optimal fluid type for resuscitation in head trauma is not established, the goals of fluid resuscitation are rapid reversal of hypovolemia, prevention of hypotension, and maintenance of CBF while avoiding intracranial hypertension. Patients should not be purposefully dehydrated to reduce cerebral edema. Permissive hypotension or hypotensive resuscitation is often used in trauma, but is inappropriate for head trauma. Human guidelines recommend targeting a systolic blood pressure of at least 90 mm Hg. A retrospective study of people with severe brain injury found that a single episode of hypotension (systolic blood pressure <90 mm Hg) was associated with a 150% increase in mortality.[21]

Head trauma presents challenges regarding fluid therapy. In health, the blood–brain barrier (BBB) tightly regulates changes in intracranial volume. After trauma, disruption of the BBB may lead to pathologic fluid shifts, vasogenic edema, and cytotoxic edema. Until BBB disruptions heal, the brain may be less tolerant of fluids and at increased risk for fluid overload. Impaired autoregulation increases the brain sensitivity to changes in volume status. Fluid therapy is further complicated by the lack of specific monitoring for ICP. Striking a balance between optimizing cardiac output and minimizing tissue edema remains a challenge. Numerous fluid choices are available, with their own sets of advantages and disadvantages.[22]

Isotonic crystalloids

Isotonic crystalloids should be titrated to reach goals as discussed. Dose recommendations start with a one-quarter of the shock volume of fluids (20 mL/kg in dogs, 15 mL/kg in cats). Some support 0.9% NaCl because it contains the least amount of free water, but it also an acidifying solution and may worsen acid–base imbalance. Isotonic crystalloids redistribute over the intravascular and interstitial spaces, so large volumes can exacerbate tissue edema.[7]

Hypertonic saline

HTS offers several benefits in head trauma. By rapidly increasing blood osmolality, HTS expands the intravascular space by shifting fluid from the interstitial and intracellular spaces, allowing administration of smaller volumes. Other theoretic benefits of HTS are discussed elsewhere in this article in the hyperosmolar therapy section. Dosage recommendations for 7.5% and 3% NaCl are 4 mL/kg and 5.3 mL/kg, respectively. Although the response to HTS is rapid, fluid redistribution limits duration of action to less than 75 minutes.[7,23]

Colloids

The rationale for colloid administration in head trauma is compelling. By supporting plasma oncotic pressure, colloids should minimize extravasation of fluid from the intravascular space and tissue edema. The duration of action of colloids is longer than crystalloids. However, large metaanalyses have failed to demonstrate a clear benefit of any colloids in any patient group.[24] Post hoc analysis of the landmark SAFE trial (Saline versus Albumin Fluid Evaluation) found that resuscitation with 4% albumin significantly increased mortality compared with 0.9% NaCl in TBI.[25] Although the exact mechanism is unknown, leakage of albumin through a disrupted BBB may create oncotic shifts, promoting edema formation and leading to increased ICP and mortality. There are no large randomized trials regarding synthetic colloids in TBI. The authors infer similar disadvantages as albumin for synthetic colloids until further studies are performed. Other investigators recommend the use of synthetic colloids and some consider them the fluid of choice for head trauma.[4,7] Regardless of fluid type, frequent reassessment and titrating to effect to avoid overload is essential.

Hyperosmolar Therapy

Hyperosmolar agents create an osmotic gradient across the intact BBB to shift water from the interstitial space to the intravascular space to decrease ICP. Mannitol and HTS are routinely used to reduce ICP. Some recent metaanalyses favor HTS, but the choice remains controversial.[26–28]

Mannitol

Mannitol, a sugar molecule, acts as an osmotic diuretic. Immediately, the osmotic effect expands the plasma volume reducing viscosity and improving microcirculatory flow. Persisting for an estimated 75 minutes, the reduction in viscosity causes a reflex vasoconstriction of pial arterioles as does hyperventilation. The osmotic gradient across the BBB forms slowly over 15 to 30 minutes, persists for 2 to 5 hours, and shifts fluid from the brain into the intravascular space. Mannitol may also act as a free radical scavenger.[7] The diuretic effect is not desirable in hypotensive patients and the loss of fluids must be addressed. Patients should be volume resuscitated before mannitol administration.

Extravasation of mannitol owing to ongoing cerebral hemorrhage leading to increased ICP is a common concern, but remains unproven. In people, no difference in outcome has been found between patients with intracerebral hemorrhage that did or did not receive mannitol.[29]

Accumulation of mannitol in the extravascular space leading to a “reverse osmotic shift” is unlikely with appropriate dosing. The benefits of mannitol far outweigh the potential risks. Recommended dosing is 0.5 to 1.0 g/kg intravenously over 15 to 20 minutes.[4] Historically, furosemide was administered concurrently in hopes of decreasing cerebrospinal fluid production, counteracting the initial plasma expansion, and potentiation of the osmotic gradient.[30] However, these benefits are unproven and furosemide may increase the risk of dehydration and hypovolemia.[31]

Hypertonic Saline

HTS shares similar mechanisms with mannitol including expanding the plasma volume and reducing viscosity. Proposed advantages of HTS over mannitol include volume expansion leading to improved cardiac output and blood pressure, a reduced likelihood of HTS crossing the BBB, improved regional CBF by reducing endothelial swelling, and modulation of neuroinflammatory pathways.[32–34] HTS is less desirable in a hyponatremic patient. Recommended dosing is 4 mL/kg and 5.4 mL/kg for 7.5% and 3% NaCl, respectively.[7] Although the debate continues between mannitol versus HTS, HTS seems ideal for the hypovolemic patient; both are reasonable in the euvolemic patient. If the patient fails to respond to one, the other should be considered.

Anesthetics, Analgesics, and Sedatives

Analgesia is essential in management of head trauma, and anesthesia is often required for procedures such as surgery, diagnostic imaging, and mechanical ventilation. Because pressure autoregulation may be lost after trauma, the brain is particularly vulnerable to hypotension and alterations in $Paco_2$. A balanced approach minimizes the risk of secondary injury and provides analgesia without excessive sedation.[35] Inhalant anesthetics have a dose-related effect on ICP. As concentrations increase greater than 1.0 to 1.5 the minimum effective alveolar concentration, ICP increases.[36] Anesthesia-induced hypoventilation and hypercapnia also increases ICP. The risk of increasing ICP can be minimized by titrating inhalants to effect and providing adequate ventilator and cardiovascular support. At lower concentrations, the vasodilatory effects of inhalants may improve cerebral perfusion.[37]

If the ICP is increased, inhalants are contraindicated and total intravenous anesthesia is recommended.[35] Direct comparison studies have shown that injectable anesthetics such as propofol improve cerebral perfusion and maintain pressure autoregulation better than inhalant anesthetics.[38–41] Propofol may also be neuroprotective via modulation of GABA receptors and antioxidant effects.[42] However, propofol may also cause hypotension and hypoventilation. Careful titration, meticulous monitoring, and supportive care are essential.

Analgesia is essential for patient comfort and preventing further increases in ICP. Pain and anxiety increase cerebral metabolic rate, which increases CBF, cerebral blood volume, and ultimately ICP. Opioids are the analgesic of choice because they are cardiovascular sparing and easily reversible. Respiratory depression is possible, but minimized with careful titration. The patient's ability to protect their airway (gag reflex and/or ability to swallow) should be assessed frequently to decrease the risk of aspiration pneumonia. Continuous rate infusions of full mu agonists such as fentanyl are recommended to provide consistent analgesia and to avoid the adverse effects seen at higher blood levels. Recommended dosing for fentanyl is 2 to 6 μg/kg/h. Opioid agonist/antagonists such as buprenorphine cause less cardiovascular, respiratory, and central nervous system depression, but provide only moderate analgesia and are more difficult to reverse.[35] Having less sedation allows more accurate patient assessment and may be particularly important in patients with subtle changes or at risk for rapid changes in neurologic status.

Benzodiazepines are a valuable adjunct to the balanced approach. They provide anxiolysis and sedation with minimal intracranial, cardiovascular, and respiratory effects. They also enable dose reduction of other agents, such as propofol, minimizing adverse effects.[35] Midazolam, but not diazepam, significantly reduced the propofol dose required for intubation in dogs, whereas both were effective in cats.[43,44]

Ketamine is an anesthetic drug with potent analgesic and hypnotic action. By inhibiting the NMDA receptor, ketamine may have neuroprotective effects as NMDA receptor signaling plays a key role in neuronal death.[45] Other potential advantages are stimulation of the cardiovascular system and minimal respiratory depression. The benefits of ketamine have led to reexamination of its role in neurotrauma. Historically, ketamine was contraindicated owing to drug-induced increases in ICP. Older literature performed in patients with nontraumatic intracranial lesions showed an increase in ICP, and ketamine's supposed effect on ICP was perpetuated in anesthetic texts and literature.[46–49] However, recent studies of ketamine use in TBI do not support the increase in ICP.[45] Other studies in human TBI show higher mean CPP and lower vasopressor requirements with ketamine.[50,51] Ketamine may be a useful adjunct in veterinary head trauma, but further studies are warranted before specific recommendations can be made.

Alpha-2 agonists are easily reversible and provide sedation, anxiolysis, and analgesia without respiratory depression. However, their use in head trauma is controversial. Although dexmedetomidine may have neuroprotective properties, clinical studies in human patients with severe TBI have been mixed.[52–55] A 2016 metaanalysis of dexmedetomidine concluded that although the literature was limited in quantity and quality, dexmedetomidine seems to be both efficient and safe as a sole or adjunct agent in human neurocritical care patients.[56] However, dexmedetomidine was associated with significantly more hypotension in a prospective human study with 198 patients.[57] In a study with isoflurane-anesthetized dogs, dexmedetomidine significantly decreased

CBF and cardiac output, but without evidence of global cerebral ischemia.[58] Medetomidine did not increase ICP in healthy dogs under isoflurane anesthesia.[59] Given the mixed results and the risk of clinically significant reductions in heart rate and cardiac output, alpha-2 agonists should be avoided unless analgesics with fewer adverse effects are unavailable or are providing inadequate pain relief.[7] Recommended dosing is listed in **Table 1**.

Anticonvulsants

In human medicine, there is an established correlation between the severity of TBI and the development of posttraumatic seizures as well as an increased incidence of epilepsy in TBI patients compared with the general population.[60–62] In veterinary patients, the incidence is less well-documented, but a recent study found a higher epilepsy rate in dogs (3.5%–6.8%) with head trauma as compared with a standard population epilepsy rate of 1.4%.[63]

Seizures may occur at different time points relative to the injury, either early (within 7 days) or late (after 7 days). Preventing seizure development may limit the detrimental effects of seizure activity such as increased ICP and increased metabolic demands.

A recent Cochrane review evaluated prophylactic antiepileptic medications for the prevention of early and late seizures and impact outcome in humans.[64] There was minimal evidence that seizure prophylaxis reduced early seizures and no evidence in reduction of late seizures or improvements in outcome. The current recommendation is treatment for 1 week.[65] There are no studies in veterinary medicine investigating the use of seizure prophylaxis in a population of TBI patients. If seizures develop, it is reasonable to initiate emergency treatment with benzodiazepines followed by a maintenance antiepileptic medication. In the authors' experience, continued neurologic assessment may be easier to facilitate with levetiracetam.

Corticosteroids

Based on previous experimental evidence, steroids were often used in the treatment of TBI.[66,67] However, the results of the CRASH trial demonstrated an increased risk of death at both 2 weeks and 6 months in human adults.[68] Corticosteroids are not recommended for TBI patients.

Gastric Ulcer Prophylaxis

Patients with neurologic injury, including TBI, are at an increased risk of gastric ulceration and bleeding.[69] A recent metaanalysis concluded that ulcer prophylaxis with

Table 1
Recommended doses for anesthetics, analgesics, and sedatives

Drug	Recommended Dose
Propofol	1–6 mg/kg, then 100–400 μg/kg/min
Fentanyl	Dogs: 2–6 μg/kg, then 2–6 μg/kg/h Cats: 1–3 μg/kg, then 1–3 μg/kg/h
Buprenorphine	0.01–0.02 mg/kg q8h
Midazolam	0.1–0.5 mg/kg
Ketamine	0.1–1.0 mg/kg, then 2–10 μg/kg/min
Dexmedetomidine	0.5–3 μg/kg/h, then 0.5–1 μg/kg/h

either proton pump inhibitors or histamine-2 receptor antagonists was effective in preventing gastrointestinal bleeding in humans. There was no increase in the risk of nosocomial pneumonia.[70] In veterinary medicine, drugs including proton pump inhibitors, such as pantoprazole or omeprazole, and histamine-2 receptor antagonists, such as famotidine may be used.

NONPHARMACOLOGIC TREATMENT OPTIONS

Oxygen and Ventilation

Respiratory compromise may result from pneumothorax, pulmonary contusion, aspiration pneumonia, or an abnormal respiratory drive. Normal oxygenation and ventilation are the goals of treatment. Hyperoxygenation and hyperoxemia may worsen reperfusion injury. Oxygen should be titrated to achieve normoxemia (Pao_2 >80 mm Hg and SpO_2 >94%).[7]

Oxygenation supplementation should be individualized. Most patients tolerate flow-by with or without a mask during initial assessment and stabilization. Nasal cannulas are effective, but may cause sneezing or coughing, which can increase ICP. Nasal cannulas should be used as a last resort. Apply care when placing nasal cannulas in patients with head trauma. The distal tip of the catheter should not extend past the medial canthus because possible fractures may allow communication with the cranial vault. Oxygen cages may be ineffective if frequent or constant monitoring is required. Intubation or temporary tracheostomy should be considered in stuporous or comatose patients and those lacking a gag reflex.[4]

Under normal conditions, $Paco_2$ is the most powerful determinant of CBF. CO_2 affects ICP by regulating vessel tone and diameter. Between 20 and 80 mm Hg, CBF changes linearly with $Paco_2$.[71] Decreases in $Paco_2$ lead to vasoconstriction, with a $Paco_2$ of less than 30 mm Hg causing excessive vasoconstriction, low CBF, and cerebral ischemia. Conversely, high $Paco_2$ leads to excessive CBF, increased CBF, and worsened ICP.[7] Hypoventilation and increased CO_2 may occur from damage to the respiratory center, oversedation, thoracic pain, mechanical airway obstruction, or respiratory muscle fatigue or paralysis.[72]

Prophylactic hyperventilation is not recommended. After trauma, ischemia from excessive vasoconstriction is common.[73] Hyperventilation worsens ischemia and secondary injury by promoting vasoconstriction. Subsequent alkalosis with a leftward shift in the oxygen–hemoglobin dissociation curve decreases oxygen delivery. Numerous studies have shown a poorer outcome with prophylactic hyperventilation during initial resuscitation in humans.[74,75] Normoventilation ($Paco_2$ 35–40 mm Hg) is recommended. Short-term conservative hyperventilation ($Paco_2$ >30 mm Hg) should only be used to reduce increased ICP. Guidelines for human patients recommend avoiding hyperventilation in the first 24 hours after trauma when CBF may be critically reduced.[71]

Nutrition

Head trauma is associated with a hypermetabolic and hypercatabolic state and early nutritional support is essential. Early enteral nutrition maintains gastrointestinal integrity, improves immune function, and attenuates the metabolic response to stress.[76] A retrospective study of 797 humans with severe TBI found that early nutrition (within 5 days) reduced 2-week mortality and the amount of nutrition was inversely correlated with mortality.[77]

The patient's ability to protect their airway, tolerance of a tube placement procedure, and anticipated duration of use must be considered when choosing the method of providing nutrition. In stable patients, esophagostomy tubes are well-tolerated and associated with few complications.[78] Owners can be trained to use and maintain these tubes at home, allowing for at-home care.

Parenteral nutrition should be considered in patients at risk for aspiration.[4] Commercial products are available and well tolerated in hospitalized dogs in intensive care.[79]

Head Elevation

Mild head elevation of less than 30° is associated with decreases in ICP and increases in CPP without affecting MAP. Mild head elevation does not compromise cerebral oxygenation.[80] In veterinary patients, a rigid back board may be used to avoid kinking the neck and compressing the jugular veins, which could lead to increased ICP. See **Fig. 2** for an example of head elevation.

Therapeutic Hypothermia

The mechanisms that lead to secondary brain injury are inhibited by hypothermia. Apoptosis, excitotoxicity, increases in inflammatory mediators, free radical formation, microcirculatory dysfunction, and other mechanisms are implicated.[81] Therapeutic hypothermia (32°C–34°C), may protect against secondary injury. In humans, therapeutic hypothermia is the standard of care for patients after cardiac arrest and stroke and may be used in TBI with intracranial hypertension and status epilepticus.[82,83] However, a recent study of humans with intracranial hypertension treated with therapeutic hypothermia in addition to standard care failed to demonstrate benefit.[84] At this time, there is only 1 report of a veterinary TBI patient treated with therapeutic hypothermia.[85] At the authors' institution, hypothermic TBI patients are allowed to passively rewarm, but are not actively cooled.

Glycemic Control

In human patients, hyperglycemia leads to increases in mortality and duration of hospitalization, and worse neurologic outcome owing to accelerated secondary brain injury.[86] In veterinary patients, hyperglycemia is an indication of the severity of the injury, but not necessarily a prognostic indicator.[87] Studies do not support the use of insulin protocols owing to possible hypoglycemia.[88] See **Fig. 3** for an overview of patient stabilization.

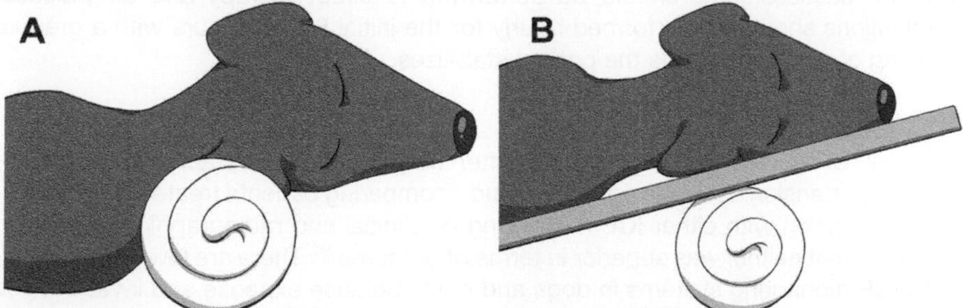

Fig. 2. Elevation of the head and neck is associated with decreases in intracranial pressure and increased cerebral perfusion pressure. (*A*) Inappropriate head elevation using a rolled up towel may lead to kinking of the neck, which can compress the jugular veins and increase intracranial pressure. (*B*) A rigid backboard allows head elevation without risk of compressing the jugular veins. (*Courtesy of* Silas Lee, Department of Information and Instructional Technology, Auburn, AL.)

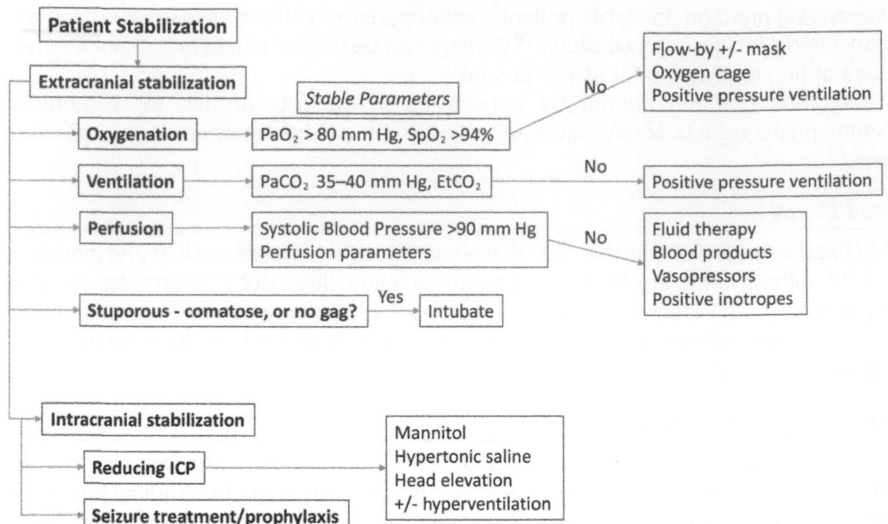

Fig. 3. Overview of patient stabilization after head trauma. $EtCO_2$, end-tidal carbon dioxide; ICP, intracranial pressure.

SURGICAL TREATMENT OPTIONS

Decompressive craniectomy may be performed in patients with refractory intracranial hypertension at risk for cerebral herniation.[89] A recent trial in human TBI patients comparing decompressive craniectomy with standard medical therapy for intracranial hypertension resulted in a lower mortality rate in the surgery group.[90] In veterinary patients, decompressive craniectomy should be considered in those failing aggressive medical therapy or a compressive lesion from fracture or hemorrhage.[91]

MONITORING

Repeated Physical and Neurologic Examinations

Frequent reassessments should be performed to direct therapy and diagnostics. Examinations should be performed hourly for the initial 6 to 12 hours with a gradual lessening of assessments as the patient stabilizes.

Intracranial Pressure

In human TBI patients, ICP monitoring is often used in titrating therapies to treat intracranial hypertension. However, a recent study comparing patients treated for intracranial hypertension with either ICP monitoring or clinical and radiographic information concluded that neither was superior in terms of outcome.[92] There are few studies evaluating ICP monitoring systems in dogs and cats, because expense and invasiveness preclude widespread use.[93–95]

Electrocardiography

Traumatic myocarditis causing arrhythmias is common in blunt trauma patients.[1,96] Patients presenting with evidence of concurrent thoracic trauma should be monitored for 24 to 48 hours.

Blood Pressure

Blood pressure should be monitored to ensure a minimum systolic blood pressure of 100 mm Hg to promote cerebral perfusion. Blood pressure should also be monitored if the patient becomes bradycardic to determine if the patient is experiencing a Cushing's reflex.

ACKNOWLEDGMENTS

The authors would like to thank Sonya Hansen for help with the creation of **Box 1**.

REFERENCES

1. Simpson S, Syring R, Otto C. Severe blunt trauma in dogs: 235 cases (1997–2003). J Vet Emerg Crit Care (San Antonio) 2009;19(6):588–602.
2. Platt S, Radaelli S, McDonnell J. The prognostic value of the Modified Glasgow Coma Scale in head trauma in dogs. J Vet Intern Med 2001;15(6):581–4.
3. Sorjonen DC, Thomas WB, Myers LJ, et al. Radical cerebral cortical resection in dogs. Prog Vet Neurol 1991;2(4):225–36.
4. Dewey CW. Emergency management of the head trauma patient. Principles and practice. Vet Clin North Am Small Anim Pract 2000;30(1):207–25.
5. Platt SR, Radaelli ST, McDonnell JJ. Computed tomography after mild head trauma in dogs. Vet Rec 2002;151(8):243.
6. Dewey CW, Downs MO, Aron DN, et al. Acute traumatic intracranial haemorrhage in dogs and cats. Vet Comp Orthop Traumatol 1993;6(3):29–35.
7. DiFazio J, Fletcher DJ. Updates in the management of the small animal patient with neurologic trauma. Vet Clin North Am Small Anim Pract 2013;43(4):915–40.
8. Sande A, West C. Traumatic brain injury: a review of pathophysiology and management. J Vet Emerg Crit Care (San Antonio) 2010;20(2):177–90.
9. Siegel JH. The effect of associated injuries, blood loss, and oxygen debt on death and disability in blunt traumatic brain injury: the need for early physiologic predictors of severity. J Neurotrauma 1995;12(4):579–90.
10. Lisciandro G, Lagutchik M, Mann K, et al. Evaluation of a thoracic focused assessment with sonography for trauma (TFAST) protocol to detect pneumothorax and concurrent thoracic injury in 145 traumatized dogs. J Vet Emerg Crit Car 2008;18(3):258–69.
11. Sharma D, Holowaychuk M. Retrospective evaluation of prognostic indicators in dogs with head trauma: 72 cases (January–March 2011). J Vet Emerg Crit Care (San Antonio) 2015;25(5):631–9.
12. Rockar R, Drobatz K, Shofer F. Development of a scoring system for the veterinary trauma patient. J Vet Emerg Crit Care (San Antonio) 1994;4(2):77–83.
13. Streeter EM, Rozanski EA, Laforcade-Buress Ad, et al. Evaluation of vehicular trauma in dogs: 239 cases (January–December 2001). J Am Vet Med Assoc 2009;235(4):405408.
14. Hall K, Holowaychuk M, Sharp C, et al. Multicenter prospective evaluation of dogs with trauma. J Am Vet Med Assoc 2014;244(3):300–8.
15. Boysen SRR, Rozanski EA, Tidwell AS, et al. Evaluation of a focused assessment with sonography for trauma protocol to detect free abdominal fluid in dogs involved in motor vehicle accidents. J Am Vet Med Assoc 2004;225(8):1198–204.
16. Lisciandro GR. Abdominal and thoracic focused assessment with sonography for trauma, triage, and monitoring in small animals. J Vet Emerg Crit Care (San Antonio) 2011;21(2):104–22.

17. Kim J, Gean A. Imaging for the diagnosis and management of traumatic brain injury. Neurotherapeutics 2011;8(1):39–53.
18. Caputo N, Stahmer C, Lim G, et al. Whole-body computed tomographic scanning leads to better survival as opposed to selective scanning in trauma patients: a systematic review and meta-analysis. J Trauma Acute Care Surg 2014;77(4):534.
19. Lagares A, Ramos A, Pérez-Nuñez A, et al. The role of MR imaging in assessing prognosis after severe and moderate head injury. Acta Neurochir 2009;151(4): 341–56.
20. Beltran E, Platt SR, McConnell JF, et al. Prognostic value of early magnetic resonance imaging in dogs after traumatic brain injury: 50 cases. J Vet Intern Med 2014;28(4):1256–62.
21. Chesnut RM, Marshall LF, Klauber MR, et al. The role of secondary brain injury in determining outcome from severe head injury. J Trauma 1993;34(2):216–22.
22. van der Jagt M. Fluid management of the neurological patient: a concise review. Crit Care 2016;20(1):126.
23. Smith GJ, Kramer G, Perron P, et al. A comparison of several hypertonic solutions for resuscitation of bled sheep. J Surg Res 1985;39(6):517–28.
24. Perel P, Roberts I, Ker K. Colloids versus crystalloids for fluid resuscitation in critically ill patients. Cochrane Database Syst Rev 2013;(2):CD000567.
25. SAFE Study Investigators, Australian and New Zealand Intensive Care Society Clinical Trials Group, Australian Red Cross Blood Service, George Institute for International Health, Myburgh J, Cooper DJ, Finfer S, et al. Saline or albumin for fluid resuscitation in patients with traumatic brain injury. N Engl J Med 2007; 357(9):874–84.
26. Li M, Chen T, Chen S, et al. Comparison of equimolar doses of mannitol and hypertonic saline for the treatment of elevated intracranial pressure after traumatic brain injury: a systematic review and meta-analysis. Medicine 2015;94(17):e736.
27. Mortazavi M, Romeo A, Deep A, et al. Hypertonic saline for treating raised intracranial pressure: literature review with meta-analysis. J Neurosurg 2012;116(1): 210–21.
28. Fink M. Osmotherapy for intracranial hypertension: mannitol versus hypertonic saline. Continuum (Minneap Minn) 2012;18(3):640–54.
29. Misra UK, Kalita J, Ranjan P, et al. Mannitol in intracerebral hemorrhage: a randomized controlled study. J Neurol Sci 2005;234(1–2):41–5.
30. Roberts A, Pollay M, Engles C, et al. Effect on intracranial pressure of furosemide combined with varying doses and administration rates of mannitol. J Neurosurg 1987;66(3):440–6.
31. Todd M, Cutkomp J, Brian J. Influence of mannitol and furosemide, alone and in combination, on brain water content after fluid percussion injury. Anesthesiology 2006;105(6):1176.
32. Shackford SR, Schmoker JD, Zhuang J. The effect of hypertonic resuscitation of pial arteriolar tone after brain injury and shock. J Trauma Acute Care Surg 1994; 37(6):899.
33. Angle N, Hoyt DB, Coimbra R, et al. Hypertonic saline resuscitation diminishes lung injury by suppressing neutrophil activation after hemorrhagic shock. Shock 1998;9(3):164.
34. Doyle J, Davis D, Hoyt D. The use of hypertonic saline in the treatment of traumatic brain injury. J Trauma Acute Care Surg 2001;50(2):367.
35. Armitage-Chan E, Wetmore L, Chan D. Anesthetic management of the head trauma patient. J Vet Emerg Crit Car 2007;17(1):5–14.

36. Artru A. Relationship between cerebral blood volume and CSF pressure during anesthesia with isoflurane or fentanyl in dogs. Anesthesiology 1984;60(6):575.
37. Newberg LA, Milde JH, Michenfelder JD. The cerebral metabolic effects of isoflurane at and above concentrations that suppress cortical electrical activity. Anesthesiology 1983;59(1):23.
38. McCulloch T, Visco E, Lam A. Graded hypercapnia and cerebral autoregulation during sevoflurane or propofol anesthesia. Anesthesiology 2000;93(5):1205.
39. Cenic A, Craen R, Lee T-Y, et al. Cerebral blood volume and blood flow responses to hyperventilation in brain tumors during isoflurane or propofol anesthesia. Anesth Analg 2002;94(3):661.
40. Holzer A, Winter W, Greher M, et al. A comparison of propofol and sevoflurane anaesthesia: effects on aortic blood flow velocity and middle cerebral artery blood flow velocity. Anaesthesia 2003;58(3):217–22.
41. Strebel S, Lam A, Matta B, et al. Dynamic and static cerebral autoregulation during isoflurane, desflurane, and propofol anesthesia. Anesthesiology 1995; 83(1):66.
42. Hans P, Bonhomme V. Why we still use intravenous drugs as the basic regimen for neurosurgical anaesthesia. Curr Opin Anaesthesiol 2006;19(5):498.
43. Robinson R, Borer-Weir K. The effects of diazepam or midazolam on the dose of propofol required to induce anaesthesia in cats. Vet Anaesth Analg 2015;42(5): 493–501.
44. Robinson R, Borer-Weir K. A dose titration study into the effects of diazepam or midazolam on the propofol dose requirements for induction of general anaesthesia in client owned dogs, premedicated with methadone and acepromazine. Vet Anaesth Analg 2013;40(5):455–63.
45. Zeiler FA, Teitelbaum J, West M, et al. The ketamine effect on ICP in traumatic brain injury. Neurocrit Care 2014;21(1):163–73.
46. Wyte SR, Shapiro HM, Turner P, et al. Ketamine-induced intracranial hypertension. Anesthesiology 1972;36(2):174.
47. Shapiro H, Wyte S, Harris A. Ketamine anaesthesia in patients with intracranial pathology. Br J Anaesth 1972;44(11):1200–4.
48. Gardner A, Olson B, Lichticer M. Cerebrospinal-fluid pressure during dissociative anesthesia with ketamine. Anesthesiology 1971;35(2):226.
49. List WF, Crumrine RS, Cascorbi HF, et al. Increased cerebrospinal fluid pressure after ketamine. Anesthesiology 1972;36(1):98.
50. Schmittner M, Vajkoczy S, Horn P, et al. Effects of fentanyl and S(+)-ketamine on cerebral hemodynamics, gastrointestinal motility, and need of vasopressors in patients with intracranial pathologies: a pilot study. J Neurosurg Anesthesiol 2007;19(4):257.
51. Kolenda H, Gremmelt A, Rading S, et al. Ketamine for analgosedative therapy in intensive care treatment of head-injured patients. Acta Neurochir 1996;138(10): 1193–9.
52. Zornow M, Scheller M, Sheehan P, et al. Intracranial pressure effects of dexmedetomidine in rabbits. Anesth Analg 1992;75(2):232.
53. Maier C, Steinberg G, Sun G, et al. Neuroprotection by the [alpha]2-adrenoreceptor agonist dexmedetomidine in a focal model of cerebral ischemia. Anesthesiology 1993;79(2):306.
54. Cosar M, Eser O, Fidan H, et al. The neuroprotective effect of dexmedetomidine in the hippocampus of rabbits after subarachnoid hemorrhage. Surg Neurol 2009;71(1):54–9.

55. Aryan H, Box K, Ibrahim D, et al. Safety and efficacy of dexmedetomidine in neurosurgical patients. Brain Inj 2009;20(8):791–8.
56. Tsaousi G, Lamperti M, Bilotta F. Role of dexmedetomidine for sedation in neurocritical care patients: a qualitative systematic review and meta-analysis of current evidence. Clin Neuropharmacol 2016;39(3):144.
57. Pajoumand M, Kufera J, Bonds B, et al. Dexmedetomidine as an adjunct for sedation in patients with traumatic brain injury. J Trauma Acute Care Surg 2016;81(2):345.
58. Zornow M, Fleischer J, Scheller M, et al. Dexmedetomidine, an [alpha]2-adrenergic agonist, decreases cerebral blood flow in the isoflurane-anesthetized dog. Anesth Analg 1990;70(6):624.
59. Keegan RD, Greene SA, Bagley RS, et al. Effects of medetomidine administration on intracranial pressure and cardiovascular variables of isoflurane-anesthetized dogs. Am J Vet Res 1995;56(2):193–8.
60. Torbic H, Forni A, Anger K, et al. Use of antiepileptics for seizure prophylaxis after traumatic brain injury. Am J Health Syst Pharm 2013;70(9):759–66.
61. Ferguson P, Smith G, Wannamaker B, et al. A population-based study of risk of epilepsy after hospitalization for traumatic brain injury. Epilepsia 2010;51(5): 891–8.
62. Hirtz D, Thurman DJ, Gwinn-Hardy K, et al. How common are the "common" neurologic disorders? Neurology 2007;68(5):326–37.
63. Friedenberg S, Butler A, Wei L, et al. Seizures following head trauma in dogs: 259 cases (1999–2009). J Am Vet Med Assoc 2012;241(11):1479–83.
64. Thompson K, Pohlmann-Eden B, Campbell L, et al. Pharmacological treatments for preventing epilepsy following traumatic head injury. Cochrane Database Syst Rev 2015;(8):CD009900.
65. Temkin N, Dikmen S, Wilensky A, et al. A randomized, double-blind study of phenytoin for the prevention of post-traumatic seizures. N Engl J Med 1990; 323(8):497–502.
66. Maxwell R, Long D, French L. The effects of glucosteroids on experimental cold-induced brain edema. J Neurosurg 1971;34(4):477–87.
67. Hall E. The neuroprotective pharmacology of methylprednisolone. J Neurosurg 1992;76(1):13–22.
68. Edwards P, Arango M, Balica L, et al. Final results of MRC CRASH, a randomised placebo-controlled trial of intravenous corticosteroid in adults with head injury—outcomes at 6 months. Lancet 2005;365(9475):1957–9.
69. Kamada T, Fusamoto H, Kawano S, et al. Gastrointestinal bleeding following head injury: a clinical study of 433 cases. J Trauma Acute Care Surg 1977;17(1):44.
70. Liu B, Liu S, Yin A, et al. Risks and benefits of stress ulcer prophylaxis in adult neurocritical care patients: a systematic review and meta-analysis of randomized controlled trials. Crit Care 2015;19(1):1–13.
71. Carney N, Totten AM, O'Reilly C, et al. Guidelines for the management of severe traumatic brain injury, 4th edition. Neurosurgery 2017;80(1):6–15.
72. Syring R. Assessment and treatment of central nervous system abnormalities in the emergency patient. Vet Clin North Am Small Anim Pract 2005;35(2):343–58.
73. Yundt KD, Diringer MN. The use of hyperventilation and its impact on cerebral ischemia in the treatment of traumatic brain injury. Crit Care Clin 1997;13(1): 163–84.
74. Davis D, Dunford J, Poste J, et al. The impact of hypoxia and hyperventilation on outcome after paramedic rapid sequence intubation of severely head-injured patients. J Trauma Acute Care Surg 2004;57(1):1.

75. Muizelaar P, Marmarou A, Ward J, et al. Adverse effects of prolonged hyperventilation in patients with severe head injury: a randomized clinical trial. J Neurosurg 1991;75(5):731–9.
76. Marik P, Varon J, Trask T. Management of head trauma. Chest 2002;122(2):699–711.
77. Härtl R, Gerber L, Ni Q, et al. Effect of early nutrition on deaths due to severe traumatic brain injury. J Neurosurg 2008;109(1):50–6.
78. Levine P, Smallwood L, Buback J. Esophagostomy tubes as a method of nutritional management in cats: a retrospective study. J Am Anim Hosp Assoc 1997;33(5):405–10.
79. Olan NV, Prittie J. Retrospective evaluation of ProcalAmine administration in a population of hospitalized ICU dogs: 36 cases (2010–2013). J Vet Emerg Crit Care (San Antonio) 2015;25(3):405–12.
80. Ng I, Lim J, Wong H. Effects of head posture on cerebral hemodynamics: its influences on intracranial pressure, cerebral perfusion pressure, and cerebral oxygenation. Neurosurgery 2004;54(3):593–7 [discussion: 598].
81. Sadaka F, Veremakis C. Therapeutic hypothermia for the management of intracranial hypertension in severe traumatic brain injury: a systematic review. Brain Inj 2012;26(7–8):899–908.
82. Jiang JY, Yu MK, Zhu C. Effect of long-term mild hypothermia therapy in patients with severe traumatic brain injury: 1-year follow-up review of 87 cases. J Neurosurg 2000;93(4):546–9.
83. McCarthy P, Scott K, Ganta C, et al. Hypothermic protection in traumatic brain injury. Pathophysiology 2013;20(1):5–13.
84. Andrews P, Sinclair L, Rodriguez A, et al. Hypothermia for intracranial hypertension after traumatic brain injury. N Engl J Med 2015;373(25):2403–12.
85. Hayes G. Severe seizures associated with traumatic brain injury managed by controlled hypothermia, pharmacologic coma, and mechanical ventilation in a dog. J Vet Emerg Crit Car 2009;19(6):629–34.
86. Jeremitsky E, Omert L, Dunham M, et al. The impact of hyperglycemia on patients with severe brain injury. J Trauma Acute Care Surg 2005;58(1):47.
87. Syring RS, Otto CM, Drobatz KJ. Hyperglycemia in dogs and cats with head trauma: 122 cases (1997–1999). J Am Vet Med Assoc 2001;218(7):1124–9.
88. Green D, O'Phelan K, Bassin S, et al. Intensive versus conventional insulin therapy in critically ill neurologic patients. Neurocrit Care 2010;13(3):299–306.
89. Farahvar A, Gerber L, Chiu Y-L, et al. Response to intracranial hypertension treatment as a predictor of death in patients with severe traumatic brain injury. J Neurosurg 2011;114(5):1471–8.
90. Hutchinson P, Kolias A, Timofeev I, et al. Trial of decompressive craniectomy for traumatic intracranial hypertension. N Engl J Med 2016;375(12):1119–30.
91. Dewey CW, Fletcher DJ. Medical and surgical management of the brain-injured pet. In: Tobias KM, Johnston SA, editors. Veterinary surgery: small animal. St. Louis: Saunders; 2012. p. 508–9.
92. Chesnut R, Temkin N, Carney N, et al. A trial of intracranial-pressure monitoring in traumatic brain injury. N Engl J Med 2012;367(26):2471–81.
93. Dewey C, Bailey C, Haskins S, et al. Evaluation of an epidural intracranial pressure monitoring system in cats. J Vet Emerg Crit Car 1997;7(1):20–33.
94. Ilie L, Thomovsky E, Johnson P, et al. Relationship between intracranial pressure as measured by an epidural intracranial pressure monitoring system and optic nerve sheath diameter in healthy dogs. Am J Vet Res 2015;76(8):724–31.

95. Bagley RS, Keegan RD, Greene SA, et al. Intraoperative monitoring of intracranial pressure in five dogs with space-occupying intracranial lesions. J Am Vet Med Assoc 1995;207(5):588–91.
96. Marcolini E, Keegan J. Blunt cardiac injury. Emerg Med Clin North Am 2015; 33(3):519–27.

Transsphenoidal Surgery for Pituitary Tumors and Other Sellar Masses

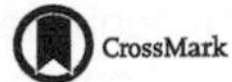

Tina J. Owen, DVM[a,*], Linda G. Martin, DVM, MS[b],
Annie V. Chen, DVM, MS[b]

KEYWORDS

- Hypophysectomy • Transsphenoidal surgery • Sellar masses
- Pituitary-dependent hyperadrenocorticism • Cushing disease • Pituitary tumor
- Acromegaly • Hypersomatotropism

KEY POINTS

- Functional and nonfunctional pituitary tumors and other sellar and parasellar masses can be treated by transsphenoidal surgery in dogs and cats.
- Diagnosis, decompression, rapid resolution of clinical signs, and a potential cure are the goals of transsphenoidal surgery.
- Imaging is indicated early in the diagnostic process because larger tumors have worse outcomes.
- Larger tumors are associated with shorter survival and remission times and have a greater chance of requiring long-term treatment of central diabetes insipidus.
- There is a steep learning curve with this surgical procedure and the postoperative management of patients with large tumors is intensive.

 **Video content accompanies this article at http://www.vetsmall.theclinics.com.**

INTRODUCTION

For many years, transsphenoidal surgery (TSS) has been the treatment of choice for humans with a pituitary tumor or a definable sellar mass. Early surgery in dogs was used primarily for research and training human surgeons. Veterinary surgical protocols for the transsphenoidal approach to the pituitary gland and subsequent

Disclosure: The authors have nothing to disclose.

[a] Department of Veterinary Clinical Sciences, College of Veterinary Medicine, Washington State University, PO Box 647060, Pullman, WA 99164-7060, USA; [b] Department of Veterinary Clinical Sciences, College of Veterinary Medicine, Washington State University, PO Box 646610, Pullman, WA 99164-6610, USA
* Corresponding author.
E-mail address: tinajoowen@vetmed.wsu.edu

Vet Clin Small Anim 48 (2018) 129–151
http://dx.doi.org/10.1016/j.cvsm.2017.08.006

hypophysectomy were refined in the late 1980s by Niebauer and Evans,[1] Niebauer and colleagues,[2] and Lantz and colleagues,[3] and transsphenoidal hypophysectomy (TSH) has been used successfully by Meij and colleagues[4] and others to treat dogs with pituitary-dependent hyperadrenocorticism (PDH) since 1993.[4–8]

Thirty-five percent of secondary intracranial neoplasia in dogs is attributed to pituitary tumors or other sellar masses.[9] A retrospective study of skull-base neoplasia in dogs found pituitary adenomas to be the most common sellar mass, followed by meningiomas. Less common tumors in this location included craniopharyngioma, oligodendroglioma, and pituitary adenocarcinoma.[10] Sellar masses may be a functional pituitary adenoma (FPA), nonfunctional pituitary adenoma (NFPA), or another nonfunctional sellar mass (NFSM). The most common clinically recognized FPA in dogs is an adrenocorticotropic hormone (ACTH)-secreting tumor causing PDH.[11] FPAs in cats can be corticotroph or somatotroph in origin causing PDH or hypersomatotropism (acromegaly), respectively.[12,13] A double adenoma both corticotroph and somatotroph in origin has been identified in a cat.[14] A growth hormone–secreting adenoma causing acromegaly is the more common feline FPA. It is estimated that approximately 32% of diabetic cats have increased insulinlike growth factor 1 (IGF-1) concentrations[15] and the overall prevalence of acromegaly in diabetic cats in the United Kingdom is 25%.[16]

Although PDH is usually attributed to pituitary microadenomas (tumors <1 cm in diameter), the prevalence of visible pituitary tumors reaches 52% when magnetic resonance (MR) imaging is used to screen affected dogs.[17] In the authors' experience, TSH can also be used to successfully treat NFPA and other NFSMs in dogs and cats.

Pituitary or sellar masses in dogs and cats can present as (1) incidentalomas, (2) a cause of endocrine abnormalities, or (3) a cause of neurologic signs secondary to a mass effect. An incidentaloma is a mass found on computed tomography (CT)/MR imaging that is performed for reasons unrelated to the pituitary or sellar mass.[18] Incidentalomas are usually monitored for further growth and surgery is rarely recommended.

CASE SELECTION

Dogs and cats with MR image/CT definable pituitary or other sellar masses can be considered for TSS. Functional sellar masses are more likely to have a successful surgical outcome because the tumor is likely of pituitary origin. Patients with large pituitary tumors or sellar masses, which typically present for severe neurologic signs, may be appealing candidates. Some clinicians have discouraged surgery for large tumors because the smaller the tumor, the better the prognosis.[8,19,20] However, patients with large tumors do not have many options for care. In our experience, a good outcome is possible if an owner is well informed of the surgical risks and wishes to pursue surgical treatment.

An MR imaging–based classification system may help assess suitability of TSH in canine PDH by evaluating the extent and vascular involvement of the tumor.[19] Surgery for tumors that touch the interthalamic adhesion, occupy the third ventricle, or involve the arterial circle of Willis or the cavernous sinus should be approached with caution. For a large tumor, debulking surgery followed by radiation may be preferred.[19] Debulking of a pituitary or sellar mass should only be pursued when an owner is well informed of the surgical risks and is preoperatively planning to follow surgery with radiation.

Patients considered for TSS must not only be evaluated by the family veterinarian but must have a thorough work-up by an internist and neurologist to ensure they are good surgical candidates. The owner and the pituitary team must have a discussion about all available treatment options and the owner must be well informed of the potential complications of TSS as well as postoperative recovery and long-term management.

Algorithms for case selection and treatment considerations for pituitary tumors and other sellar masses are outlined in **Fig. 1**. **Fig. 1**A outlines the treatment options for tumors in dogs and **Fig. 1**B for cats. The goals of surgery include diagnosis; decompression; rapid resolution of clinical signs, whether endocrine or neurologic; and to treat the underlying source, be it the pituitary tumor or sellar mass (see **Fig. 1**).

CLINICAL PRESENTATION

Endocrine Presentation

Clinical signs of canine PDH, feline PDH, and feline acromegaly have been outlined in the literature. Please refer to other sources for more detailed information.[11,21,22]

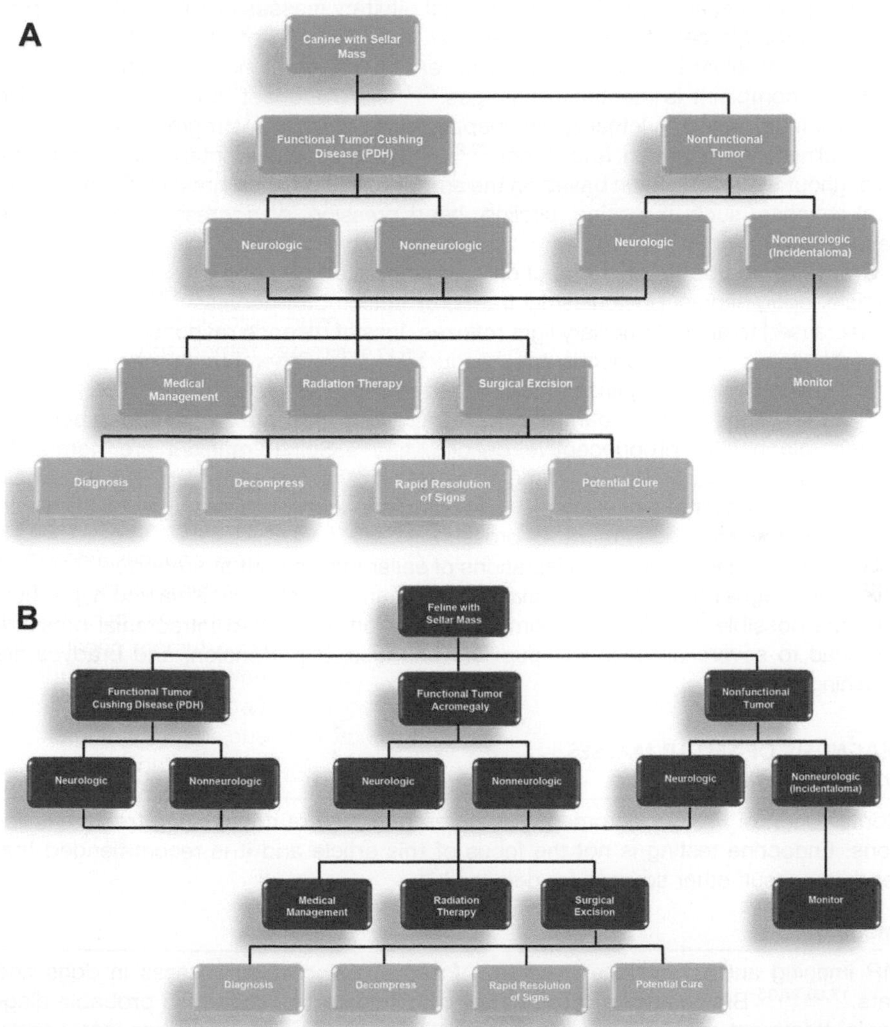

Fig. 1. Canine (*A*) and feline (*B*) sellar mass algorithm: case selection and treatment options for functional and nonfunctional pituitary and sellar masses. The green boxes represent the goals and benefits of surgery.

Neurologic Presentation

Animals with sellar masses can present with normal neurologic examinations.[17,23–26] Although larger masses can lead to more neurologic deficits,[20,24] the size of the sellar mass does not always correlate with the degree of neurologic disease[23,25,27] because these slow-growing masses allow the brain to compensate over time.[27] Central nervous system dysfunction may also be related less to tumor size and more to tumor type.[27] Tumors with a rapid growth rate may enlarge so quickly that the surrounding brain cannot compensate, causing neurologic signs.[27] Sometimes these masses acutely bleed, causing secondary mass effect from hemorrhage and edema, leading to neurologic deterioration.

Most animals with functional pituitary masses are neurologically sound at initial presentation, because their endocrine imbalance is the primary clinical complaint.[12,17,27] In our experience, animals with nonfunctional pituitary masses present with more profound neurologic deficits, and present later in the course of disease for a primary neurologic problem because there are no endocrine imbalances to note. The most common complaint is mentation changes.[23,25–29] The onset is usually nonspecific and insidious, including lethargy and inappetence, which may progress to disorientation, dullness, obtundation, and stupor.[23,25–29] The degree of mental dullness can vary throughout the examination based on the amount of stimulation present. Other behavioral changes, such as pacing, circling, head pressing, or aggression, can also be seen.[23,25–29]

Cranial nerve deficits are rare but can be associated with compression of the optic chiasm, optic nerves, postchiasmal tracts, or oculomotor nerves[25,27,28,30–32] leading to decreased to absent pupillary light reflexes, loss of menace response, with associated blindness, and anisocoria may occur.[25,27,31,32] Other cranial nerves can be affected secondary to significant cerebral edema or mass effect.[25,27,28,30]

Gait alterations such as paraparesis, tetraparesis, and ataxia have also been reported, along with proprioceptive deficits.[23,27–30] Spinal reflexes are normal to increased, consistent with upper motor neuron dysfunction. Animals usually remain ambulatory even if the gait is altered. Head and cervical spinal pain may be observed secondary to increased intracranial pressure.

Seizures are uncommon manifestations of sellar masses but are reported.[25,27–29] In rare cases, signs related to hypothalamic disturbance, such as adipsia and hyperthermia, are possible.[30,33] Acute decompensation from increased intracranial pressure can lead to severe obtundation, pupillary changes, hypertension, and bradycardia (Cushing reflex).

DIAGNOSIS OF SELLAR MASSES

Endocrine Testing

Confirmation of PDH or acromegaly is paramount before considering treatment options. Endocrine testing is not the focus of this article and it is recommended that readers consult other sources for details.[26,34]

Imaging

MR imaging and CT are the mainstays for diagnosing sellar masses in dogs and cats.[17,26,27,35] Brain imaging provides valuable information regarding probable diagnosis, treatment options, and prognosis. With both imaging modalities increasingly available to clinicians, early diagnosis can lead to better prognosis with treatment.

MR imaging gives better intracranial anatomic resolution and soft tissue contrast than CT.[28,30] It is the modality of choice for evaluation of sellar masses in humans.[18]

Intravenous (IV) injection of contrast further increases the sensitivity and specificity of MR imaging by delineating the extent of tumor expansion into the parasellar tissues.[28,36,37] Use of CT for evaluation of the brain is limited because of poor soft tissue contrast and artifact from surrounding bone.[30] However, CT can be helpful for surgical planning by providing the exact location of the sellar mass relative to important bony surgical landmarks.[6,38]

Pituitary Imaging

- The pituitary gland lies outside of the blood-brain barrier. Following IV contrast, the pituitary gland enhances on CT and MR.[39,40]
- In healthy dogs, the pituitary gland is 6 to 10 mm in length, 5 to 9 mm in width, and 4 to 6 mm in height.[40] These values are highly variable, depending on breed, size, and individual variation.[41,42]
- Classification of pituitary adenomas in humans into microadenomas (≤10 mm) and macroadenomas (>10 mm) is not helpful in dogs because canine pituitary adenomas that are between 6 to 10 mm in height enlarge the gland and are not classified technically as microadenomas.[40] Some clinicians have defined macroadenomas as anything that extends out of the sella turcica.[43,44] Pituitary height to brain area (P/B) ratio allows correction for the size of the dog. The P/B ratio, measured on CT or MR imaging containing the largest pituitary cross section, was developed to standardize the measurement across dog breeds. P/B ratio = height of the pituitary (mm)/area of brain (cm^2). Kooistra and colleagues[44] used a cutoff P/B ratio of less than or equal to 0.31 to differentiate normal from enlarged pituitary glands. Using this ratio, it is appropriate in dogs to adjust the definition of microadenoma to adenomas that do not affect the size or shape of the pituitary gland.[39,44]
- Pituitary tumors are classified as adenoma, invasive adenoma, or adenocarcinoma. Invasive adenoma is suspected if the dog is less than 7.7 years of age and the mass greater than 1.9 cm in vertical height. Adenomas tend to be round instead of oval or irregular. Mineralization of the mass may indicate an invasive adenoma. Tumor functionality does not predict tumor type.[45]
- A 5-point MR imaging classification system based on tumor extension has been developed, with grade 1 having no extension and grade 5 having the most extension. Cases were then classified as type A if there was no arterial circle of Willis or cavernous sinus involvement and type B if these blood vessels were involved. Dogs with grade 1 to 3, type A classifications had better prognoses following TSH.[19]
- Dorsal extension of the macroadenoma can cause compression of the hypothalamus and interthalamic adhesion, displacement of the third ventricle, and dilation of the lateral and third ventricles secondary to obstruction.[17,24,28,30] Cranial extension of the macroadenoma can displace the optic chiasm and optic tracts.[19,28,31]
- MR imaging features of pituitary adenomas include isointensity to hyperintensity on T2-weighted (T2-W) images, isointensity to hypointensity on T1-weighted (T1-W) images, and avid homogeneous contrast enhancement on T1-W post-contrast images[17,24,27,35,46] (**Fig. 2**). Gradient echo T2*-weighted images may identify hemorrhage within the mass. MR may detect pituitary tumors as small as 3 mm.[17]
- With MR imaging, microadenomas may have delayed enhancement, appearing hypointense to normal pituitary immediately after contrast; however, macroadenomas often have rapid enhancement after contrast, caused by their increased vascularity.[37,47]

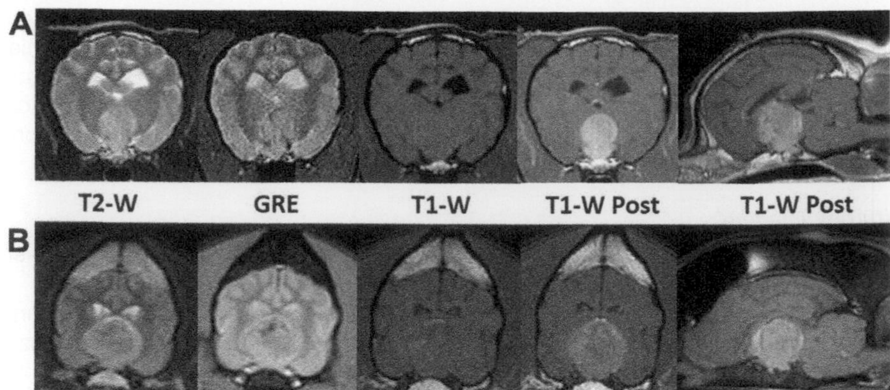

Fig. 2. MR images of a dog with a pituitary adenoma (*A*) and a meningioma (*B*). The MR imaging features are very similar between the 2 diagnoses. The masses are predominately hyperintense on T2-W images, have areas of hypointensity on the gradient-recalled echo (GRE) images indicating hemorrhage, are predominately isointense on the T1-W images, and contrast enhance avidly delineating a discrete, well-marginated circular mass in the area of the pituitary with dorsal extension into the thalamus creating mass effect.

- The posterior lobe (neurohypophysis) can have a high signal intensity on noncontrast T1-W images, representing the secretory granules containing arginine vasopressin. The posterior lobe is located slightly to the dorsal side of the center of the pituitary. Displacement of the posterior lobe dorsally may suggest the presence of an adenoma.[48]
- With conventional CT, 40% of dogs with microadenomas have normal-appearing pituitary gland.[44] Microadenomas and small macroadenomas often cannot be localized on routine contrast-enhanced CT images because of isoattenuation and because the enhancement represents the secondary capillary phase, which is less visible.[39,49,50]
- Dynamic contrast-enhanced CT can identify a so-called pituitary flush: the arterial blood supply of the neurohypophysis is seen slightly earlier than the enhancement of the adenohypophysis through the portal blood supply. The displacement, distortion, reduction, or disappearance of the pituitary flush sign in the early phase of dynamic CT can be used to identify microadenomas or nonenlarged pituitary tumors.[39,41]
- Frontal bone thickness and soft tissue accumulation in the nasal cavity, sinuses, and pharynx have been reported with acromegalic cats with CT and MR imaging–confirmed pituitary tumors.[51]

Imaging of Other Sellar Masses

- Tumors with nonpituitary origins, such as meningiomas, ependymomas, craniopharyngiomas, oligodendrogliomas, lymphomas, and metastatic disease, can involve the sella.[10,46,52]
- These tumors often have MR imaging characteristics indistinguishable from pituitary tumors.[46] Associated hemorrhage can also be seen, similar to pituitary tumors (see **Fig. 2**).
- The P/B ratio is often larger in these nonfunctional tumors because these animals present later in the disease course with neurologic signs.[46]

- Expansion of the sella and compression of the parasellar tissues in the rostral, caudal, and dorsal directions is often noted. This condition can lead to obstructive hydrocephalus with dilatation of the lateral and third ventricles.[46]
- Imaging diagnosis is presumptive and often more difficult with NFSMs. Definitive diagnosis can only be made with tissue histopathology.

TREATMENT OPTIONS FOR SELLAR MASSES

Medical Management

Medical management of sellar masses differs with functional or nonfunctional status and histologic type. Several drugs are available for the treatment of PDH, including drugs that chemically destroy the adrenal glands (mitotane),[53] inhibit the release of ACTH from the pituitary gland (Anipryl or selegiline),[54] or inhibit synthesis of steroid hormones (trilostane, ketoconazole).[55–58] Trilostane is most often used, with a median survival time of 549 to 930 days, depending on the study.[56,57] Dogs treated with somatostatin analogues, Som230 (pasireotide) and cabergoline, have shown favorable response.[59,60] Somatostatin analogues may be useful in treating feline acromegaly.[61] Prednisone is used to treat neurologic signs attributed to large functional or nonfunctional pituitary or sellar masses. Although medical treatment can improve the clinical signs in 40% to 80% of patients, medications need to be chronically administered, necessitate frequent monitoring, and do not address the primary cause of the disease (the pituitary tumor). Disadvantages of medical treatment include vomiting and diarrhea (from drug reaction or adrenocortical insufficiency), and relapse rates are as high as 50%. One-year survival with medical management can range from 45% to 80%.[53,55–57] Withholding treatment in dogs with PDH may be associated with a higher risk of death (506 days in untreated dogs vs median survival not reached during study period for treated dogs).[62] Chemotherapeutic drugs such as hydroxyurea for meningioma may be useful in treating sellar masses.[63]

Radiation Therapy

Dogs and cats diagnosed with sellar masses can be treated with radiation therapy (RT). Radiation generally shrinks the tumor by 25% to 50%[64,65] and may not completely control the neurologic signs associated with a large tumor. Dogs with pituitary masses treated with radiation had a 93% survival at 1 year with a mean survival of 1405 days.[25] Mariani and colleagues[66] reported a median survival of 118 days in 3 dogs with a presumptive pituitary tumor and 1 dog with a histologically confirmed pituitary adenocarcinoma treated with stereotactic radiosurgery. Smaller macroadenomas treated early respond more favorably to RT.[25] It is difficult to gain complete control of endocrine-related clinical signs associated with functional tumors with radiation alone.[64] Sixty percent of cats with pituitary tumors treated with RT[67–69] improved, with 50% to 60% no longer needing insulin or having improved insulin response and partial or complete remission of neurologic signs.[68,69]

Surgical Therapy

Remission rates for dogs with PDH treated with TSH are 86% to 95%, with a recurrence of 25% and mortality of 12% to 20%.[6,8,70] Survival at 1, 2, 3, and 4 years was 86%, 79%, 74%, and 72% respectively for dogs undergoing TSH.[8] In 7 cats treated with TSH for PDH, 70% went into remission, with a recurrence rate of 20%.[12]

Dogs with large pituitary (P/B ratio >0.31) tumors had a significantly shorter survival and disease-free interval (DFI) than dogs with small tumors (P/B ratio <0.31).[8] Large tumors (>1.9 cm vertical height) in a young dog (<7.7 years) should raise suspicion of an invasive adenoma.[45] Twenty-one acromegalic cats were treated with TSH; 78% had diabetic remission and 22% had a reduction in insulin requirement.[71]

Surgery is more effective than medical management or RT at controlling endocrine-related signs associated with a FPA and can also address neurologic signs associated with the mass effect. Reported survival time and DFI are correlated negatively with pituitary size,[8] adding support to the recommendation that pituitary imaging should be done at the time of diagnosis of PDH.[26] Veterinarians should consider TSH a viable option for treatment of PDH and other pituitary or sellar masses. As Meij and colleagues[4] stated, "Early diagnosis of PDH, pituitary imaging and treatment at the pituitary level should be the hallmarks of a successful treatment protocol for canine PDH as there are few treatment options left once pituitary macroadenomas have resulted in neurologic signs."

Serial monitoring of pituitary size is important to successful treatment of pituitary adenomas. Both RT and hypophysectomy are more effective in treating smaller tumors.[8,25] Although many clinicians in the United States reserve surgery for patients that have failed medical management or have neurologic signs, Feldman and Nelson[72] state that TSH is the treatment of choice for dogs with PDH, limited only by availability of experienced pituitary teams. In the Netherlands, TSH is the first line of treatment of PDH in dogs.

Compared with FPA and NFPA, the benefits of surgery for NFSM are less well defined. The authors have experience in treating 10 known cases of dogs with a NFSM (discussed later).

Combination Therapy

At present there are no published reports of adjunctive therapy post-TSH for functional or NFSMs in small animals. van Rijn and colleagues[8] discuss the potential for identifying patients at higher risk for relapse, monitoring them, and following hypophysectomy with RT. In humans, alternative modalities for recurrent or persistent PDH after surgery include pituitary reintervention (second surgery), ketoconazole, radiotherapy, and bilateral adrenalectomy. Interventions to control recurrent or persistent PDH are tailored to the individual patient to achieve a long-lasting remission. In our practice, 5 dogs (2 FPA, 3 NFPA) all with a P/B ratio of greater than 0.74, have been treated with adjunct therapy (various RT protocols, n = 4; trilostane, n = 1) post-TSH with survival times ranging from 371 days to 1190 days, with 2 dogs still alive.

PREOPERATIVE TESTING AND DIAGNOSTICS

Preoperative diagnostics should confirm the presence of PDH or acromegaly, establish a baseline database, identify comorbidities, provide surgical planning, and be tailored to the individual patient. Diagnostics to establish the baseline and identify comorbidities may include the following:

- Complete blood count (CBC), serum chemistry profile, and urinalysis
- Urine culture and susceptibility
- Abdominal ultrasonography
- Three-view thoracic radiographs
- Echocardiogram and electrocardiogram (ECG)
- Coagulation screening (prothrombin time, activated partial thromboplastin time, thromboelastography)
- Blood type and cross match

Comorbidities (eg, chronic renal failure, cardiac disease, aspiration pneumonia, neoplasia) may alter overall surgical prognosis or exclude surgery from consideration.

Additional MR imaging using 1-mm slices for better visualization of vascular structures may be necessary.

TRANSSPHENOIDAL SURGERY (HYPOPHYSECTOMY)

This procedure has previously been published with illustrations.[6,38]

Patient Positioning

After localization of the pituitary fossa is complete,[6] the patient is placed in sternal recumbency with the maxilla suspended over a rubber-covered bar and taped in position.[38] The mandible is held open with roll gauze fixed to the table, and released every 30 minutes allowing passive range of motion for 1 minute.

Surgical Technique

The soft palate incision is retracted laterally using hook retractors (Lone Star, Stafford, TX). The oropharynx is packed with radiopaque gauze. The remainder of the surgery is performed using the VITOM system, a high-definition (HD) exoscope, for better magnification and visualization (Karl Storz-Endoskope, Tuttlingen, Germany), held in position by a pneumatic scope holder (Wingman Stryker, San Jose, CA). The surgeon operates looking at the HD screen during the remainder of the surgery (**Fig. 3**). Drilling of the basisphenoid bone is progressively enlarged using a high-speed drill with an elongated angled tip with a 2-mm diamond burr (Saber drill, Stryker, Kalamazoo, MI). The drilling typically creates an ovoid or rectangular opening of 1 to 1.5 cm in the rostrocaudal plane, and 4 to 6 mm in the lateral plane. The size of the defect is determined based on preoperative imaging. Lateral drilling is extended to the edges of the cavernous sinuses, although large tumors can make visualization of the cavernous sinus difficult. Drilling continues until a thin shelf of inner cortical bone remains over the pituitary fossa and dura. The remaining bone is removed with a ball-tipped probe, cup curettes (Tew Dissectors, KLS Martin, Jacksonville, FL) (**Fig. 4**), and 1-mm upbiting and downbiting 40° forward Kerrison rongeurs (Karl Storz-Endoskope). Bleeding is controlled with Gelfoam, bone wax, and micro–cotton-tipped applicators. Once the pituitary fossa is exposed, dura is

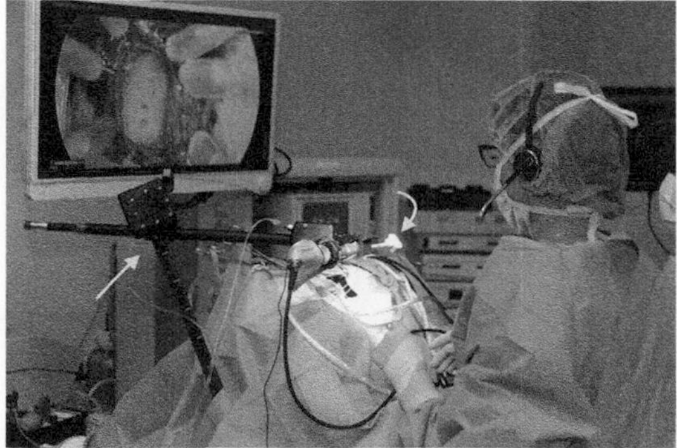

Fig. 3. Intraoperative view. Pneumatic scope holder, the Wingman (Stryker, San Jose, CA) (*straight arrow*), is holding a 90° VITOM exoscope (STORZ, Karl Storz-Endoskope, Tuttlingen, Germany) (*curved arrow*). The surgeon is drilling while using the HD screen and the VITOM exoscope, which increases visualization and magnification. (*Courtesy of* Karl Storz-Endoskope; with permission from STORZ; *Courtesy of* Stryker (San Jose, CA); with permission; and *Courtesy of* Henry Moore Jr, College of Veterinary Medicine/Biomedical Communications Unit, Washington State University, Pullman, WA.)

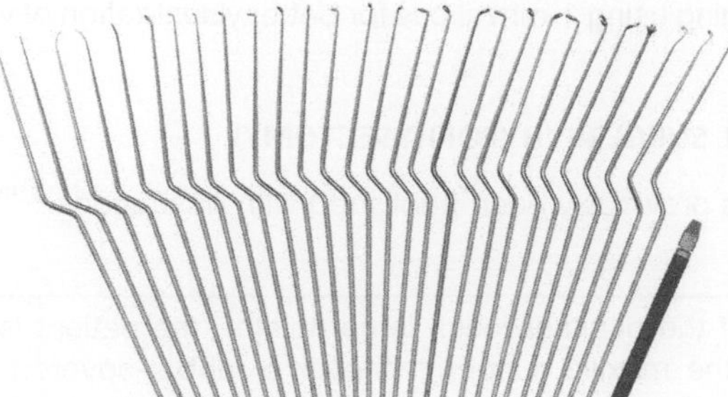

Fig. 4. Tew (KLS Martin) elongated and bayonetted neurosurgical instruments used for navigating around and in front of the exoscope while resecting tumor tissue. (*Courtesy of* the KLS Martin Group, Jacksonville, FL; with permission.)

opened using a microblade (Feather Safety Razor, Osaka, Japan) and the tumor is removed using small biopsy forceps, cup curettes, and suction (**Fig. 5**). Fine-diameter neurosurgical suction tips (2–7 Fr) with a slight curve and ports along the side of the cannula are useful in drawing tumor toward the center of the cavity. The NICO Myriad (NICO corporation, Indianapolis, IN), an aspiration device with side ports, is also useful in drawing tumor to midline away from the lateral and rostral margins, and assists in removing tumor without damaging the surrounding tissue.

The third ventricle and lateral walls of the hypothalamus are important landmarks to indicate complete tumor removal. Palpation of the dorsum sellae caudally is useful to determine whether the caudal aspect of the tumor has been removed. After tumor resection, the surgical site is lavaged with sterile saline (0.9% NaCl) solution and hemostasis is obtained by packing the site with Gelfoam. The bony defect is filled with a single layer of ACell Vet Scaffold corneal disc, 15 mm, porcine urinary bladder (ACell, Inc, Columbia, MD) tucked under the lip of the bone window. The soft palate is released from the LoneStar retractor and the edges are debrided and closed in 2 layers. The radiopaque gauze sponges are removed from the oropharynx (Video 1).

INTRAOPERATIVE MONITORING AND MANAGEMENT

Anesthetic protocols are tailored to the individual patient while avoiding increased intracranial pressure.[73] A coiled, cuffed endotracheal tube with a Murphy eye should

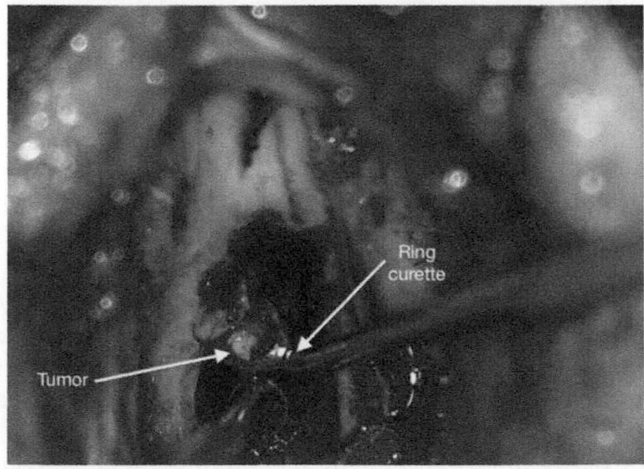

Fig. 5. Using a Tew ring curette to remove tumor.

be used to prevent the airway from becoming occluded from head positioning. To decrease aspiration, the pharynx and nasopharynx are intermittently suctioned during surgery. Anesthetic monitoring should include ECG, pulse oximetry, capnography, direct arterial blood pressure, central venous pressure (CVP), body temperature, urine output, urine specific gravity, packed cell volume (PCV), total solids (TS), lactate level, and serum electrolyte concentrations. Urine output, urine specific gravity, PCV, TS, lactate, and serum electrolytes are monitored hourly during surgery and intraoperative therapies modified as indicated. A balanced electrolyte solution such as lactated Ringer solution is recommended during surgery[73] and fluid rates of 5 to 10 mL/kg/h IV are titrated to effect. Fluids delivered at a rate of 10 mL/kg/h or higher may cause hypokalemia and potassium supplementation should be instituted. Central diabetes insipidus (CDI) can occur early in the postoperative period, which may worsen hypokalemia (discussed later). During surgery, pain, arrhythmias, hypotension, and increased intracranial pressure are treated appropriately. Before extubation, the oral cavity and pharynx are suctioned and the gauze is removed from the oropharynx.

POSTHYPOPHYSECTOMY MANAGEMENT

Patients are recovered in an intensive care unit and extubated when breathing spontaneously and able to protect their airways.[4,6] Postoperative management includes monitoring of vital signs, neurologic status, fluid intake and output, serum electrolyte concentrations, incision site, and tear production. Fluid balance can be assessed by measuring fluid intake, urine output, urine specific gravity, body weight, PCV, TS, lactate level, and CVP. Comorbidities (diabetes mellitus, chronic renal failure, or cardiac disease) are closely monitored. In the immediate postoperative period, patients are administered glucocorticoids, desmopressin acetate, antibiotics, analgesia, artificial tears, and IV fluid therapy (discussed later). Eating and drinking are encouraged, and, when the patient is able to tolerate oral medications, thyroid hormone supplementation is started and injectable formulations of glucocorticoids, antibiotics, and analgesics are converted to oral medications. Neurologic status, visual capabilities, and tear production are assessed and monitored at regular intervals following surgery.

POSTHYPOPHYSECTOMY COMPLICATIONS

Metabolic and Endocrine Complications

Central diabetes insipidus

Selective resection of pituitary masses is difficult in animals undergoing TSH and, therefore, the entire pituitary gland, including normal tissue, is frequently resected.[74] Following complete TSH, there is a sudden cessation of antidiuretic hormone (ADH) secretion from the neurohypophysis, which results in the development of CDI. The development of CDI following TSH may also reflect the sensitivity of the hypothalamic-neurohypophysis to surgical alterations in blood flow, edema, and manipulation of the pituitary stalk when there is incomplete resection of the pituitary gland and/or pituitary mass.[4] Most, if not all, animals develop CDI following TSH. It is usually a transient condition because ADH produced in the hypothalamus can still be secreted into the systemic circulation via the portal capillaries in the median eminence,[4,20] and CDI typically resolves within days to months following TSH.[4,6,20,74,75] Permanent disturbance of ADH secretion has also been documented,[4,20,74] can be caused by direct damage to the neurohypophysis or hypothalamic nuclei, and can depend on the size and location of the tumor and extent of the surgical resection.[4,20,74] Pituitary tumor extension that occurs in the dorsal direction and results in a prolonged mass effect of the tumor on the hypothalamic nuclei may result in damage to the ADH-producing nuclei, such as the paraventricular and supraoptic nuclei.[20] Efforts to completely remove dorsally located tumor tissue in animals with large pituitary tumors may also lead to damage to the pituitary stalk and cell bodies in the hypothalamic nuclei, leading to the development of permanent CDI.[20,76] The incidence of permanent CDI seems to be higher in dogs with a P/B ratio greater than 0.31 than in dogs with a P/B ratio less than or equal to 0.31.[20,74]

The preferred agent for treating postoperative CDI is desmopressin acetate (DDAVP), a synthetic vasopressin analogue. Compared with the natural hormone, DDAVP has a greater antidiuretic activity, longer duration of action, fewer pressor actions and adverse effects, and a greater capacity to cause platelet aggregation and the release of hemostatic factors.[77,78] DDAVP is a highly selective agonist for vasopressin V2 receptors, making it an effective treatment of CDI.[79] When given intravenously or subcutaneously to human patients with CDI, DDAVP induces antidiuresis that lasts from 8 to 24 hours.[80] The duration of action is similar in dogs and cats.[81,82] DDAVP is available for clinical use via nasal or conjunctival sac administration as well as orally, subcutaneously, and via IV administration.[79,83] Although administration of medication to dogs and cats via the intranasal route is possible, it is not well tolerated in many cases. Therefore, the intranasal drops placed in the conjunctival sac are a more suitable alternative. Poor or erratic response in some dogs and cats can be caused by incomplete absorption caused by conditions that alter the absorptive capacity of the nasal mucosa, or by atresia or blockage of the nasolacrimal duct,[79] as well as concurrent administration of ophthalmic artificial tear ointment for the treatment of keratoconjunctivitis sicca (KCS), which can occur following TSH. Because of individual differences in absorption and metabolism, the dose required to achieve complete, around-the-clock control varies from animal to animal. Usually 1 to 4 drops of the intranasal solution (0.01%) administered 2 to 3 times daily in the conjunctival sac is sufficient to control the signs of CDI.[79] The maximal effect of the drug is evident 6 to 10 hours after the administration and the duration of effect of DDAVP varies from 8 to 24 hours.[81,82,84–86] The oral preparation of DDAVP is available as 0.1-mg and 0.2-mg tablets. Each 0.1-mg tablet of DDAVP is comparable with 5 μg (1 large drop) of the intranasal DDAVP preparation and it is generally dosed at 0.1 to 0.2 mg orally every 8 to 12 hours.[79] The parenteral dose of DDAVP for CDI is 0.5 to 2 μg subcutaneously or IV every 12 to 24 hours.[79] The dose range given can be used as a starting point for the treatment of CDI following TSS. The dose is then adjusted based on changes in urine output, urine specific gravity, body weight, PCV, TS, and sodium concentrations. DDAVP therapy is titrated over time to the lowest dose that controls the patient's clinic signs and is continued until the polyuria is resolved, the patient is able to concentrate urine, and serum sodium concentrations remain in the normal reference range.

DDAVP is generally safe for dogs and cats with CDI. The main complications of administration are the development of water intoxication and hyponatremia. These complications can result from overzealous administration of DDAVP in conjunction with failure to reduce IV fluid administration. Serum sodium concentrations should be monitored after the initiation of DDAVP therapy. If hyponatremia develops, treatment with DDAVP should be delayed or temporarily stopped.[79]

Hypernatremia

Hypernatremia can occur following TSH because of ADH deficiency and results from hypotonic or pure water loss via polyuria. In the immediate postoperative period, increasing serum sodium concentrations can reflect the presence of CDI and the development of hypernatremia can be prevented by the administration of DDAVP and appropriate fluid therapy. Prompt diagnosis and treatment of CDI are essential to prevent the extreme alterations in sodium and water balance that accompany this disorder. CDI is easily recognized by the polyuria that develops early in the postoperative period, commonly occurring within the first 24 hours after TSS.[75] The authors' have noted that the development of CDI can occur rapidly following TSS, within 1 to 4 hours after surgery. Urine output can be dramatic (>10 mL/kg/h) and urine specific gravity quickly becomes hyposthenuric (frequently <1.005); serum sodium concentrations can also rapidly increase (>160 mEq/L).[74,75] Basic requirements of successful management of CDI include meticulous assessment of fluid intake and output, measurement of body weight, and assessment of serum electrolyte concentrations. A urinary catheter with a closed collection system is placed preoperatively to monitor urine output intraoperatively and postoperatively. Initially in the postoperative period fluid intake, urine output, urine specific gravity, body weight, PCV, TS, CVP, and serum electrolyte concentrations are monitored every 3 hours. Once CDI develops, the volume and/or rate of IV fluid therapy may need to be increased to keep up with urinary losses. IV replacement of fluid losses is typically done with lactated Ringer solution, 0.45% NaCl, 5% dextrose in water, or a combination of these fluid solutions. Patients that can take oral fluids should be allowed to regulate their own intake and water balance. This regulation helps to normalize fluid and sodium imbalances.[4,6,74] Serum sodium concentrations should be checked every 3 hours until a consistent trend of change has been established, and then sodium monitoring can be adjusted accordingly.

Hypokalemia

Hypokalemia can be seen postoperatively if the patient is on a high rate of IV fluids or with the development of CDI and resultant polyuria that develops.[75] Potassium chloride is typically supplemented in the patient's IV fluids on an as-needed basis based on the patient's serum potassium concentration. Serum potassium concentrations should be monitored every 6 to 24 hours based on the degree of abnormality and desired rate of supplementation. Once a consistent trend of change has been established, then potassium monitoring can be adjusted accordingly.

Hypoadrenocorticism

The total resection of the pituitary gland that occurs with TSH not only induces CDI but also hypoadrenocorticism, which requires careful postoperative management primarily by hormone supplementation therapy.[7] Treatment consists of hydrocortisone sodium succinate (Solu-Cortef) at a dose of 1 mg/kg IV before the start of surgery and is continued at the same dose every 6 hours for the first 48 to 72 hours. When the patient is able to tolerate oral medications, it is then switched to cortisone acetate at a dose of 0.5 to 1 mg/kg orally every 12 to 24 hours. Over the next 4 weeks the dose of cortisone acetate is gradually tapered to 0.25 mg/kg orally every 12 to 24 hours. Long term, the dose can generally be further reduced to 0.10 to 0.5 mg/kg orally every 24 hours. Dose adjustments are based on endocrine monitoring and clinical status. Therapy is likely to be lifelong unless there is regrowth of the FPA.

Hypothyroidism

Complete resection of the pituitary gland also results in hypothyroidism and requires postoperative management and monitoring. Treatment consists of starting levothyroxine at a dose of 0.02 mg/kg orally every 12 to 24 hours, once the patient is able to tolerate oral medications. The dose of levothyroxine is titrated based on thyroid function testing and typically this is a lifelong therapy for the patient.

Neurologic Complications

Increased intracranial pressure

Postoperatively each patient is monitored for signs of increased intracranial pressure. Initially, repeat assessments of mental status, cranial nerve status, pupil size, pupillary light reflexes, and signs of the Cushing reflex are monitored every 3 to 6 hours until neurologic status is deemed stable for 24 hours. Serial neurologic examinations are crucial to a successful outcome because neurologic status can change rapidly and dramatically in the first 24 hours postsurgery, which may require medical intervention. If there are concerns that increased intracranial pressure is present, mannitol is given at a dose of 1 g/kg IV over 15 to 30 minutes and/or hypertonic saline (7.5% solution) can be given at a dose of 3 to 5 mL/kg IV over 5 to 10 minutes. Because of the likelihood that CDI and subsequent hypernatremia could develop, mannitol is generally the preferred treatment in this situation to avoid the development or worsening of hypernatremia.

In the authors' experience, most patients recover neurologically fairly rapidly assuming there are no secondary complications. Patients are usually ambulatory shortly after surgery but may have worsening of proprioception and paresis. These deficits are usually transient and patients are often back to their initial presentation statuses within the first week after surgery.

Blindness

The optic chiasm and optic nerves are parasellar structures that can be damaged while performing TSS, which can lead to blindness. Blindness can result from direct damage, neuropraxia, or secondary damage via postoperative hemorrhage or cerebral edema causing compression of the optic chiasm or nerves. As long as the optic chiasm or optic nerves have not been directly damaged, the condition is typically transient and resolves within a few days.[6,70]

Procedural-related Complications

Keratoconjunctivitis sicca

Keratoconjunctivitis sicca is a complication that can occur following TSS. Its development has been attributed to direct (traumatic) or indirect (ischemic) neuropraxia of the major petrosal nerves, resulting in decreased tear production from the lacrimal glands.[38] Previous investigators have reported that decreased tear production occurred more frequently in the left eye than in the right eye.[4,20,38] A theory for the occurrence of KCS following TSH is that it is caused by ischemic damage to the pterygopalatine ganglion from long-standing pressure on the mandibular coronoid process in the retrobulbar area caused by the open-mouth approach of the surgery.[20] However, this does not explain the predominance of KCS in the left eyes.[20]

In most cases, the decrease in tear production is transient following TSS.[4,20] At present there does not seem to be a relationship between the frequency of KCS development and size of the pituitary mass.[20]

Routine preoperative and postoperative monitoring of Schirmer tear test values should be performed on each patient. Tear production can be monitored on the first day following TSH and then every 2 days while the patient is hospitalized. Ophthalmologic treatment with artificial tears is started postoperatively and continued until tear production has normalized. Initially, artificial tears are instilled into each eye every 6 hours and the frequency of administration is reduced as tear production improves.

Aspiration pneumonia

Aspiration pneumonia has been documented in patients following TSH,[4,20,87] and this complication can potentially be life threatening. It is unknown why this complication occurs; however, it is possible that the cause is multifactorial. Possible causes include immunosuppression of dogs with PDH, medications given to the patient that predispose to vomiting and/or regurgitation, copious lavage of the oral cavity during surgery, and prolonged length of surgery and time under anesthesia. If aspiration pneumonia develops postoperatively, broad-spectrum antibiotic therapy should be instituted and supplemental oxygen therapy should be started if the patient is hypoxemic. Nebulization, coupage, and recumbency care can also be considered as additional therapies.

Soft palate dehiscence

Complete dehiscence of the soft palate or development of an oronasal fistula are also potential complications of TSS.[12,73] Complete dehiscence can be seen on the second to fourth day following surgery[73] and the oronasal fistula typically reveals itself several days postoperatively. The soft palate incision is monitored daily until the patient is discharged from the hospital to assess for dehiscence of the surgical site. Clinical signs that may indicate the presence of soft palate dehiscence include nasal discharge, sneezing, and food or water coming from the nose after eating or drinking. If untreated, the patient may develop rhinitis, middle ear infections, or aspiration pneumonia.[12,73] The incidence of dehiscence can be minimized by not placing undue traction on the soft palate edges when the retractor is inserted during surgery. In small dogs, the use of retention sutures instead of instrument retractors is recommended.[73] Debridement of the edges of the soft palate before closure is important to decrease the incidence of dehiscence, as well as a 2-layer closure. If soft palate dehiscence occurs, debridement and resuturing are done as soon as possible.

Surgical site infection

Patients are typically placed on antibiotic therapy following TSS because of the surgical location (mouth/soft palate) being contaminated with bacteria. Antibiotics with a spectrum appropriate for oral flora should be used. The authors use ampicillin and sulbactam at a dose of 30 to 50 mg/kg IV every 6 to 8 hours or clindamycin at a dose of 5 to 10 mg/kg IV every 12 hours for 48 to 72 hours following TSS. When the patient can tolerate oral medication, amoxicillin and clavulanic acid at a dose of 13.75 mg/kg by mouth every 12 hours or clindamycin at a dose of 5 to 10 mg/kg by mouth every 12 hours is given for 10 days.

Pain

Following TSS it is vital that all postoperative pain be adequately controlled and the analgesia protocol be tailored to the individual patient. Options include, but are not limited to, buprenorphine, butorphanol, methadone, fentanyl, or sufentanil. It is the authors' clinical impression that most patients experience mild pain and discomfort following TSS. Analgesia should be titrated to adequately treat the patient's pain but also to prevent excessive sedation postoperatively (which can make neurologic assessment difficult) and the other side effects of opioids (vomiting, regurgitation, inappetence, ileus, and constipation). When able to tolerate oral medication, the patient can be transitioned to tramadol or gabapentin. Other oral analgesics can be administered as well, as long as there are no contraindications for their use.

Inappetence

Eating and drinking the day following surgery is encouraged. As previously mentioned, oral water intake helps to normalize any hypernatremia and fluid imbalances that are present. Because of the location of the surgical site, only soft food and no chew toys are recommended for 4 weeks following TS to allow healing of the soft palate incision.

If caloric or fluid intake is inadequate, feeding tube placement can be considered to facilitate the patient being discharged from the hospital.

Fluid overload

Cardiac abnormalities such as left ventricular concentric hypertrophy, left atrial enlargement, and diastolic dysfunction have been noted in cats with hypersomatotropism.[88,89] Therefore, these cats are at risk for the development of fluid overload and subsequent pulmonary edema and/or pleural effusion. Kenny and colleagues[71] reported that 4 of 19 cats (21%) developed congestive heart failure after hypophysectomy. All 4 cases occurred before the reduction of postoperative IV fluid volume.[71] To prevent the development of fluid overload, fluid intake and output, urine specific gravity, body weight, PCV, TS, CVP, respiratory rate and effort, and auscultation of the lungs should be closely monitored and assessed. If fluid overload develops, appropriate therapies can include reducing or discontinuing IV fluid therapy, furosemide administration, and supplemental oxygen therapy.

LONG-TERM FOLLOW-UP

Consistent and long-term follow-up is vital to ensure the best outcome for each patient. The authors recommend reevaluation following hospital discharge at 1 week and at 1, 3, 6, 9, and 12 months postoperatively and yearly thereafter. Reevaluation includes physical examination, CBC, serum chemistry profile, urinalysis, and Schirmer tear test until tear production has normalized. Except for the 1-week recheck, thyroid function (serum total T4, free T4, and TSH concentrations 12 hours after previous dose of levothyroxine given) and hypothalamic adrenocortical function (urinary corticoid/creatinine ratio [UCCR] 24 hours after previous dose of cortisone given and endogenous ACTH concentrations) are assessed at every reevaluation for dogs and cats that present with PDH, acromegaly, or NFSM. For cats with acromegaly, IGF-1 concentrations are also reevaluated. These cats may also need blood glucose monitoring and insulin dose assessment when they are reevaluated. At 3, 6, 9, and 12 months, and then yearly thereafter, MRI is recommended to monitor for regrowth of the tumor. If tumor regrowth is noted, RT may be indicated. Long-term follow-up should be tailored to each patient and additional diagnostics may be necessary.

PROGNOSIS

Survival data were gathered from a literature search and authors' experience. Survival is defined in these studies as patients surviving 4 weeks postsurgery.[4]

Dogs with Pituitary-dependent Hyperadrenocorticism

From 1993 to 2003, Meij and his group at Utrecht University performed surgery in 306 dogs with PDH (median P/B ratio of 0.43) with a remission rate of 92%, a procedural mortality of 9%, and a recurrence rate of 28%.[8] Survival and DFI correlated negatively with pituitary size, making the P/B ratio an important preoperative prognosticator. However, with increasing experience for larger tumors, TSH remains an option to debulk the mass and control neurologic signs and hypercortisolism.[8] Prognostic factors for dogs associated with increased risk of PDH-related death are old age, large pituitary size, and high preoperative concentrations of plasma ACTH.[5] Factors associated with disease recurrence, and therefore predictors of long-term remission, are large pituitary size, thick sphenoid bone, high UCCR, and high concentration of plasma α-melanocyte–stimulating hormone.[5] Mortality in humans treated for

Cushing's disease was higher than for patients treated for NFPA, suggesting that overexposure to cortisol is associated with increased mortality.[90]

Thirty-four dogs from West Los Angeles Animal Hospital and Washington State University Veterinary Teaching Hospital with PDH associated with an enlarged pituitary tumor (median P/B ratio, 0.74; range, 0.35–1.54) undergoing TSH using an HD video telescope had a median survival of 471 days (range, 0–1095 days; 5 still alive) with a procedural mortality of 20%.[91] Twenty-five of 26 of these cases reported by Mamelak and colleagues[6] had sustained remission at 1-year follow-up.

Cats with Pituitary-dependent Hyperadrenocorticism

Meij and colleagues[12] described 7 cats with PDH that underwent TSH. Two cats died within 4 weeks of surgery from nonrelated disease. All 5 remaining cats went into remission. Recurrence occurred in 1 cat after 19 months and the cat died 28 months after surgery. One cat died of anemia and 1 from complications secondary to soft palate dehiscence. Remission in the 2 remaining cats was sustained at 15 months and 46 months.

Cats with Hypersomatotropism (Acromegaly)

Kenny and colleagues[71] reported on 21 cats with acromegaly treated with TSH. Eighteen of the 21 (86%) survived the surgery and perioperative period. Fourteen of the surviving 18 (78%) went into diabetic remission with the remaining 4 having a lower insulin requirement.[71] After TSH, 8 cats with hypertrophic cardiac changes associated with acromegaly had mostly reversible changes on repeat echocardiography.[89]

Nonfunctional Sellar Mass

Our pituitary group has performed TSS in 10 dogs with an NFSM (median P/B ratio, 1.1; range, 0.66–1.38).[91] Seven had an NFPA and 1 each had meningioma, ependymoma, and a craniopharyngioma.[91,92] Overall survival rate was 60%. The survival rate of the dogs with NFPA was 86% (6 out of 7) with a median survival time of 207 days (range, 0–1190 days; 2 still alive). The dog with the meningioma survived 232 days. The dogs with the ependymoma and craniopharyngioma did not recover from anesthesia. It would be important to be able to predict which NFSMs are pituitary adenomas or meningiomas compared with other sellar masses because survival post-surgery may be dramatically different. Survival of dogs with NFPA and meningioma combined was 80% compared with 0% with other sellar masses. It is important to remember that the most common NFSM is a pituitary adenoma and the second most common is meningioma.[10] To the authors' knowledge there are no reported cases of cats treated for NFSM.

SUMMARY

TSS is a viable option with excellent outcomes possible in dogs and cats with functional or nonfunctional pituitary or sellar masses. Dogs and cats with a functional pituitary mass can be treated medically, with RT, or with surgery. These decisions are made between client and veterinarian with the best interests of the patient in mind. Surgery addresses both the endocrine disturbances of a functional mass and the mass effect, if present, that can eventually lead to neurologic dysfunction. A patient with a nonfunctional mass is usually not presented until the mass is large enough to cause neurologic deficits by compressing the surrounding brain. Surgery in this situation addresses the mass effect and neurologic signs associated with the space-occupying tumor. Overall, surgery does carry a risk and may be cost-prohibitive to some owners; however, it is the only way to treat the pituitary or sellar mass directly. Patient selection and an experienced surgical and medical team are imperative to a successful outcome.

SUPPLEMENTARY DATA

Supplementary data related to this article can be found online at https://doi.org/10.1016/j.cvsm.2017.08.006.

REFERENCES

1. Niebauer GW, Evans SM. Transsphenoidal hypophysectomy in the dog. A new technique. Vet Surg 1988;17:296–303.
2. Niebauer GW, Eigenmann JE, Van Winkle TJ. Study of long-term survival after transsphenoidal hypophysectomy in clinically normal dogs. Am J Vet Res 1990;51:677–81.
3. Lantz GC, Ihle SL, Nelson RW, et al. Transsphenoidal hypophysectomy in the clinically normal dog. Am J Vet Res 1988;49:1134–42.
4. Meij BP, Voorhout G, van den Ingh TS, et al. Results of transsphenoidal hypophysectomy in 52 dogs with pituitary-dependent hyperadrenocorticism. Vet Surg 1998;27:246–61.
5. Hanson JM, Teske E, Voorhout G, et al. Prognostic factors for outcome after transsphenoidal hypophysectomy in dogs with pituitary-dependent hyperadrenocorticism. J Neurosurg 2007;107:830–40.
6. Mamelak AN, Owen TJ, Bruyette D. Transsphenoidal surgery using a high definition video telescope for pituitary adenomas in dogs with pituitary dependent hypercortisolism: methods and results. Vet Surg 2014;43:369–79.
7. Hara Y, Teshima T, Taoda T, et al. Efficacy of transsphenoidal surgery on endocrinological status and serum chemistry parameters in dogs with Cushing's disease. J Vet Med Sci 2010;72:397–404.
8. van Rijn SJ, Galac S, Tryfonidou MA, et al. The influence of pituitary size on outcome after transsphenoidal hypophysectomy in a large cohort of dogs with pituitary-dependent hypercortisolism. J Vet Intern Med 2016;30:989–95.
9. Snyder JM, Lipitz L, Skorupski KA, et al. Secondary intracranial neoplasia in the dog: 177 cases (1986-2003). J Vet Intern Med 2008;22:172–7.
10. Rissi DR. A retrospective study of skull base neoplasia in 42 dogs. J Vet Diagn Invest 2015;27:743–8.
11. Melian C, Perez-Alenza MD, Peterson ME. Hyperadrenocorticism in dogs. In: Ettinger SJ, Feldman EC, editors. Textbook of veterinary internal medicine. 7th edition. St Louis (MO): Elsevier Saunders; 2010. p. 1816–40.
12. Meij BP, Voorhout G, van den Ingh TSGAM, et al. Transsphenoidal hypophysectomy for treatment of pituitary-dependent hyperadrenocorticism in 7 cats. Vet Surg 2001;30:72–86.
13. Meij BP, Auriemma E, Grinwis G, et al. Successful treatment of acromegaly in a diabetic cat with transsphenoidal hypophysectomy. J Feline Med Surg 2010;12:406–10.
14. Meij BP, van der Vlugt-Meijer RH, van den Ingh TS, et al. Somatotroph and corticotroph pituitary adenoma (double adenoma) in a cat with diabetes mellitus and hyperadrenocorticism. J Comp Pathol 2004;130:209–15.
15. Niessen SJ, Petrie G, Gaudiano F, et al. Feline acromegaly: an underdiagnosed endocrinopathy? J Vet Intern Med 2007;21:899–905.

16. Niessen SJ, Forcada Y, Mantis P, et al. Studying cat (*Felis catus*) diabetes: beware of the acromegalic imposter. PLoS One 2015;10:e0127794.
17. Bertoy EH, Feldman EC, Nelson RW, et al. Magnetic resonance imaging of the brain in dogs with recently diagnosed but untreated pituitary-dependent hyperadrenocorticism. J Am Vet Med Assoc 1995;206:651–6.
18. Famini P, Maya MM, Melmed S. Pituitary magnetic resonance imaging for sellar and parasellar masses: ten-year experience in 2598 patients. J Clin Endocrinol Metab 2011;96:1633–41.
19. Sato A, Teshima T, Ishino H, et al. A magnetic resonance imaging-based classification system for indication of trans-sphenoidal hypophysectomy in canine pituitary-dependent hypercortisolism. J Small Anim Pract 2016;57:240–6.
20. Hanson JM, van 't HM, Voorhout G, et al. Efficacy of transsphenoidal hypophysectomy in treatment of dogs with pituitary-dependent hyperadrenocorticism. J Vet Intern Med 2005;19:687–94.
21. Graves TK. Hypercortisolism in cats (feline Cushing's syndrome). In: Ettinger SJ, Feldman EC, editors. Textbook of veterinary internal medicine. 7th edition. St Louis (MO): Elsevier Saunders; 2010. p. 1840–7.
22. Kooistra HS. Growth hormone disorders: acromegaly and pituitary dwarfism. In: Ettinger SJ, Feldman EC, editors. Textbook of small animal internal medicine. 7th edition. St Louis (MO): Saunders Elsevier; 2010. p. 1711–6.
23. Kipperman BS, Feldman EC, Dybdal NO, et al. Pituitary tumor size, neurologic signs, and relation to endocrine test results in dogs with pituitary-dependent hyperadrenocorticism: 43 cases (1980-1990). J Am Vet Med Assoc 1992;201: 762–7.
24. Bertoy EH, Feldman EC, Nelson RW, et al. One-year follow-up evaluation of magnetic resonance imaging of the brain in dogs with pituitary-dependent hyperadrenocorticism. J Am Vet Med Assoc 1996;208:1268–73.
25. Kent MS, Bommarito D, Feldman E, et al. Survival, neurologic response, and prognostic factors in dogs with pituitary masses treated with radiation therapy and untreated dogs. J Vet Intern Med 2007;21:1027–33.
26. Behrend EN, Kooistra HS, Nelson R, et al. Diagnosis of spontaneous canine hyperadrenocorticism: 2012 ACVIM consensus statement (small animal). J Vet Intern Med 2013;27:1292–304.
27. Wood FD, Pollard RE, Uerling MR, et al. Diagnostic imaging findings and endocrine test results in dogs with pituitary-dependent hyperadrenocorticism that did or did not have neurologic abnormalities: 157 cases (1989-2005). J Am Vet Med Assoc 2007;231:1081–5.
28. Duesberg CA, Feldman EC, Nelson RW, et al. Magnetic resonance imaging for diagnosis of pituitary macrotumors in dogs. J Am Vet Med Assoc 1995;206: 657–62.
29. Sarfaty D, Carrillo JM, Peterson ME. Neurologic, endocrinologic, and pathologic findings associated with large pituitary tumors in dogs: eight cases (1976-1984). J Am Vet Med Assoc 1988;193:854–6.
30. Ihle SL. Pituitary corticotroph macrotumors. Diagnosis and treatment. Vet Clin North Am Small Anim Pract 1997;27:287–97.
31. Lynch GL, Broome MR, Scagliotti RH. What is your diagnosis? Mass originating from the pituitary fossa. J Am Vet Med Assoc 2006;228:1681–2.
32. Seruca C, Rodenas S, Leiva M, et al. Acute postretinal blindness: ophthalmologic, neurologic, and magnetic resonance imaging findings in dogs and cats (seven cases). Vet Ophthalmol 2010;13:307–14.

33. Moore SA, O'Brien DP. Canine pituitary macrotumors. Compend Contin Educ Vet 2008;30:33–40 [quiz: 41].
34. Church D, Niessen S. Acromegaly in cats. In: Rand J, editor. Clinical endocrinology of companion animals. Ames (IO): Wiley-Blackwell; 2013. p. 427–35.
35. Kraft SL, Gavin PR, DeHaan C, et al. Retrospective review of 50 canine intracranial tumors evaluated by magnetic resonance imaging. J Vet Intern Med 1997;11: 218–25.
36. Nakamura T, Schorner W, Bittner RC, et al. The value of paramagnetic contrast agent gadolinium-DTPA in the diagnosis of pituitary adenomas. Neuroradiology 1988;30:481–6.
37. Macpherson P, Hadley DM, Teasdale E, et al. Pituitary microadenomas. Does gadolinium enhance their demonstration? Neuroradiology 1989;31:293–8.
38. Meij BP, Voorhout G, Van den Ingh TS, et al. Transsphenoidal hypophysectomy in beagle dogs: evaluation of a microsurgical technique. Vet Surg 1997;26:295–309.
39. van der Vlugt-Meijer RH, Meij BP, van den Ingh TS, et al. Dynamic computed tomography of the pituitary gland in dogs with pituitary-dependent hyperadrenocorticism. J Vet Intern Med 2003;17:773–80.
40. Meij B, Voorhout G, Rijnberk A. Progress in transsphenoidal hypophysectomy for treatment of pituitary-dependent hyperadrenocorticism in dogs and cats. Mol Cell Endocrinol 2002;197:89–96.
41. van der Vlugt-Meijer RH, Voorhout G, Meij BP. Imaging of the pituitary gland in dogs with pituitary-dependent hyperadrenocorticism. Mol Cell Endocrinol 2002; 197:81–7.
42. Hullinger R. The endocrine system. In: Evans HE, editor. Miller's anatomy of the dog. 3rd edition. Philadelphia: WB Saunders; 1993. p. 559–85.
43. Kippenes H, Gavin PR, Kraft SL, et al. Mensuration of the normal pituitary gland from magnetic resonance images in 96 dogs. Vet Radiol Ultrasound 2001;42: 130–3.
44. Kooistra HS, Voorhout G, Mol JA, et al. Correlation between impairment of glucocorticoid feedback and the size of the pituitary gland in dogs with pituitary-dependent hyperadrenocorticism. J Endocrinol 1997;152:387–94.
45. Pollard RE, Reilly CM, Uerling MR, et al. Cross-sectional imaging characteristics of pituitary adenomas, invasive adenomas and adenocarcinomas in dogs: 33 cases (1988-2006). J Vet Intern Med 2010;24:160–5.
46. Chen AV, Owen TJ, Martin LG, et al. Magnetic resonance imaging characteristics of histopathologically confirmed non-functional sellar masses in dogs. J Vet Intern Med 2016;30:1939.
47. Dwyer AJ, Frank JA, Doppman JL, et al. Pituitary adenomas in patients with Cushing disease: initial experience with Gd-DTPA-enhanced MR imaging. Radiology 1987;163:421–6.
48. Taoda T, Hara Y, Masuda H, et al. Magnetic resonance imaging assessment of pituitary posterior lobe displacement in dogs with pituitary-dependent hyperadrenocorticism. J Vet Med Sci 2011;73:725–31.
49. Hasegawa T, Ito H, Shoin K, et al. Diagnosis of an "isodense" pituitary microadenoma by dynamic CT scanning. Case report. J Neurosurg 1984;60:424–7.
50. Escourolle H, Abecassis JP, Bertagna X, et al. Comparison of computerized tomography and magnetic resonance imaging for the examination of the pituitary gland in patients with Cushing's disease. Clin Endocrinol (Oxf) 1993;39:307–13.
51. Fischetti AJ, Gisselman K, Peterson ME. CT and MRI evaluation of skull bones and soft tissues in six cats with presumed acromegaly versus 12 unaffected cats. Vet Radiol Ultrasound 2012;53:535–9.

52. Tamura S, Tamura Y, Suzuoka N, et al. Multiple metastases of thyroid cancer in the cranium and pituitary gland in two dogs. J Small Anim Pract 2007;48:237–9.
53. den Hertog E, Braakman JC, Teske E, et al. Results of non-selective adrenocorticolysis by o,p'-DDD in 129 dogs with pituitary-dependent hyperadrenocorticism. Vet Rec 1999;144:12–7.
54. Bruyette DS, Ruehl WW, Entriken T, et al. Management of canine pituitary-dependent hyperadrenocorticism with l-deprenyl (Anipryl). Vet Clin North Am Small Anim Pract 1997;27:273–86.
55. Lien YH, Huang HP. Use of ketoconazole to treat dogs with pituitary-dependent hyperadrenocorticism: 48 cases (1994-2007). J Am Vet Med Assoc 2008;233: 1896–901.
56. Alenza DP, Arenas C, Lopez ML, et al. Long-term efficacy of trilostane administered twice daily in dogs with pituitary-dependent hyperadrenocorticism. J Am Anim Hosp Assoc 2006;42:269–76.
57. Neiger R, Ramsey I, O'Connor J, et al. Trilostane treatment of 78 dogs with pituitary-dependent hyperadrenocorticism. Vet Rec 2002;150:799–804.
58. Mellett Keith AM, Bruyette D, Stanley S. Trilostane therapy for treatment of spontaneous hyperadrenocorticism in cats: 15 cases (2004-2012). J Vet Intern Med 2013;27:1471–7.
59. Castillo VA, Gallelli MF. Corticotroph adenoma in the dog: pathogenesis and new therapeutic possibilities. Res Vet Sci 2010;88:26–32.
60. Castillo V, Theodoropoulou M, Stalla J, et al. Effect of SOM230 (pasireotide) on corticotropic cells: action in dogs with Cushing's disease. Neuroendocrinology 2011;94:124–36.
61. Gostelow R, Scudder C, Keyte S, et al. Pasireotide long-acting release treatment for diabetic cats with underlying hypersomatotropism. J Vet Intern Med 2017;31: 355–64.
62. Nagata N, Kojima K, Yuki M. Comparison of survival times for dogs with pituitary-dependent hyperadrenocorticism in a primary-care hospital: treated with trilostane versus untreated. J Vet Intern Med 2017;31:22–8.
63. Tamura S, Tamura Y, Ohoka A, et al. A canine case of skull base meningioma treated with hydroxyurea. J Vet Med Sci 2007;69:1313–5.
64. Goossens MM, Feldman EC, Theon AP, et al. Efficacy of cobalt 60 radiotherapy in dogs with pituitary-dependent hyperadrenocorticism. J Am Vet Med Assoc 1998; 212:374–6.
65. de Fornel P, Delisle F, Devauchelle P, et al. Effects of radiotherapy on pituitary corticotroph macrotumors in dogs: a retrospective study of 12 cases. Can Vet J 2007;48:481–6.
66. Mariani CL, Schubert TA, House RA, et al. Frameless stereotactic radiosurgery for the treatment of primary intracranial tumours in dogs. Vet Comp Oncol 2013;13: 409–23.
67. Goossens MM, Feldman EC, Nelson RW, et al. Cobalt 60 irradiation of pituitary gland tumors in three cats with acromegaly. J Am Vet Med Assoc 1998;213: 374–6.
68. Brearley MJ, Polton GA, Littler RM, et al. Coarse fractionated radiation therapy for pituitary tumours in cats: a retrospective study of 12 cases. Vet Comp Oncol 2006;4:209–17.
69. Sellon RK, Fidel J, Houston R, et al. Linear-accelerator-based modified radiosurgical treatment of pituitary tumors in cats: 11 cases (1997-2008). J Vet Intern Med 2009;23:1038–44.

70. Hara Y, Tagawa M, Masuda H, et al. Transsphenoidal hypophysectomy for four dogs with pituitary ACTH-producing adenoma. J Vet Med Sci 2003;65:801–4.
71. Kenny P, Scudder C, Keyte S, et al. Treatment of feline hypersomatotropism. Efficacy, morbidity and mortality of hypophysectomy. J Vet Intern Med 2015;29: 1271.
72. Feldman E, Nelson R. Canine hyperadrenocorticism (Cushing's syndrome). In: Feldman E, Nelson R, editors. Canine and feline endocrinology and reproduction. 3rd edition. St Louis (MO): Saunders; 2004. p. 252–357.
73. Niebauer GW. Hypophysectomy. In: Slatter D, editor. Textbook of small animal surgery. 3rd edition. Philadelphia: WB Saunders; 2003. p. 1677–94.
74. Teshima T, Hara Y, Taoda T, et al. Central diabetes insipidus after transsphenoidal surgery in dogs with Cushing's disease. J Vet Med Sci 2011;73:33–9.
75. Hara Y, Masuda H, Taoda T, et al. Prophylactic efficacy of desmopressin acetate for diabetes insipidus after hypophysectomy in the dog. J Vet Med Sci 2003;65: 17–22.
76. Nemergut EC, Zuo Z, Jane JA Jr, et al. Predictors of diabetes insipidus after transsphenoidal surgery: a review of 881 patients. J Neurosurg 2005;103:448–54.
77. Sawyer WH, Acosta M, Manning M. Structural changes in the arginine vasopressin molecule that prolong its antidiuretic action. Endocrinology 1974;95: 140–9.
78. Kimbrough RD Jr, Cash WD, Branda LA, et al. Synthesis and biological properties of 1-desamino-8-lysine-vasopressin. J Biol Chem 1963;238:1411–4.
79. Nichols R, Hohenhaus AE. Use of the vasopressin analogue desmopressin for polyuria and bleeding disorders. J Am Vet Med Assoc 1994;205:168–73.
80. Richardson DW, Robinson AG. Desmopressin. Ann Intern Med 1985;103:228–39.
81. Krause KH. The use of desmopressin in diagnosis and treatment of diabetes insipidus in cats. Compend Contin Educ Vet 1986;9:752–8.
82. Greene CE, Wong PL, Finco DR. Diagnosis and treatment of diabetes insipidus in two dogs using two synthetic analogs of antidiuretic hormone. J Am Anim Hosp Assoc 1979;15:371–7.
83. Rado JP, Marosi I, Fisher J. Comparison of the antidiuretic effects of single intravenous and intranasal doses of DDAVP in diabetes insipidus. Pharmacology 1977;15:40–5.
84. Feldman E, Nelson R. Water metabolism and diabetes insipidus. In: Feldman E, Nelson R, editors. Canine and feline endocrinology and reproduction. 3rd edition. St Louis (MO): Saunders; 2004. p. 2–44.
85. Burnie AG, Dunn AK. A case of central diabetes insipidus in the cat: diagnosis and treatment. J Small Anim Pract 1979;24:569–73.
86. Nicohols R. Clinical use of the vasopressin analogue DDAVP for the diagnosis and treatment of diabetes insipidus. In: Bonagura JD, editor. Kirk's current veterinary therapy XIII small animal practice. Philadelphia: WB Saunders; 2000. p. 325–6.
87. Fracassi F, Mandrioli L, Shehdula D, et al. Complete surgical removal of a very enlarged pituitary corticotroph adenoma in a dog. J Am Anim Hosp Assoc 2014;50:192–7.
88. Myers JA, Lunn KF, Bright JM. Echocardiographic findings in 11 cats with acromegaly. J Vet Intern Med 2014;28:1235–8.
89. Borgeat K, Niessen S, Scudder C, et al. Feline hypersomatotropism is a naturally occurring, reversible cause of myocardial remodeling. J Vet Intern Med 2015;29: 1263.

90. Dekkers OM, Biermasz NR, Pereira AM, et al. Mortality in patients treated for Cushing's disease is increased, compared with patients treated for nonfunctioning pituitary macroadenoma. J Clin Endocrinol Metab 2007;92:976–81.
91. Owen TJ, Chen AV, Martin LG. Why, when, how and post-operative care of dogs undergoing transsphenoidal hypophysectomy for large sellar masses. J Vet Intern Med 2016;30:1939.
92. Martin LG, Owen TJ, Chen AV, et al. Clinical characteristics and outcome in dogs treated with transsphenoidal hypophysectomy for non-functional sellar masses. J Vet Intern Med 2016;30:1941.

Minimally Invasive Spine Surgery in Small Animals

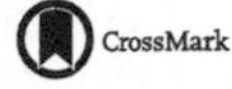

Bianca F. Hettlich, Dr med vet

KEYWORDS

• Spine • Veterinary • Approach • Minimally invasive • Open

KEY POINTS

- Minimally invasive spine surgery (MISS) in humans leads to shorter surgery times, decreased intraoperative blood loss, shorter durations of hospital stay, and decreased complications.
- MISS uses intraoperative imaging, magnification, and special instrumentation, and applies minimally invasive access strategies.
- Few veterinary studies have evaluated MISS, most using standard approaches with video assistance for improved visualization; few apply MISS access strategies using special retractors.
- Although MISS in small animals is currently not commonplace, modifying one's approach from open to miniopen procedures is the first step toward applying minimally invasive principles.

The goal of minimally invasive surgery (MIS) is to perform a surgical procedure with the least iatrogenic trauma as possible. The minimally invasive approach must not compromise the goal of the procedure, and should be applicable regardless of the underlying disease. MIS has become popular in human spine surgery and has been used for cervical, thoracolumbar, and lumbosacral (LS) procedures. Such approaches require modifications in access strategies to the different anatomic locations of the spine. Using specialized retractors and either endoscopic or magnification assistance, decompressive and stabilization procedures are performed successfully in humans through MIS approaches, while still being able to adhere to orthopedic fixation principles. The application of MIS to the vertebral column of veterinary patients is still at its early stages, with only few experimental and rare clinical reports available. The increasing availability of instrumentation necessary for MIS will allow veterinary surgeons to further develop minimally invasive techniques for veterinary patients and their specific spinal diseases.

Disclosure Statement: The author has nothing to disclose.
Department of Small Animal Surgery, Vetsuisse Faculty, University of Bern, Laenggassstrasse 128, Bern 3012, Switzerland
E-mail address: bianca.hettlich@vetsuisse.unibe.ch

Vet Clin Small Anim 48 (2018) 153–168
http://dx.doi.org/10.1016/j.cvsm.2017.08.008
vetsmall.theclinics.com

The application of MIS to the spine (minimally invasive spinal surgery [MISS]) requires careful preoperative planning and intraoperative imaging, as well as the use of specialized instrumentation and surgical techniques.[1] After the anatomic location of the pathology has been identified, the type of procedure required and thereby type of MIS approach can be determined. Correct positioning of the patient is paramount for MIS to ensure adequate instrument placement and avoid movement of landmarks during surgery. Using positioning aids such as sandbags or beanbags, and tape, belts, or metal holding frames, the patient is maintained in a fixed position so that approach trajectories can be maintained. Entry areas for instruments are localized using intraoperative imaging such as fluoroscopy or computed tomography (CT). Then, MIS surgical techniques are used, often using specialized retractors, to approach the spine and perform the required procedure.

ACCESS STRATEGIES

Most open approaches use subperiosteal dissection of tissues, where muscles, tendons, and ligaments are elevated or cut away from their osseous attachments. In human spine surgery, specific concerns are associated with traditional open approaches. Experimental models and clinical studies have shown that such approaches to lead to direct effects on soft tissues such as denervation of elevated musculature with subsequent atrophy, increased intraoperative bleeding, reduction of segmental innervation to the area owing to damage to the local nerves, and compromised local blood supply owing to damage to local vessels.[2] Studies using MRI to evaluate changes in paraspinal musculature after lumbar decompressive surgery found significantly fewer negative changes in cases with MISS versus open approaches.[3,4] Postoperative sequelae from a larger approach are increased scar tissue formation, which may impair the function of local musculature. In humans, local pain syndrome is a well-recognized postoperative complication from spinal surgery. Traditional approaches to the vertebral column seem to be associated with longer postoperative need for analgesia and immobilization, leading to longer durations of recovery and disability. These undesirable effects have an economic effect on people and efforts are made to reduce them through minimally invasive approaches.

To decrease the undesirable effects of extensive tissue dissection, MISS approaches are aimed at being muscle sparing and maintaining soft tissue attachments as much as possible.[5] There are 2 types of muscle sparing approaches: intermuscular and intramuscular.

The intermuscular approach uses anatomically defined tissue planes to access parts of the spine. Although such tissue planes are separated, an effort is made to spare tissue attachments to bone. The intramuscular approach uses muscle-splitting techniques to gain access and achieve a direct path to the area of interest. Because the target area can be approached via the most direct route, tissue dissection can be kept to a minimum. The intramuscular approach is the standard approach for MIS techniques such as percutaneous procedures or procedures using tubular retractors. Both procedures use dilating trochars and intraoperative imaging to determine accurate positioning of instruments. The learning curve for the application of these procedures to the spine is high.

INTRAOPERATIVE IMAGING

To avoid the need for visualization of identifiable landmarks and use a targeted muscle-sparing approach to a specific location, some form of imaging must confirm localization of instrument placement. Although conventional radiography can be used intraoperatively, fluoroscopy is the most commonly used imaging modality in human spinal MIS for identification of the appropriate access portal location. Intraoperative CT is primarily used to determine proper implant trajectory rather than for location identification. With the development of MISS, the use of intraoperative imaging modalities has increased significantly. Care must be taken to consider intraoperative radiation exposure to the patient and operating staff, and use of fluoroscopy and CT should be limited.

The development of spinal navigation systems has increased the feasibility of MIS approaches for complex spinal procedures, where a larger approach was previously necessary to visualize bony anatomy. By using preoperative CT linked to the patient's vertebral anatomy intraoperatively, MIS approaches can be used to perform advanced spinal fixation (ie, deformity correction, trauma). Ultimately, the use of navigation systems will also drive the further development of robotic spine surgery, where approaches will be even more limited compared with what a human surgeon would require.

ACCESS TO THE SPINE IN MINIMALLY INVASIVE SURGERY

There are 2 methods to access the vertebral column in a minimally invasive fashion: percutaneous access and access via tubular or expandable retractors. For pathologies affecting a small area, requiring focal treatment, percutaneously placed rigid spinal endoscopes can be used to gain access and perform certain procedures (**Fig. 1**). Such endoscopes have several working portals for lavage, suction, drill, and probing instruments. In humans, spinal endoscopes are commonly used to treat disk pathologies and perform limited decompression. Accurate placement of the endoscope is guided and confirmed using intraoperative fluoroscopy. Magnified images are displayed on an external screen, thereby allowing multiple people to view the surgical field. Working space is limited with this approach and drilling of bone requires frequent cleaning of the endoscopy lens from bone debris.

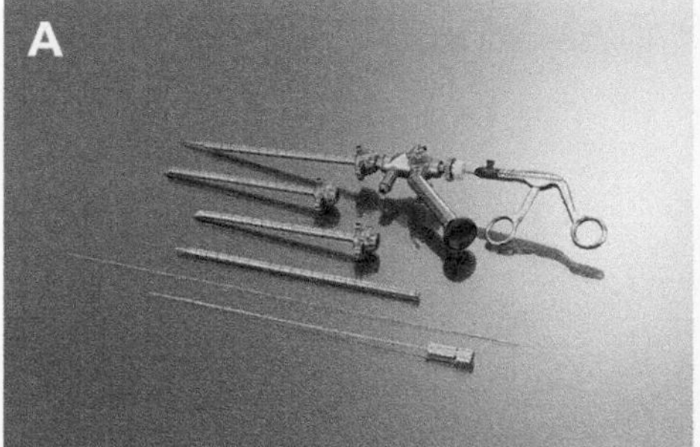

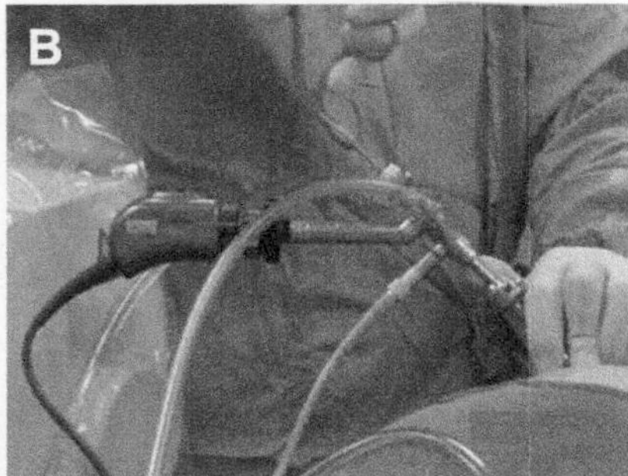

Fig. 1. (*A*) Instrument set up of the Endospine endoscope by Karl Storz (©Karl Storz GmbH & Co. KG, Germany). A guidewire and cannulated sleeve are used under imaging guidance to locate target position. Cannulated dilators are then used before the endoscope sleeve is placed, through which the spinal endoscope is inserted. (*B*) Intraoperative use of the Endospine endoscope by Karl Storz (©Karl Storz GmbH & Co. KG, Germany). A camera head is attached to the endoscope. The working portal of the endoscope is being used by the surgeon. Bayoneted instruments (images copied from website) have contacted company to obtain permission for use but despite multiple attempts have not heard from them. (Used with permission from Karl Storz GmbH & Co. KG, Germany.)

For procedures requiring a larger working area than provided by a spinal endoscope or for application of implants, special MIS retractors are used. These can be rigid tubular or have adjustable retraction blades. The precise location is documented using intraoperative fluoroscopy. Retractors are used with some form of intraoperative magnification, most commonly an operating microscope, although use of surgical magnification loupes or videoendoscopy is also possible.

MAGNIFICATION AND ILLUMINATION

Owing to the limited access of MIS approaches, magnification of the surgical field is extremely important. The simplest form of magnification is the use of surgical loupes, providing 2-dimensional enlargement to the wearer. Although loupes do not obstruct the access portal by adding an additional instrument, they limit visual access to the area to a single observer. Video-assisted spinal endoscopy is another form of magnification. Although most spinal endoscopes are used to perform percutaneous procedures, they can also be combined with a tubular access port to provide magnification and display via a monitor. Some tubular retractors have an integrated endoscope, whereas with others the endoscope is simply passed along the inside of the tubular retractor. A disadvantage of the endoscope use in tubular retractors is the space requirement and possible interference with other instruments. One distinct benefit of video assistance is the ability to visualize the periphery of the surgical field owing to the angled lens of the endoscope.

The highest quality of magnification can be achieved using an operating microscope (**Fig. 2**). This modality allows multiple observers to visualize the surgical field through the microscope directly and via monitors. It also removes potentially interfering video assistance instruments from the tubular portal. Modern operating microscopes have the ability to display images 3-dimensionally, which may be beneficial to the surgeon.

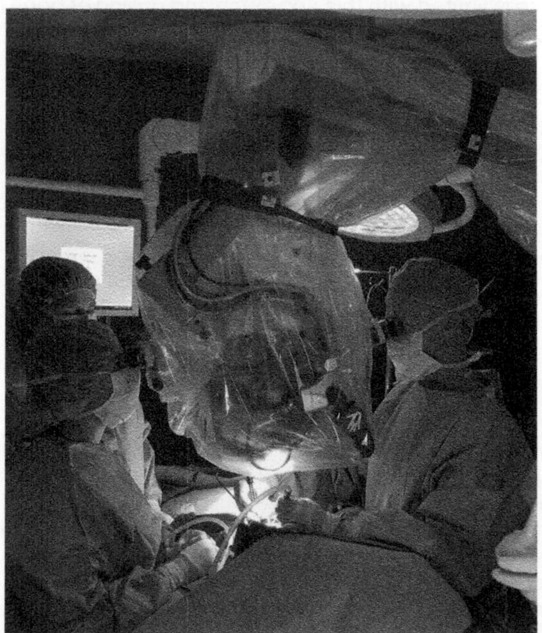

Fig. 2. Operating room set up of the Zeiss OPMI Neuro MultiVision operating microscope.

As with surgical loupes, the field of view is limited to the tissues in the direct line of view.

INSTRUMENTATION

Fixed diameter, rigid tubular retractors are the standard for most MIS spinal procedures in humans (**Fig. 3**). Most of these retractors place a series of atraumatic dilators of increasing diameter using intramuscular approaches (**Fig. 4**). Rigid tubular retractors come in various diameters and lengths, to be used according to anatomic location and working space required. Many of them can be used with an inbuilt fiber optic light source, and some may have specific working portals for various instruments and for video-endoscopy. Expandable retractors are made of several components and have expandable blades for tissue retraction. Some of these retractors use atraumatic dilators, whereas others require a small surgical approach before placement. They are often used for miniopen approaches and allow variation in size of surgical exposure.

The instruments used for MISS differ in shape to regular ones in that they are bayoneted. The bayonet shape allows the surgeon's hand to be positioned out of the line of view along the long axis of the instrument, thereby decreasing visual obstruction of

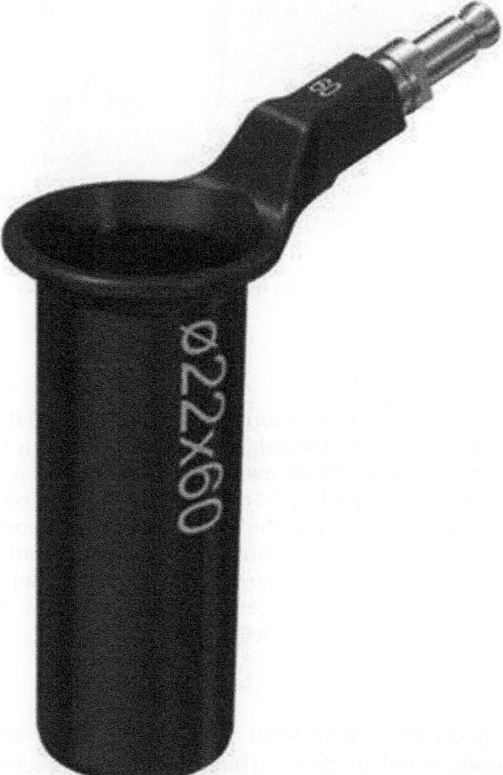

Fig. 3. Example of a tubular retractor (INSIGHT, DePuy Synthes, Inc). Tubular retractors are available in different diameters and lengths, depending on patient and procedural requirements. (Used with permission from DePuy Synthes, Inc, West Chester, PA. SPOTLIGHT and INSIGHT are trademarks of DePuy Systems, Inc.)

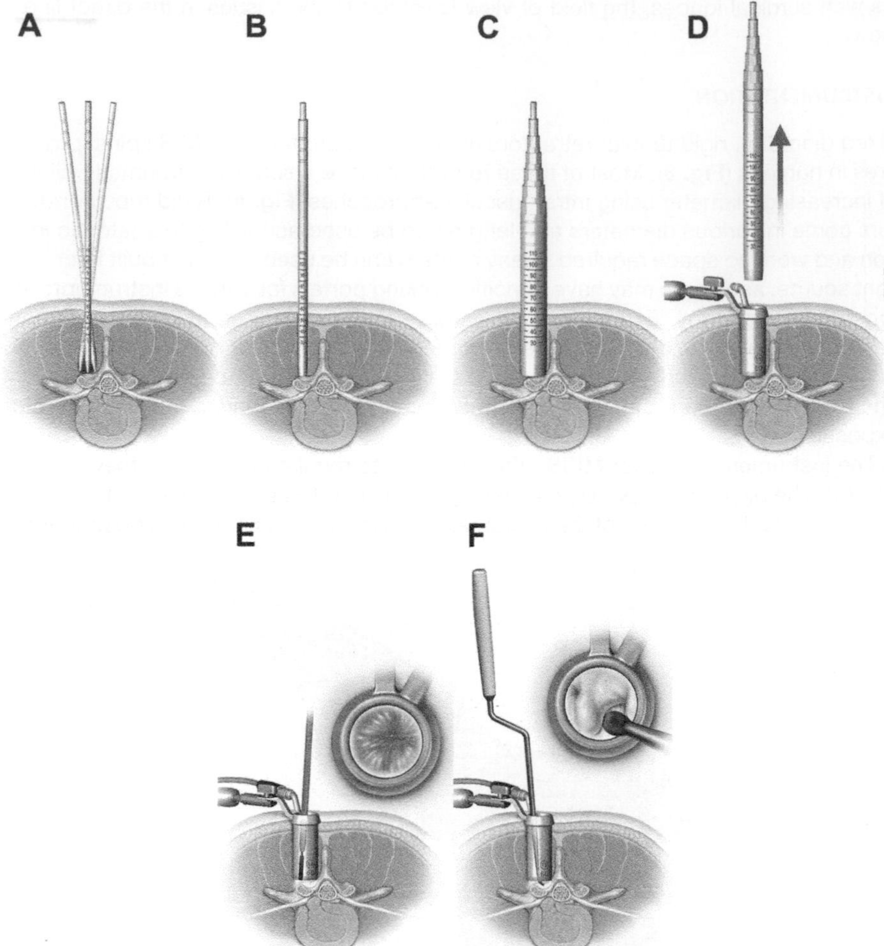

Fig. 4. Use of the Spotlight tubular retractor system (SPOTLIGHT DePuy Synthes, Inc). (*A*) A guide pin has been inserted percutaneously and correct position is determined by probing. (*B*) The first dilator has been placed over the guide pin. (*C*) A series of dilators of increasing diameters has been placed. (*D*) The Spotlight tubular retractor is positioned over the dilators, which are removed, and the retractor is fixed in position with an adjustable holding frame attached to the surgical table. (*E*) Soft tissues covering the articular facet are removed. (*F*) The articular facets have been cleared of soft tissue and a bayoneted instrument is used for probing. (Used with permission from DePuy Synthes, Inc, West Chester, PA. SPOTLIGHT and INSIGHT are trademarks of DePuy Systems, Inc.)

the surgical field (**Fig. 5**). MIS instruments are also long handled to allow their use through potentially deep working portals. This applies to rongeurs, such as bayonetted Kerrison rongeurs, nerve root retractors, bipolar cautery handles, forceps, among others. To allow working through a limited portal, MIS drills are narrower with a longer tip than traditional drills. As with bayonetted instruments, the drill hand piece can cause visual impairment of the limited field of view, which led to the development of angled hand pieces. With the introduction of specialized MISS approach instruments,

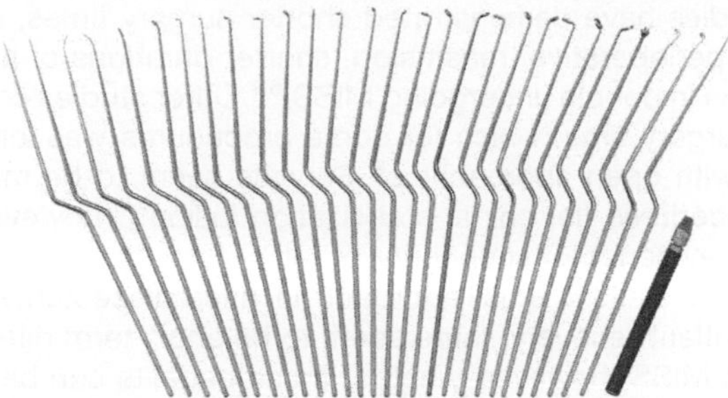

Fig. 5. Example of a bayoneted instrument set of various probes and curettes (Tew dissector set, KLS Martin LP). (*Courtesy of* KLS Martin LP, Jacksonville, FL; with permission.)

there was also a development of instrumentation to allow application of spinal implants in a minimally invasive fashion.

LEARNING CURVE

When switching from standard open approaches to MISS, the learning curve can be substantial, because most aspects of the approach are different and unfamiliar instrumentation is used. The adjustments of only changing the type of approach are much easier to accomplish than changing the entire method of the procedure. When switching from an open to a less invasive approach for a procedure, the required changes will be easier to handle if the approach is decreased to a miniopen or MIS via a retractor, while the actual procedure is still performed in the same manner as before. More dramatic changes in procedural technique, that is, executing the procedure via a spinal endoscope versus through an opening with routine equipment, will require learning of a new technique and naturally require more time and experience.

EVIDENCE IN HUMAN MINIMALLY INVASIVE SPINE SURGERY

The proposed benefits of MIS in human spine surgery are multiple. The direct effects on the tissues and wound healing seem to be logical when comparing large with small approaches. Smaller approaches lead to decreased tissue trauma, which in turn lead to decreased scar tissue formation. Less trauma should decrease bleeding and, therefore, the need for blood transfusions. Decreasing tissue dissection and preserving muscle, tendinous, and ligamentous attachments should increase perispinal stability. Procedural benefits such as decreased operating times not only depend on the type of approach, but also on the procedure performed. Learning curve and time requirements for procedures unrelated to the approach must be taken into consideration. If MISS were to decrease surgical time, then this may lead to a potentially decreased infection rate, because surgical and anesthesia times are contributing factors. Suggested postoperative benefits for the patient include decreased immediate postoperative and long-term pain and faster return to function, allowing faster return to normal personal and work life. From a hospital standpoint, shorter durations of hospital stay may lead to decreased institutional costs.

Concrete evidence for many of these proposed benefits for human MISS is limited. Few prospective, randomized, clinical trials have been performed and other studies need to be carefully evaluated for possible bias and confounding factors. Many human clinical studies have demonstrated shorter surgery times, decreased blood loss and need for perioperative transfusion, shorter durations of hospital stay, and fewer complications in people undergoing MISS.[6,7] Other studies confirm these benefits, except for surgery time, which for some procedures was longer in the MISS group compared with open approaches.[8] Benefits seem to be more prominent in more invasive procedures (ie, spinal stabilization/fusion[9]); however, other studies do not show clear evidence of superiority of MISS for procedures that traditionally already only require a relatively small approach (ie, microdiscectomy[10] or lumbar laminectomy[11]). For patient recovery, there seem to be short-term differences reported between open and MISS; however, whether these benefits can be maintained long term remains uncertain.[6,12,13] Regarding MISS with intraoperative imaging versus open approaches, a recent study comparing MISS using intraoperative fluoroscopy, CT integrated navigation, and open surgery found reduced surgery time, blood loss, duration of hospital stay, and improved function outcome with the use of CT integrated navigation.[14] Not surprisingly, the use of intraoperative imaging modalities using radiographs also increases the radiation dose for the patient and operating team.[12]

When evaluating studies, one must also recognize that statistical differences are not always clinically important differences. Also, many studies are based on a small patient population. Another postoperative evaluation challenge is that quantification of spinal pain is very difficult, which is true not just for humans, but even more so for veterinary patients. With the increase in use of MISS in humans, future studies will help to provide stronger evidence.

WHY MINIMALLY INVASIVE SPINE SURGERY IN VETERINARY SURGERY?

With the many proposed and documented benefits of MISS in humans, the application of such techniques to veterinary spine surgery should be beneficial for our patients. However, not all benefits should be extrapolated with the same significance. For example, a main clinical difference between humans and small animals is that significant blood loss is not common during routine approaches to the spine in cats and dogs. The requirement to give blood transfusions is rare in cats and dogs and mostly a result of complications instead of the approach. Postoperatively, it is more difficult to recognize subtle changes in wound pain status, possible denervation, effects of fibrosis, and chronic pain in veterinary patients. Although possibly upsetting to owners, pets do not carry the emotional burden of a disfiguring scar. There are also limited socioeconomic implications owing postoperative sequelae during healing from a specific surgical approach to the spine.

Whereas in human spine surgery, MISS seems to be particularly beneficial for more invasive surgeries and less so for simple decompressive procedures, the latter is the most common indication for small animal spinal surgery. Depending on the location and extent of disk disease, and the signalment of the patient, the standard surgical approach can be limited or extensive. The approach for a T12 to T13 hemilaminectomy in a thin miniature breed dog will naturally be small and using tubular retractors may not be practical. However, when performing an L7 to S1 dorsal laminectomy in an obese, large breed dog, the benefits of MIS become much more obvious. Although no comparative studies have been done in veterinary spine surgery, the benefits of MIS will likely be greater in larger and heavier patients.

Stabilization procedures are being more commonly used as treatment for degenerative conditions such as cervical spondylomyelopathy or LS degenerative stenosis.

Although there is evidence of the clinical benefit in using MIS for stabilizing spinal procedures in humans, no such studies have been performed in dogs. It is currently rare to perform extensive, multilevel spinal procedures in dogs and comparative studies will be challenging, particularly single-center studies.

VETERINARY MINIMALLY INVASIVE SPINE SURGERY: ACCESS STRATEGIES

Although the use of specialized MIS instrumentation and, with that, true MIS spine approaches are not common practice, much can be done during veterinary spinal surgery to apply the general principles. Surgeons can convert standard open to miniopen approaches using available retractors. This change does not require specialized MIS equipment, only an adjustment of technique, and it would limit soft tissue dissection. The goal would be to approach as little as possible while still being able to execute the procedure in a routine fashion. To aid retraction, deep angle (right angle) Gelpi retractors or similar can be used that allow retraction of deep tissues through a limited approach. Although not used frequently, the increasing availability and feasibility of MIS retractors and the rising use of magnification makes muscle-splitting techniques a realistic option for veterinary patients.

VETERINARY MINIMALLY INVASIVE SPINE SURGERY: IMAGING AND NAVIGATION

Currently, many spinal procedures are performed with intraoperative localization by palpation or visual identification of certain anatomic landmarks. This may require extension of the surgical approach to identify such structures. To allow a limited approach directly over the target location, several relatively simple methods can be used. For the thoracolumbar spine, popular techniques to aid in identification of target location are preoperative placement of a needle or pin with subsequent radiography, or marking of the target with methylene blue.

To apply percutaneous or MISS retractor techniques, the precise location has to be determined intraoperatively. Intraoperative fluoroscopy is becoming more commonplace in veterinary surgery for this purpose. Benefits of using intraoperative fluoroscopy include not only the ability to locate the target area, but also ensure proper placement of the MIS retractor and possible implants.

It is not commonplace in veterinary spine surgery to use intraoperative CT, and spinal navigation devices are currently only investigated experimentally.

VETERINARY MINIMALLY INVASIVE SPINE SURGERY: MAGNIFICATION AND ILLUMINATION

Owing to the limited exposure of the surgical target area, magnification is an important requirement for MISS. Surgical loupes with magnification between 2.5 and 4.5 are common tools in veterinary neurosurgery. Loupes are often worn with an additional light source, which greatly facilitates illumination of the small, frequently deeply located surgical field. One downside of surgical loupes is that magnification is only available for the wearer and images cannot be displayed. Also, with increasing magnification, effective assistance during surgery is required because it can be difficult for the surgeon to switch between different focal lengths during the procedure.

Recently gaining in popularity is the use of magnification using an externally positioned scope (ie, VITOM, Karl Storz, Tuttlingen, Germany; **Fig. 6**). The exoscope is positioned over the surgical field and fixed by a holding device to the surgical table.

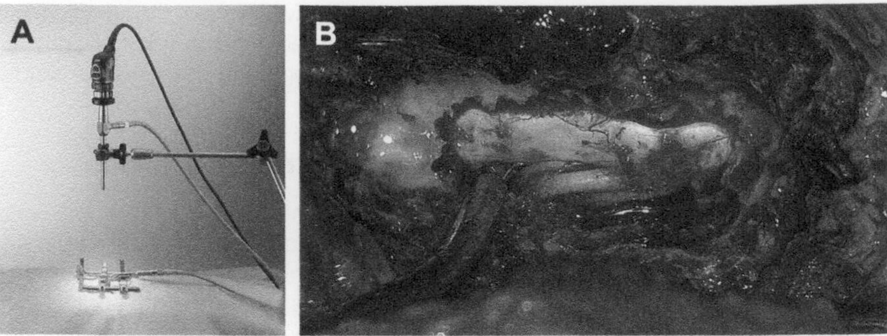

Fig. 6. (*A*) Intraoperative setup using the video telescope operating monitor VITOM by Karl Storz (©Karl Storz GmbH & Co. KG, Germany). It consists of a rigid lens telescope and fiber optic light source, a high-definition digitized camera with connection to a video monitor (not shown), and an adjustable mechanical endoscope holder affixed to the surgical table. (*B*) Intraoperative image of a VITOM-assisted lateral decompression at C6-C7 in a dog. For size reference, the instrument is a 7-Fr Frazier suction tip. ([*A*] Used with permission from Karl Storz GmbH & Co. KG, Germany; and [*B*] *Courtesy of* Dr Fred Wininger, Veterinary Specialty Services, Manchester, MO.)

Often, exoscope assistance is used after a traditional open approach has been made to improve visualization during the actual surgical procedure. It can also be used through approaches using MIS retractors. Apart from magnification, the use of an exoscope also allows the display of images on a screen, facilitating recording and multiperson viewing for teaching. Obstruction of the view through debris during drilling has been reported to be an issue.

Specialized spinal endoscopes use a scope with working portals, which is introduced to the surgical target area using endoscope specific trochars. Spinal endoscopes were developed for percutaneous MISS and their use in veterinary medicine is currently rare. Images are displayed on screen allowing multiperson viewing and recording. Endoscopes can also be used through MISS retractors. Because their field of view is often angled, they can also be used to visualize the periphery of the surgical field. This ability to "look around the corner" is one benefit of using an endoscope.

Operating microscopes are slowly gaining traction in veterinary spine surgery. The surgeon and assistant can both visualize the surgical field, and the on-screen display and recording ability facilitate teaching. The microscope is usually in position from the beginning to the end of surgery. Owing to the fixed angle of the magnifying lens, the visual field is limited to a straight view. Approaches can be traditional open or MIS depending on the equipment available and choice by the surgeon.

VETERINARY MINIMALLY INVASIVE SPINE SURGERY: INSTRUMENTATION AND IMPLANTS

Currently, there are no veterinary MISS specific implants and, unless human instruments are used, most veterinary surgeons rely on standard neurosurgical instruments. Many veterinary spine instruments can be used for MISS, but most are not bayonetted. Veterinary rongeurs such as Kerrison or pituitary rongeurs can still be used through a miniopen or MIS approach. Ball probes and nerve root retractors need to be of sufficient lengths to reach the surgical site without interfering with view or other instrumentation. Standard pneumatic or electric surgical drills can pose a problem when being used for MISS. They may not fit through MIS retractors or may obliterate the view owing to the required hand position on the device. Hand pieces with an extended narrow and angled tip can be used through very small approaches with decreased impairment of view.

Human MISS access ports have been developed by a variety of companies and come in a selection of diameters and lengths to fit different locations along the spine, and can be rigid or adjustable. The main limitation for the use of the great variety of human MISS retractors is cost. Other retractors such as the deep angle Gelpi or the Caspar retractor are commonly used in veterinary spine surgery and can certainly be used for miniopen approaches.

VETERINARY MINIMALLY INVASIVE SPINE SURGERY EVIDENCE

To date, only a small number of publications have reported the use of MISS in small animals and, because of this, evidence for its superiority is still lacking. Most studies were cadaveric, assessing the feasibility of certain techniques, and only a few were reports on clinical cases without comparison to a control group. Also, most evaluated the use of video assistance to improve visualization of neuroanatomical structures through standard approaches rather than specific MIS approaches.[15–19] Only 2 studies so far have specifically evaluated and compared MIS approaches in cadaveric dogs.[20,21]

Specific Techniques Described

Cervical vertebral column

Ventral access to the cervical spine is a prime location for the conversion of a standard open to miniopen approach. Blunt palpation for landmarks through the limited approach can usually identify the desired location. Alternatively, imaging guidance can be used for definitive target localization. There are no reports on the use of MIS retractors for cervical procedures in veterinary patients. When approaching the ventral aspect of the cervical vertebral column through intermuscular or intramuscular techniques, care must be taken to avoid injury to important anatomic structures, such as the trachea, esophagus, carotid artery, jugular vein, and vagosympathetic trunk. The use of percutaneous equipment would require even more careful maneuvering during placement of the instrument. Leperlier and colleagues[17] successfully performed video-assisted ventral slots using the Destandau Endospine device (Karl Storz, Germany; **Fig. 7**) in cadaver and clinical dogs; however, despite describing the approach as minimally invasive and using a spinal endoscope, routine approaches were used and the device was only used for the ventral slot part of the procedure. A proceedings report by Rossetti and associates[18] described the use of a video telescope operating monitor (VITOM, Karl Storz, Germany) for clinical dogs undergoing ventral slot and compared this group to standard ventral slot. Improved visualization was found in the VITOM group with smaller ventral slot dimensions and similar surgery times. No MIS-specific aspects were evaluated regarding soft tissue approach and no MIS retractors were used. A further clinical study described the use of the VITOM in 30 dogs undergoing cervical ventral slot decompression.[22] Although concluding that the VITOM procedures were fast and easy with improved spinal cord visualization, spinal approaches and ventral slots were conventional, without MISS access strategies.

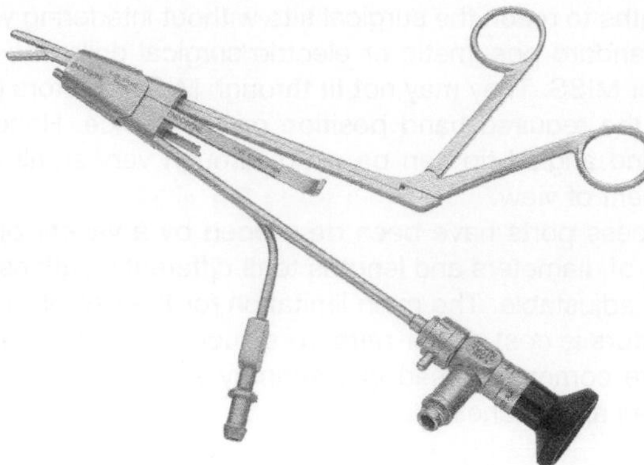

Fig. 7. Instrument set up of the Destandau Endospine device by Karl Storz (©Karl Storz GmbH & Co. KG, Germany). It consists of an operating tube with various working portals for an endoscope, instruments, and suction. The portals are angled 12° so that instrument tips can be visualized within the surgical field. (Used with permission from Karl Storz GmbH & Co. KG, Germany.)

There are no reports on the use of MIS techniques for dorsal or lateral approaches to the cervical vertebral column. Depending on the breed, there can be massive soft tissue coverage and exposure of the target area often requires large open approaches. Particularly for these locations, application of MIS techniques, that is, through tubular retractors, could significantly decrease patient morbidity, provided the desired procedure can still be performed.

Thoracolumbar vertebral column

As with the cervical approach, the first step toward minimizing iatrogenic tissue trauma would be conversion of the standard open to a miniopen approach. Once the target location is identified using preoperative or intraoperative imaging, the area can be approached directly. The most common surgical procedure in the thoracolumbar spine is spinal cord decompression after intervertebral disk extrusion. Approaches for decompression can be dorsal, dorsolateral, or lateral. The standard dorsal approach represents a subperiosteal approach and as such would be considered not ideal for MISS. If the procedure required true dorsal access (ie, dorsal laminectomy), it should be possible to convert this approach to a miniopen or even use MISS retractors. The lateral approach would be considered an intermuscular approach and mainly uses natural tissue planes to gain access. The dorsolateral approach uses mostly intramuscular access via muscle splitting. Both the lateral and dorsolateral approaches would, therefore, be more in line with the principles of MISS. However, both approaches still require removal of tendinous attachments from the articular processes for standard hemilaminectomy. Conversion to a minihemilaminectomy with preservation of the articular processes and attaching soft tissues would on principle be most appropriate for MISS. More laterally oriented approaches enable effective access to the ventrolateral aspect of the vertebral canal for minihemilaminectomy and/or partial corpectomy, which have been shown to adequately relieve spinal cord compression by extruded disk material, provided the compression is in a ventrolateral location.[23–25] Both procedures should be amenable to MIS approaches.

The apparently only published veterinary study specifically comparing MIS to traditional approach was a cadaveric study performed by Lockwood and coworkers[21] on the canine thoracolumbar spine. Here, the standard dorsal approach to the thoracolumbar vertebral column was compared with foraminotomy using a tubular retractor with a positioning arm and either endoscopy assistance or an illuminated port to aid in visualization. Incision lengths were smaller in the MIS groups compared with the standard approach. Simulated extruded disk material was successfully removed through all approaches. The endoscopy-assisted approach took significantly longer (more than twice as long as the illuminated port and standard approach) and view obstruction during burring from debris burring seemed to be a problem in both MIS groups. Carozzo and colleagues[16] performed video-assisted thoracolumbar corpectomy in cadaver dogs for which a Caspar cervical retractor was used. The procedure could be performed successfully through a limited approach, but no comparison was made with traditional approaches.

Lumbosacral spine

LS surgery is commonly performed in dogs suffering from LS degenerative stenosis. These dogs are often large breed and can be overweight. Owing to the depth of soft tissues (including fat) at which the LS space is located, standard surgical approaches are quite large, routinely exposing the L7 (and even L6) spinous process and sacral crest to provide access for dorsal laminectomy. Owing to the dimensions of the open approach, change in technique to a miniopen or MIS approach can significantly decrease soft tissue dissection, and minimally invasive retractors can provide exposure to perform the required procedures. To avoid the need for exposing landmarks through a large approach to correctly localize the LS space, imaging is used to identify the target location. Using simple retractors such as deep-angle Gelpis or Caspar, a standard open approach can be modified to a miniopen. To achieve appropriate exposure to perform a dorsal laminectomy with dimensions sufficient to work within the vertebral canal (ie, for partial discectomy), the L7 spinous process can usually be maintained and only the cranial aspect of the sacral crest be removed. Using standard neurosurgical equipment, the procedure can be performed through this limited approach; however, the use of MIS-specific equipment improves visualization along the working arm of the instruments.

Specialized human MIS retractors for the LS space are available; however, the cost of these can be prohibitively high. A study by Dent and colleagues[20] assessed the efficacy of a human MIS retractor in the canine LS spine in a cadaveric study comparing MIS and standard approaches for dorsal laminectomy and partial discectomy. Using the Pipeline Expandable Access System by DePuy Synthes (Raynham, MA), the retractor was inserted over a series of dilators and, once in place, adjustable retractor arms were deployed to increase exposure at the bone interface (**Fig. 8**). In this cadaveric model, the MIS approach had significantly smaller incision lengths and allowed successful laminectomy and discectomy with comparable dimensions to the open approach. The MIS approach using this retractor required more time to complete; however, the median time difference was 4 minutes, making this of questionable clinical relevance.

Clinically relevant, but not assessing specific MIS approaches, is a study by Wood and associates[19] on LS foraminotomies where video assistance was used to perform the foraminotomy but without a minimally invasive approach to the LS spine. Carozzo and coworkers[15] described a novel transiliac approach to the LS intervertebral disk and foramen and the use of endoscopy to visualize structures, allowing for a less invasive approach to this difficult to reach anatomic location.

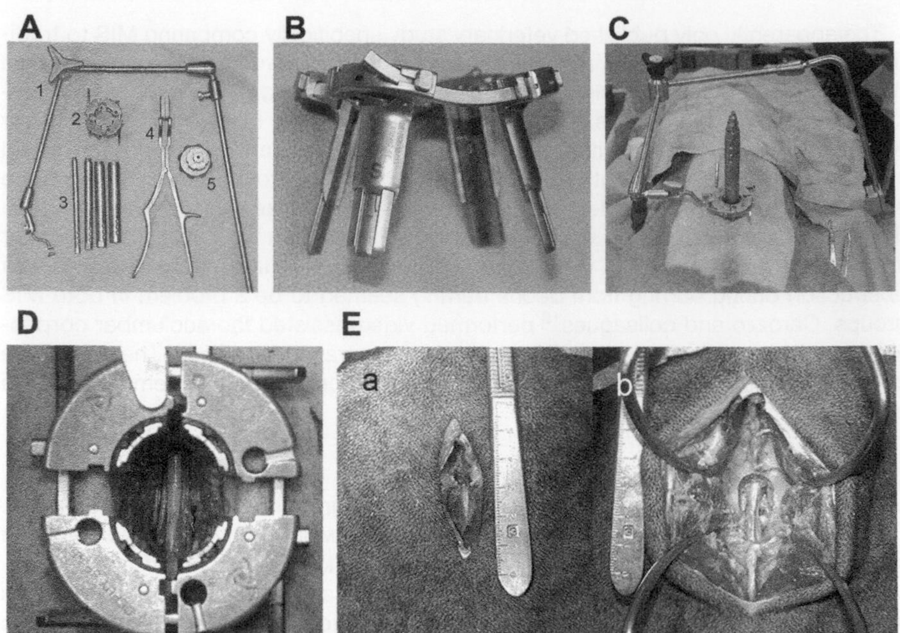

Fig. 8. (*A*) Components of the DePuy Synthes Pipeline Expandable Access System with fixation arm (1), expandable retractor (2), progressive dilators (3), retractor blade expander, (4) and depth gauge (5). (*B*) Small DePuy lumbar Pipeline retractor at maximum retraction and extended retractor blades. (*C*) Placement of the DePuy Synthes Pipeline Expandable Access System at the lumbosacral space in a canine cadaver. The expandable retractor is in place over a series of tissue dilators. Retractor position is locked in place by a fixation arm connected to the surgery table. (*D*) DePuy lumbar Pipeline retractor in situ. A dorsal laminectomy at L7-S1 has been performed through the retractor and the caudal equina is visible. (*E*) Differences in soft tissue approach dimensions between a minimally invasive approach using a lumbar retractor (*a*) and a traditional open approach (*b*) to the lumbosacral space for dorsal laminectomy. (*Courtesy of* DePuy Synthes, Inc; with permission.)

SUMMARY

The benefits of decreasing the size of surgical approaches are multiple. Although true minimally invasive approaches for veterinary spinal procedures are still in the early stages, adjusting one's traditional open to a miniopen approach would already decrease soft tissue morbidity without requirements for specialized equipment. With adequate magnification, illumination, and instrumentation to allow safe and effective execution of procedures, veterinary spinal surgeons can adjust their procedures toward minimizing surgical access. The increasing use of exoscopes and operating microscopes trains surgeons in the performance of procedures using on-screen images, which should allow for an easier transition to using exoscopes or endoscopes through MISS access portals. There is a need for the development of veterinary MISS equipment and of MIS techniques for specific veterinary spine diseases. At that point, clinical studies can be performed to critically evaluate procedural and patient benefits of MISS.

REFERENCES

1. Härtl R. The four pillars of minimally invasive spine surgery. In: Härtl R, Korge A, editors. AOSpine: minimally invasive spine surgery - techniques, evidence, and controversies. Stuttgart, Germany: Thieme; 2012. p. 23–49.

2. Stevens KJ, Spenciner DB, Griffiths KL, et al. Comparison of minimally invasive and conventional open posterolateral lumbar fusion using magnetic resonance imaging and retraction pressure studies. J Spinal Disord Tech 2006;19(2):77–86.
3. Bresnahan LE, Smith JS, Ogden AT, et al. Assessment of paraspinal muscle cross-sectional area after lumbar decompression: minimally invasive versus open approaches. Clin Spine Surg 2017;30(3):E162–8.
4. Kim DY, Lee SH, Chung SK, et al. Comparison of multifidus muscle atrophy and trunk extension muscle strength: percutaneous versus open pedicle screw fixation. Spine 2005;30(1):123–9.
5. Kim CW, Siemionow K, Anderson DG, et al. The current state of minimally invasive spine surgery. J Bone Joint Surg Am 2011;93a(6):582–96.
6. McGirt MJ, Parker SL, Mummaneni P, et al. Is the use of minimally invasive fusion technologies associated with improved outcomes after elective interbody lumbar fusion? Analysis of a nationwide prospective patient-reported outcomes registry. Spine J 2017;17(7):922–32.
7. Rahman M, Summers LE, Richter B, et al. Comparison of techniques for decompressive lumbar laminectomy: the minimally invasive versus the "classic" open approach. Minim Invasive Neurosurg 2008;51(2):100–5.
8. Park Y, Ha JW. Comparison of one-level posterior lumbar interbody fusion performed with a minimally invasive approach or a traditional open approach. Spine 2007;32(5):537–43.
9. Wang H, Zhou Y, Li C, et al. Comparison of open versus percutaneous pedicle screw fixation using the sextant system in the treatment of traumatic thoracolumbar fractures. Clin Spine Surg 2017;30(3):E239–46.
10. Arts MP, Brand R, van den Akker ME, et al. Tubular diskectomy vs conventional microdiskectomy for sciatica a randomized controlled trial. J Am Med Assoc 2009;302(2):149–58.
11. Skovrlj B, Belton P, Zarzour H, et al. Perioperative outcomes in minimally invasive lumbar spine surgery: a systematic review. World J Orthop 2015;6(11):996–1005.
12. Zhang W, Li H, Zhou Y, et al. Minimally invasive posterior decompression combined with percutaneous pedicle screw fixation for the treatment of thoracolumbar fractures with neurological deficits: a prospective randomized study versus traditional open posterior surgery. Spine 2016;41(Suppl 19):B23–9.
13. Djurasovic M, Rouben DP, Glassman SD, et al. Clinical outcomes of minimally invasive versus open TLIF: a propensity-matched cohort study. Am J Orthop (Belle Mead NJ) 2016;45(3):E77–82.
14. Wu MH, Dubey NK, Li YY, et al. Comparison of minimally invasive spine surgery using intraoperative computed tomography integrated navigation, fluoroscopy and conventional open surgery for lumbar spondylolisthesis: a prospective registry-based cohort study. Spine J 2017;17(8):1082–90.
15. Carozzo C, Cachon T, Genevois JP, et al. Transiliac approach for exposure of lumbosacral intervertebral disk and foramen: technique description. Vet Surg 2008;37(1):27–31.
16. Carozzo C, Maitre P, Genevois JP, et al. Endoscope-assisted thoracolumbar lateral corpectomy. Vet Surg 2011;40(6):738–42.
17. Leperlier D, Manassero M, Blot S, et al. Minimally invasive video-assisted cervical ventral slot in dogs. A cadaveric study and report of 10 clinical cases. Vet Comp Orthop Traumatol 2011;24(1):50–6.
18. Rossetti D, Ragetly G, Poncet C. Comparison of conventional and high definition video telescope assisted ventral slot decompression for cervical intervertebral

disc herniation in 51 dogs. Paper presented at: European College Veterinary Surgeons Annual Scientific Meeting. Berlin, Germany, 2015.
19. Wood BC, Lanz OI, Jones JC, et al. Endoscopic-assisted lumbosacral foraminotomy in the dog. Vet Surg 2004;33(3):221–31.
20. Dent BT, Fosgate GT, Hettlich BF. Minimally invasive approach to lumbosacral decompression in a cadaveric canine model. N Z Vet J 2016;64(2):71–5.
21. Lockwood AA, Griffon DJ, Gordon-Evans W, et al. Comparison of two minimally invasive approaches to the thoracolumbar spinal canal in dogs. Vet Surg 2014; 43(2):209–21.
22. Rossetti D, Ragetly GR, Poncet CM. High-definition video telescope-assisted ventral slot decompression surgery for cervical intervertebral disc herniation in 30 dogs. Vet Surg 2016;45(7):893–900.
23. Svensson G, Simonsson US, Danielsson F, et al. Residual spinal cord compression following hemilaminectomy and mini-hemilaminectomy in dogs: a prospective randomized study. Front Vet Sci 2017;4:42.
24. Medl SC, Reese S, Medl NS. Individualized mini-hemilaminectomy-corpectomy (iMHC) for treatment of thoracolumbar intervertebral disc herniation in large breed dogs. Vet Surg 2017;46(3):422–32.
25. Salger F, Ziegler L, Bottcher IC, et al. Neurologic outcome after thoracolumbar partial lateral corpectomy for intervertebral disc disease in 72 dogs. Vet Surg 2014;43(5):581–8.

Choices and Decisions in Decompressive Surgery for Thoracolumbar Intervertebral Disk Herniation

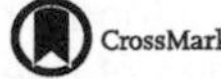

Nick D. Jeffery, BVSc, MSc, PhD, FRCVS[a,*],
Tom R. Harcourt-Brown, MA, VetMB[b], Andrew K. Barker, DVM[c],
Jonathan M. Levine, DVM[a]

KEYWORDS

- Hemilaminectomy • Decision process • Thoracolumbar intervertebral disk herniation
- Partial corpectomy

KEY POINTS

- Once decompressive surgery has been elected, the approach that maximizes the likelihood of gaining access to the herniated material for complete removal should be chosen.
- In most cases, a procedure that optimizes access to the ventrolateral aspect of the spinal cord will be advantageous but it is important to tailor the details of the surgical procedure to suit individual patients.
- Decompressive surgery for chronic (type II) herniations will frequently demand a ventral approach with partial corpectomy.

INTRODUCTION

Almost without exception, veterinary neurosurgery is concerned with decompression. Various masses can compress neural tissue, including tumors, hematomas, and, most commonly, herniated intervertebral disks. Experimentally, compression impairs conduction through axons,[1,2] perhaps by deforming the myelin sheath and altering membrane ion permeability to ions[3] and, also, by impairing normal blood flow.[4,5] Severe compression will lead to progressive atrophy of affected tissue through impairment of the blood supply.[6] For these reasons, and because it intuitively seems right to decompress compressed tissue, decompression of the spinal cord has become a routine part of veterinary surgery.[7] There are many published approaches to spinal cord decompression in veterinary surgery, and it can be difficult to choose the optimal

The authors have nothing to disclose.
[a] Department of Small Animal Clinical Sciences, Texas A&M University, 4474 TAMU, College Station, TX 77843, USA; [b] Langford Vets, University of Bristol, Bristol BS40 5DU, UK; [c] The Toronto Veterinary Emergency Hospital, 21 Rolark Drive, Scarborough, Ontario M1R 3B1, Canada
* Corresponding author.
E-mail address: njeffery@cvm.tamu.edu

Vet Clin Small Anim 48 (2018) 169–186
http://dx.doi.org/10.1016/j.cvsm.2017.08.014 vetsmall.theclinics.com
0195-5616/18/

method for each specific dog. Here we consider the decision-making process as a series of questions that a surgeon may ask before and during surgery for a herniated thoracolumbar disk.

IS THERE A NEED FOR SURGERY IN THIS SPECIFIC CASE?

The first decision is whether to carry out surgery at all. Although decompressive surgery for acute intervertebral disk herniation has become the norm in dogs that have recently become nonambulatory, the evidence in favor of a need for such surgery is not strong. For instance, for dogs with intact pain sensation to the pelvic limbs, there is an approximate 86% of recovery to walk again without surgery (see summary data in[8]). Fenestration, which is not conventionally regarded as decompressive, has a similar success rate (94%), which is comparable with that for decompressive procedures (90%).[8] Nevertheless, especially bearing in mind the recent meta-analysis comparing the results of conservative and surgical interventions for acute disk herniation in dogs,[9] for the foreseeable future it is likely that veterinary neurosurgeons will continue to use decompressive surgery for treatment of dogs that have become unable to walk following acute intervertebral disk herniation (IVDH).

In addition to the notion that decompression increases the probability of recovery, it is also often selected because it is thought that it makes recovery more rapid and/or more complete. Although these are commonly held views, there is little other than anecdotal opinion to support these assertions. On the other hand, for dogs that have lost pain perception in the hindquarters, there is some evidence to suggest that conservative therapy is not so efficacious, although this suggestion is based on very small numbers of cases and, therefore, may not be accurate.[8] It seems intuitive that the decompressed cord will recover more rapidly, and there is some experimental evidence to support this assumption[10,11] but it has not been formally proven in clinical studies in dogs. Similarly, the extent of recovery after surgery has not been formally compared with that after conservative therapy. Decompressive spinal surgery is often also appropriate for animals with intractable pain following disk herniation.[7,12]

WHEN DO I NEED TO OPERATE?

If decompressive surgery is selected as the appropriate therapy for an individual, it would seem intuitive that the procedure should be carried out as soon as possible. Although, in general, immediate surgery is usually preferable, there are other considerations. First, it is important that the animal is also suitably stable for anesthesia; this does not just imply the need to survive the anesthetic event but also that the blood pressure can be maintained at a suitable level throughout the surgery. In experimental animals, there is evidence to suggest that reduction in blood pressure after spinal cord injury is associated with a worsened outcome.[13] On the other hand, it may be that, with modern anesthetic agents and techniques, the risk of developing dangerously low blood pressure is much reduced because there is little evidence of an important clinical effect in dogs.[14,15] Second, there is evidence, at least in dogs that have lost pain perception in their hindquarters, that the time delay between the onset of paraplegia and surgery does not influence the likelihood of recovery.[16] On the other hand, there is laboratory evidence in favor of early decompression following experimental spinal cord contusion and compression in rodents.[10] In human spinal cord injury, the timing of surgery is also controversial; some studies suggest a benefit of early decompression, and others report no advantage. It is also important to note that early decompression in humans is often defined as within 24 hours of injury.[17] Humans with a spinal cord injury often have multiple other injuries (eg, those resulting from a car crash), and these other injuries take priority in treatment and/or may cause hypotension that can also have an adverse effect on neurologic outcome.

WHICH SITE IS THE PROBLEM THAT REQUIRES DECOMPRESSION?

Acute thoracolumbar disk herniations typically cause transverse myelopathy that can be readily identified through routine neurologic examination. The cutaneous trunci (panniculus) muscle reflex and careful palpation can often localize the lesion to within 1 or 2 vertebrae.[18] Subsequent imaging, nowadays, almost exclusively through cross-sectional methods, such as MRI and computed tomography (CT), will usually confirm the exact site and side of the lesion that is causing spinal cord compression (**Fig. 1**). Occasionally, there will be evidence of additional sites of spinal cord compression, often owing to previous episodes of disk herniations, some of which may have been nonsymptomatic. The differentiation of these nonactive lesions from the active site can be difficult on CT images because it is not possible to detect areas of spinal cord inflammation or edema. Magnetic resonance (MR) images are, therefore, preferable because it is possible to identify the active site because of the associated increase in hyperintensity on T2-weighted (TW) and short tau inversion recovery (STIR) images that is associated with acute spinal cord injury.[19]

Chronic thoracolumbar disk herniations will often be more problematic, mainly because affected dogs will commonly have more than 1 chronic disk herniation and, furthermore, more than 1 may be associated with evidence of spinal cord injury (T2W and STIR hyperintensity) (**Fig. 2**). The decision as to which to operate usually then rests on determining which of the lesions corresponds best to the owner description of clinical signs or in simply choosing the site where compression looks most severe. In some dogs, the pragmatic decision to operate on more than 1 disk may be necessary.

WHICH SURGICAL APPROACH SHOULD I USE?

Decompressive surgery is aimed at alleviation of spinal cord compression, but the most appropriate surgical approach needs to be determined for each individual

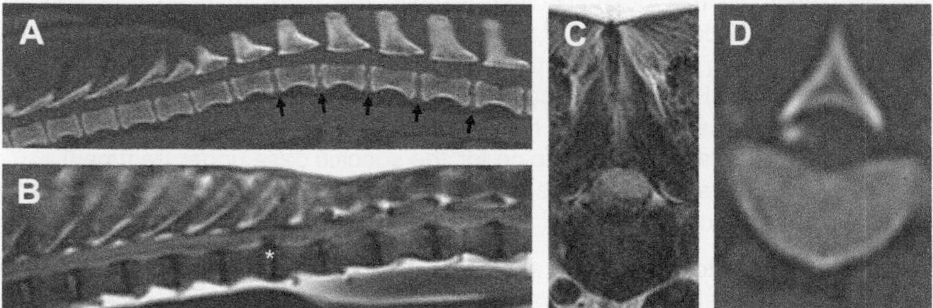

Fig. 1. CT and magnetic resonance (MR) provide complementary information, although MR is more sensitive for detection of spinal cord compression. (*A*) Midsagittal reconstructed CT scan of a dog with thoracolumbar myelopathy, revealing evidence of intervertebral disk degeneration (*arrows*) but not a site of compression. (*B*) Thoracolumbar T2-weighted (T2W) midsagittal MR scan of the same dog, revealing evidence of disk herniation and cord compression at T9/10; *asterisk*). (*C*) Transverse T2W MR scan through disk at T9/10 showing right-sided compression of the cord. (*D*) Transverse CT image through T9/10 intervertebral space showing the lateralized mineralization that, with hindsight, correlates with the MR image.

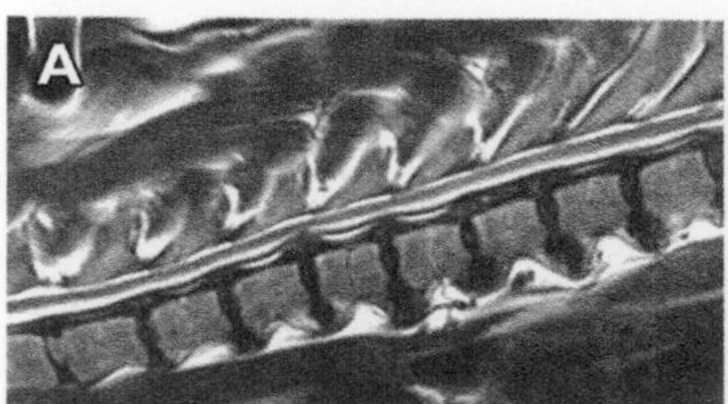

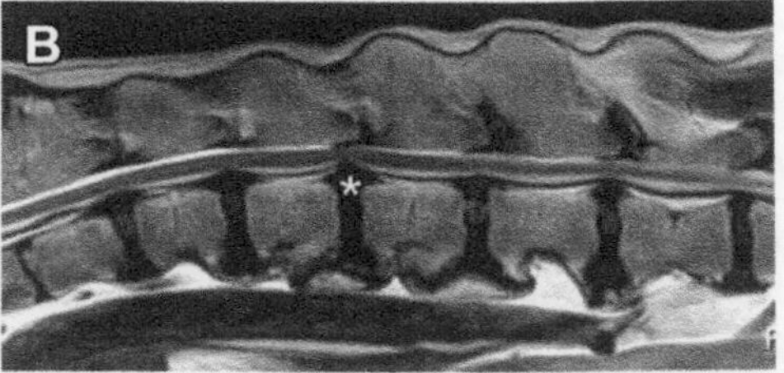

Fig. 2. Midsagittal T2W MR scans of a 10-year-old German shepherd with progressive paraparesis. Chronic disk herniation is suggested on midsagittal images of the thoracic (*A*) and thoracolumbar (*B*) regions (and was confirmed at each site on transverse images). The most compressive lesion (L1/2; *asterisk*) was selected for decompressive surgery (corpectomy).

animal. Although some investigators have suggested that a decompressive effect can be achieved through the bone removal of (dorsal) laminectomy alone, this has also been compared with removing the roof to allow water to drain from a flooded house[20] and does not affect depressed blood flow in animals with ventral spinal cord compression.[21] Therefore, decompression following disk extrusion implies removal of the herniated material. Even so, the need to remove ALL the herniated material can be questioned. For instance, although poor recovery following decompressive surgery can be associated with failure to remove all of the herniated disk,[22] substantial amounts of residual material can also be found in at least some dogs that exhibit uneventful long-term recovery.[23,24] Decision-making for acute and chronic disk herniation may differ, partly because of the character and progression (or regression) of clinical signs and partly because of the differing surgical procedures that may be most helpful.

The original procedures that were developed to decompress the spinal cord after acute disk herniation were (dorsal) laminectomy and hemilaminectomy.[25,26] Although the relative popularity of these two has altered over the decades, hemilaminectomy is now overwhelmingly preferred for most routine surgeries,[27] although laminectomy may have advantages in specific cases (see later discussion). The basic technique of hemilaminectomy has been modified to become more focused and ventrally directed through the development of the mini-hemilaminectomy/pediculectomy/foraminotomy.[28,29] During this century, the technique of (partial) lateral corpectomy for gaining access ventral to the spinal cord has also been introduced and gained popularity.[30–32] Each of these procedures has its advantages and disadvantages, and surgeons must make an appropriate choice for the specific case under treatment.

In general, the different approaches provide access to different aspects of the vertebral canal and spinal cord:

- (Dorsal) laminectomy provides access to the dorsal and lateral aspects of the vertebral canal, although removal of some of the medial aspects of the pedicles is often required to access the lateral aspect of the spinal cord.
- Hemilaminectomy provides access to the dorsolateral and lateral aspects.
- Mini-hemilaminectomy/pediculectomy provides access to the lateral and ventrolateral spinal cord.
- (Partial) corpectomy provides access to the ventrolateral and ventral aspects.

Despite the flexibility in available surgical approaches, it is (surprisingly) easy to lose focus on the aim of decompressing the spinal cord through removal of the herniated disk, mainly because the surgical procedures quickly become rote cookie-cutter procedures: it is possible for a procedure to be repeated stereotypically for each affected dog, without recognition of the specific needs of each patient. Conversely, the different procedures can often be tailored to specific patients to achieve the aim of accessing the appropriate part of the vertebral canal. For instance, hemilaminectomy is often extended ventrally to access the ventrolateral aspects of the spinal cord and corpectomy is frequently combined with mini-hemilaminectomy.[33]

The risk of indiscriminate application of hemilaminectomy to all disk herniation cases is that if herniated material lies ventral to the spinal cord, or even ventrolateral, it may be relatively inaccessible via an unmodified standard hemilaminectomy approach. The classic description of hemilaminectomy is to approach the vertebral canal from a dorsolateral direction and excise the articular processes.[34] This approach means that the dorsolateral aspect of the spinal cord is seen first, but this may not be where most of the herniated material lies (**Fig. 3**). Although extending the initial hemilaminectomy window more ventrally is well described,[34] inexperienced surgeons often feel disinclined to do so because of the risk of injuring the neurovascular structures in the foramen or the venous sinuses that lie on the floor of the canal. For this reason, it is possible to carry out the procedure as originally described and, therefore, fail to remove material that remains ventrolateral or ventral to the spinal cord because it remains invisible. Despite the natural wish to avoid encroaching on the ventral part of the vertebral canal, it may be essential to be able to decompress the cord in many cases. The modification, mini-hemilaminectomy, is designed to ensure exposure of the ventrolateral region of the vertebral canal, enabling the herniated disk at this location to be removed. Based on the commonly observed patterns of herniation, mini-hemilaminectomy would often seem to be the exposure of choice in

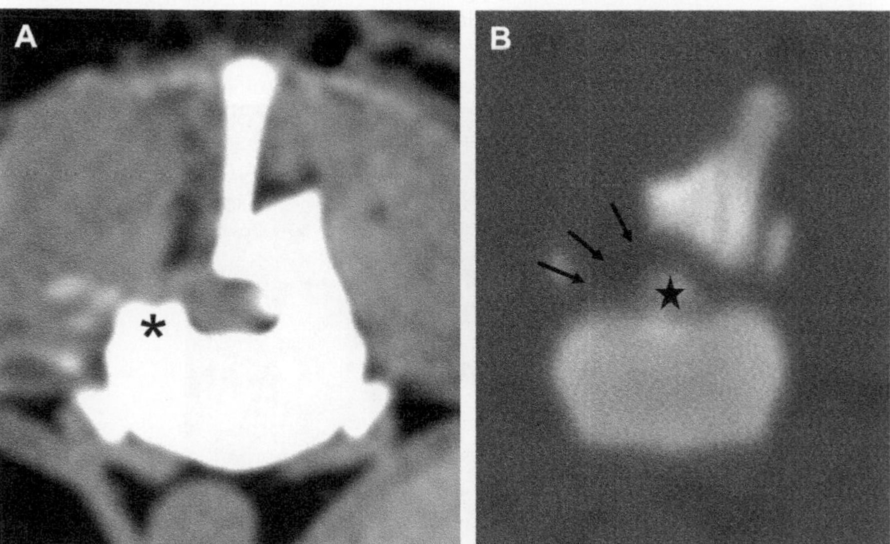

Fig. 3. Hemilaminectomy does not provide appropriate access for spinal cord decompression after acute thoracolumbar disk herniation in some dogs. (*A*) Postoperative transverse CT scan illustrating the lip of bone (*asterisk*) frequently remaining following hemilaminectomy that prevents access to the floor of the vertebral canal. (*B*) Postoperative transverse CT scan illustrating residual herniated disk (*star*) ventral to the spinal cord. Arrows indicate the lateral margin of the spinal cord; its position illustrates why the herniated disk may not be visible through this surgical window.

chondrodystrophic dogs, because herniated disk material most often lies ventrolateral or lateral to the spinal cord. Indeed, a recent study suggested that this approach was superior to conventional hemilaminectomy for spinal cord decompression.[35] Despite these advantages, hemilaminectomy is currently a far more popular choice among veterinary neurosurgeons.[27]

The location of acutely herniated disk material relative to the spinal cord often varies between different types of dogs. In chondrodystrophic dogs, the spinal cord is relatively large compared with the thoracolumbar vertebral canal,[36] which means that when a disk herniates, the material is trapped close to where it originates, implying that the compression will mostly lie ventral or ventrolateral to the spinal cord. In larger dogs, notably German shepherds and Doberman pinschers, the spinal cord has a much smaller diameter in relation to the vertebral canal, meaning that acutely herniated disk can escape from the ventral aspect of the cord and will frequently lodge lateral or even dorsal to the spinal cord. In these larger dogs, a conventional hemilaminectomy or laminectomy may be more appropriate.

Herniated material lying ventral to the spinal cord is inaccessible (unless the spinal cord is deliberately moved, which most neurosurgeons avoid doing) via most conventional approaches, including the mini-hemilaminectomy. In some cases, the material is not even visible because the spinal cord is draped over it, meaning that only by manipulating the spinal cord can it been seen (**Fig. 4**). Such cases require a ventral approach provided by partial lateral corpectomy.[30]

(PARTIAL) CORPECTOMY

This procedure was developed by Moissonnier and colleagues[30] in the early part of the 2000s. The notion was that by extending bone excision ventral to the spinal cord, it would be possible to retrieve disk herniations that lie ventral to the cord without having

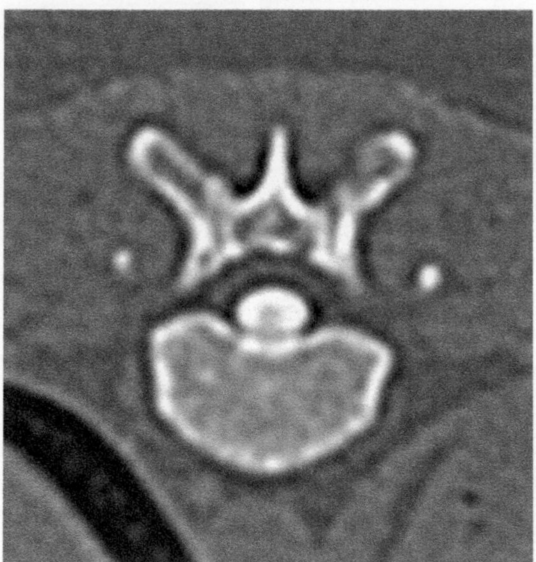

Fig. 4. Transverse CT scan illustrating large mineralized disk herniation lying directly ventral to the spinal cord. The herniated material will not be visible through a conventional lateral approach (hemilaminectomy or mini-hemilaminectomy).

to manipulate or move it. It was originally described as a procedure to remove chronic disk herniations that could not be removed through a conventional approach but has since also been widely used in the treatment of acute disk herniations.[31,32] The surgical procedure is often combined with a foraminotomy[33] because this facilitates identification of the lateral aspect of the vertebral canal and cord as a first step. After protecting the spinal nerve, usually by mobilizing it from surrounding soft tissue and retracting it cranially, the bone window is then extended ventrally. This is most conveniently done by placing the high-speed drill into the disk and extending the bone window cranially and caudally into the vertebral bodies. Cross-sectional imaging is necessary to determine the necessity for corpectomy and can also be used to measure the size of the bone window that can be made without risk of instability (**Fig. 5**). Conventionally, the bone window is restricted to about one-third of the length of the vertebrae and one-half of the depth of the vertebral end plate.[31] The lateral-lateral extent can be varied as required to remove the compressing material. During surgery, it can be difficult to be sure of the dimensions of the bone window, and so using a dental depth gauge can be useful (**Fig. 6**). These instruments have marks that show the depth of gingival pockets, and their shape facilitates their use in the confined space of a corpectomy incision.

The main difficulties with this procedure are dealing with the blood loss that can occur from the venous sinus and getting sufficient light into the surgical field. The lighting is best addressed by placing the dog in a lateral or semilateral position and then using a lateral[37] or dorsolateral[38] approach. The most lateral approach can be extremely quick for exposing the thoracolumbar junction region but, in larger dogs, the width of the lumbar musculature can make this difficult because the retracted muscle forms a tunnel in which to operate. The dorsolateral approach means that the muscle can be retracted sufficiently to gain access for using the drill in a purely lateral-lateral direction and also requires little muscle dissection. The dorsal approach (dissecting muscle from the spinous process and lateral aspect of the pedicle)[39]

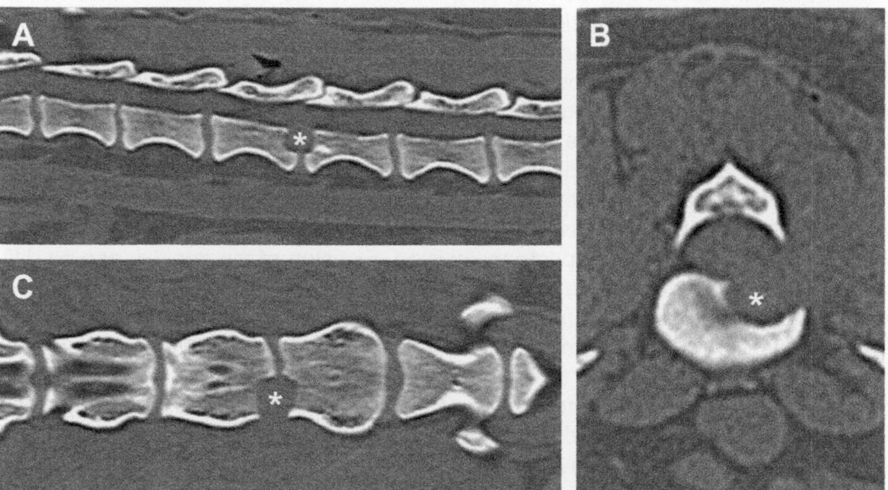

Fig. 5. Midsagittal (*A*), transverse, (*B*) and dorsal (*C*) CT scans illustrating the bone excised during a corpectomy procedure for removal of an acute disk herniation (*asterisks*). In (*B*), note the normal postoperative contour of the spinal cord. The size of the corpectomy incision can be tailored for each specific dog and disk herniation.

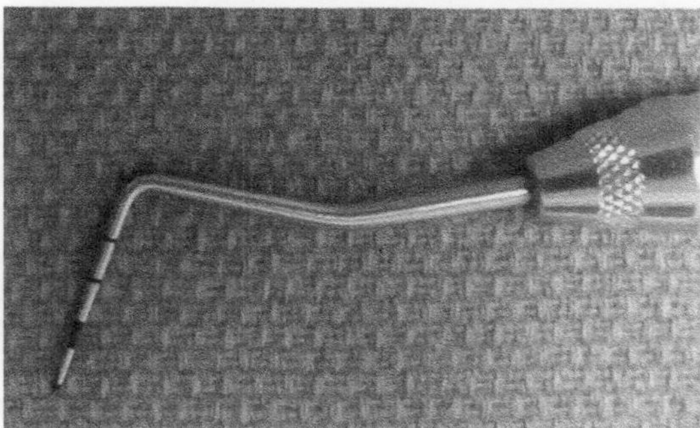

Fig. 6. Detail of one of the measuring tips of a periodontal probe, which can be inserted into the surgical site to confirm the dimensions of the corpectomy incision intraoperatively.

makes access for corpectomy problematic because it is very difficult to retract the muscle sufficiently ventrally to be able to drill parallel with the floor of the vertebral canal.

The procedure involves a gradual removal of the bone ventral to the spinal cord, leaving the dorsal longitudinal ligament intact until the last moment. The dorsal longitudinal ligament can be extremely thick in dogs that have chronic disk herniations and may need to be removed using a scalpel. In association with acute disk herniations, it is usually lacerated and thin. The approach for corpectomy necessitates opening the lateral aspect of the vertebral canal, just adjacent to the venous sinus; this can deter surgeons concerned about excessive blood loss. This blood loss can be annoying but is not likely to be life threatening, although there may also be a risk of air embolism.[40] In general, in dogs with chronic herniations, the sinus often seems to have been collapsed for a long period and may not carry any blood at all or be so compressed that it does not present a problem. In dogs with acute disk herniations, there can be some hemorrhage from this area. This hemorrhaging is usually best dealt with by rolling small pieces of absorbable gelatin sponge (Gelfoam, Pfizer Inc, New York, NY) into cigar shapes that can be pushed in a parasagittal direction into the space between the spinal cord and bone or, in some cases, the sinus can be closed using bipolar diathermy.

Once the canal is opened from the lateral direction and the soft tissue is all that remains ventrally, the dorsal longitudinal ligament and disk material can be removed, usually using strokes of a fine, sharp-tipped instrument that can tear through the soft tissue or engage the disk to pull it ventrally into the corpectomy deficit. Sharp rongeurs that can grasp the ligament and the annulus may also be useful. These procedures are repeated until there is no material ventral to the spinal cord, and it sinks ventrally to lie flat over the corpectomy incision. Excision of the annulus can be difficult; in chronic disk herniations, it is often attached firmly to the dura and may have become calcified or even resemble bone. Although usually the dura and annulus (or dorsal longitudinal ligament) can be dissected apart, on occasion it is not possible and so it becomes necessary to excise a small portion of dura to allow removal of the associated disk. This seems to be safe and without obvious adverse effects. Following completion of the decompression, the corpectomy site is lavaged and closed routinely; there is no need to place a fat graft.

IS CORPECTOMY ADVANTAGEOUS?

Corpectomy is chosen because it provides superior access to the ventral aspect of the spinal cord, and for that reason it is difficult to consider how a fair comparison with other techniques can be made: surgeons who consider it essential to approach the ventral aspect of the spinal cord would not consider randomizing their patients to another technique. However, not all surgeons agree that corpectomy is necessary for treatment of dogs that have herniated disk ventral to the spinal cord. This difference of opinion provided the authors with a set of data in which dogs were quasi-randomized to receive either corpectomy or conventional hemilaminectomy depending on the service to which they were allocated according to the day on which they presented to their clinics.

First, the authors identified dogs that had been treated by corpectomy at their clinics between 2010 and 2013 and measured the amount of spinal cord compression in these cases. We then searched the medical records to find a series of dogs that had ventral compression of similar severity but had been treated by hemilaminectomy. The authors then noted how long it had taken for these cases to recover to walk (10 consecutive steps unaided without falling) and recover voluntary urination. The question then asked was whether recovery of independent locomotion and urination was quicker in dogs that underwent corpectomy; multivariable Cox regression analysis was used to adjust for other factors that might influence recovery, such as whether the dogs had lost deep pain perception, age, weight, and the duration of clinical signs before surgery. The outcome, summarized in **Table 1**, provides support for the notion that corpectomy is advantageous in speeding the recovery after paraparesis following acute thoracolumbar disk herniation. However, these findings must be treated with caution because dogs were not randomly allocated to treatment type and so various other factors not captured in the analysis may have also influenced the outcome.

Table 1
Comparison of recovery of dogs with ventrally located acute herniated intervertebral disk following corpectomy versus conventional hemilaminectomy

	Hazard Ratio	SE	z	*P*	95% CI
Locomotion	2.610	0.962	2.60	.009	1.267–5.373
Urinary control	1.693	0.527	1.69	.090	0.920–3.115

The hazard ratio is an expression of the relative instantaneous 'risk' of recovery during the study period.

Abbreviations: CI, confidence interval; SE, standard error.

DUROTOMY, PIOTOMY, AND MYELOTOMY

Durotomy has long been advocated as a means to identify extensive myelomalacia in dogs that present with very severe clinical signs.[41] Following incision into the dura, liquefied malacic spinal cord will flow out; the assumption has been made that such cases will have a hopeless prognosis. The problem with this procedure is that it is inevitable that severely affected cases will have localized malacia and it may not be possible for the surgeon to distinguish between a localized lesion from which the animal might recover and the hopeless prognosis associated with ascending myelomalacia. For this reason, this type of exploratory/diagnostic durotomy has fallen out of favor in recent decades.

On the other hand, because the spinal cord swells after injury, it has long been thought that the meninges may form a constriction that impairs blood flow through the injured spinal cord and, therefore, that durotomy might have some therapeutic benefit. Work in experimental dogs implied that durotomy was not helpful in improving blood flow or outcome unless carried out within 2 hours of the contusive episode, and it has been suggested that the constricting membrane might in fact be the pia.[42,43] Piotomy is not an easy procedure to carry out atraumatically without also cutting the spinal cord in the sagittal direction (ie, myelotomy). Although there will be inevitable damage to the spinal cord associated with myelotomy, the procedure does not cause severe lasting neurologic deficits in normal experimental dogs.[44] Despite the theoretic benefits to carrying out myelotomy, this has not become standard practice for the treatment of even severely cord-injured dogs, perhaps because surgeons consider that the risks do not outweigh any theoretic benefits. More recently, the less invasive procedure of durotomy has been reinvestigated using Doppler to measure blood flow.[45,46] However, these studies suggested no long-term improvement of blood flow or outcome, a conclusion also supported by a more formal comparison of clinical outcomes between durotomy and control cases.[47]

Nevertheless, an ongoing series of observations made in human patients with spinal cord injuries have suggested, again, that the dura may cause spinal cord compression[48,49] and that duraplasty may improve outcomes.[50,51] The apparent difference in outcomes following durotomy in the two species seems striking and difficult to explain but might perhaps arise because (1) the human spinal cord is much larger, allowing more precise and repeatable measurements of intraspinal pressure and blood flow; (2) human durotomy is carried out from a dorsal approach, meaning that it is better located to allow decompression; and (3) the use of duraplasty rather than simple durotomy may be advantageous. A potential problem with simple durotomy is that, as the spinal cord herniates through the incision, vessels at the incision margins may be crushed, thus, impeding blood flow.

HOW MUCH BONE CAN BE REMOVED DURING DECOMPRESSIVE SURGERY?

In general, the approach for decompressive surgery is to remove the minimal amount of bone to achieve complete removal of the herniated disk. Nevertheless, there are also limits to bone removal, mainly dictated by the need to preserve adequate stability in the vertebral column. The biomechanics of the vertebral column are often analyzed in terms of the 3-column system, in which there are 3 columns that run sagittally through the length of the dog.[52] It is generally considered that disruption of 2 of the 3 columns will result in instability and so this can be used as a method to determine which dogs require surgery to stabilize vertebral column fracture-luxations.[53] It can also be used to define limits for surgical decompression after disk herniation such that more than 1 column is not disrupted as a consequence of the decompressive surgery.

Fortunately, the standard procedures do not disrupt more than 1 column, meaning that they are relatively safe when performed over any length unilaterally. However, if, for instance, a *bilateral* hemilaminectomy is performed at more than 1 consecutive space, the lamina is inevitably loosened, allowing fracture and collapse of the site. This type of problem should now be much rarer than in the past because cross-sectional imaging can identify the site and side of the lesion with greater accuracy than older techniques (ie, myelography) meaning that bilateral surgery is uncommon but, occasionally, this problem can arise when dealing with multiple disk herniations.

Instability might also be expected if a hemilaminectomy is then followed by a corpectomy because that would imply disruption of both the middle and dorsal columns[52]; indeed, cadaver studies confirm decreased stiffness after this combination of surgeries.[54] Nevertheless, although clearly not ideal, the authors know of no complications that have arisen in a small number of dogs in which corpectomy was carried out several days after a previous, unsuccessful hemilaminectomy.

A more subtle problem can arise following a standard laminectomy approach in the thoracolumbar region if a series of consecutive spinous processes are excised together with the supraspinous ligament because this removes a key part of the stabilizing elements of the vertebral column.[55] Although it is rare to encounter secondary complications in the short-term, a long-term complication of this approach can be development of kyphosis and premature disk herniation at sites of increased mobility. The problem can be avoided by preserving the supraspinous ligament by cutting and retracting the dorsal parts of the spinous processes rather than excising them (**Fig. 7**).[56]

CHOICE OF THERAPY FOR CHRONIC (TYPE II) THORACOLUMBAR DISK HERNIATIONS

Chronic disk herniations present some unique problems for decompressive surgery. The first is the difficulty in determining whether they are actually responsible for the observed clinical signs. Dogs of types that are commonly affected by chronic thoracolumbar disk herniation are also often susceptible to other disease, notably degenerative myelopathy.[57] It can be almost impossible to be sure which of these conditions is responsible for the clinical signs in an individual dog, and in some cases both may coexist. Fortunately, in many instances a negative result on the genetic screening test for the most common mutation associated with degenerative myelopathy[58] can substantially reduce the probability of this condition as a cause of the clinical signs. On the other hand, a positive test result can be difficult to interpret because a large proportion of normal individuals in some breeds may carry the mutation.[58]

The next problem is that it may be difficult to determine which one of a series of herniated disks is responsible for current clinical signs. Chronic disk herniations often develop very slowly meaning that they can be of variable size in dogs that are undergoing degeneration at several sites. Often the decision is based largely on which ones look most severe on imaging (most compression, greatest amount of T2W hyperintensity) (see **Fig. 2**), and sometimes it is necessary to operate more than one site.

The cause of clinical signs associated with chronic disk herniation is often assumed to result not only from compression but also from dynamic compression resulting from

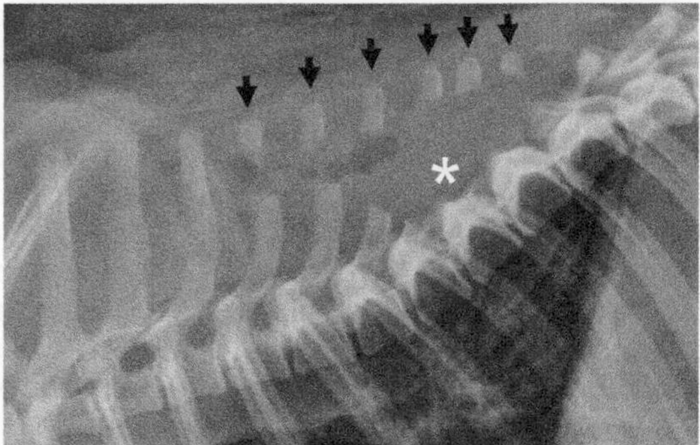

Fig. 7. Postoperative lateral radiograph of the thoracic vertebral column. A dorsal laminectomy has been carried out in the midthoracic region (*asterisk*) via a ligament-preserving approach. The spinous processes (*arrows*) were severed beneath the supraspinous ligament using an oscillating saw and, together with the ligament, retracted laterally. The remaining parts of the spinous processes were excised routinely with rongeurs to permit access to the laminae for laminectomy.

the exacerbation and alleviation of spinal cord compression that occurs during normal motion of the vertebral column.[6] This process, and the generally progressive nature of the clinical signs, suggests that chronic disk herniations are arguably more pertinent candidates for decompression than acute disks, for which there is some doubt about efficacy of decompression in restoration of function. On the other hand, the slow rate of progression associated with chronic disk herniation implies that, by the time an animal is diagnosed with the lesion, the spinal cord may have already undergone severe atrophy that cannot be reversed by decompression.

Although chronic disk herniation is almost inevitably associated with axonal loss, which is irreversible, some of the deficits in clinical patients also arise from reversible lesions, such as demyelination[59] and edema. Furthermore, there is evidence that conservative therapy is not very effective in these affected dogs,[60] whereas surgery often is,[61] therefore, implying that surgery should be strongly favored. In order to provide some reassurance to the surgeon and owner, a short trial course of glucocorticoids may determine whether the deficits are responsive to symptomatic therapy. A positive response would suggest that surgery is likely to be at least equally effective and also aid in confirming that degenerative myelopathy is not responsible for all observed neurologic deficits.

If surgery is selected, there is a choice to be made between decompression via corpectomy in which the entire dorsal annulus is excised and augmentation of the decompression achievable via hemilaminectomy with stabilization.[62] A rationale for stabilization is that it will eliminate the dynamic compression that is associated with chronic disk herniation, allowing reversal of the reversible lesions within the spinal cord. The choice is largely made by surgeon experience: orthopedic surgeons often prefer to fix the affected region, whereas neurosurgeons tend to prefer to decompress. Either technique can be effective based on published clinical reports.

IS THERE A ROLE FOR STABILIZATION FOLLOWING DECOMPRESSIVE SURGERY?

Following routine approaches to the spinal cord as outlined here, there is no need for stabilization of the vertebrae following decompressive approaches. However, as described earlier, some surgeons would consider the need for stabilization after surgery for chronic disk herniations, especially if this has not been combined with aggressive removal of the protruding disk (eg, via corpectomy). For instance, following hemilaminectomy and annulectomy for chronic disks, it might be worthwhile to eliminate the dynamic component of the compression by fixation of the vertebrae to eliminate further motion.

APPROACHES AND POSITIONING FOR SURGERY

In the earliest days of veterinary spinal surgery, the site to be approached was usually diagnosed using myelography; sometimes the images were insufficiently precise to enable the surgeon to be sure of the precise site and side of compression. This uncertainty implied that it was sometimes necessary to operate on both sides for a single disk herniation, if the herniated material was not located during the first approach. Logically, this meant that a reliance on positioning in symmetric ventral recumbency was prudent. With the widespread use of cross-sectional imaging, which provides very accurate information about the location of the material to be excised, alternative positioning of the dog may be advantageous. For instance, it can be difficult to direct sufficient light toward the ventral aspect of the spinal cord, or to use instruments ventrally to the spinal cord, when using a dorsal approach. It is difficult to retract the muscle sufficiently to provide an unobstructed light path. As described earlier, more lateral approaches, either dorsolateral[38] or lateral,[37] overcome these problems. Often, positioning in lateral recumbency and then elevating the dorsal aspect of the dog to form an angle of about 20° to the horizontal is a good compromise between adequate lighting and avoiding stress to the surgeon's neck. In some parts of the world, surgeons will operate from the dorsal aspect of the laterally recumbent dog to aid visibility and improve surgeon comfort.

ADDITION OF PROPHYLACTIC PROCEDURES

Dogs that develop disk degeneration sufficient to have a symptomatic episode are at high risk of recurrence that can be substantially reduced by fenestration.[63] However, many surgeons are dubious about the time risk-benefit ratio for doing multilevel fenestration meaning that they will frequently search for means to limit the numbers of fenestrations needed. Some suggestions include doing the one affected and 2 neighbors or fenestrating those that appear degenerate on MRI (see Nick D. Jeffery and Paul M. Freeman's article, "The Role of Fenestration in Management of Type I Thoracolumbar Disk Degeneration," in this issue). The problem with many of these other options is that the degenerative process develops over time, and so a nondegenerate-looking disk at one time point might within a few months appear degenerate. The choice may be to decide how much time is to be allocated to each animal's surgery and then decide how best to spend that time.

HOW DO I JUDGE WHETHER MY DECOMPRESSIVE SURGERY HAS ACHIEVED ITS AIM?

Finding some herniated disk material within the vertebral canal usually provides confirmation that the correct space has been operated (if it can be aged to correlate with the clinical signs), but how much material should be removed? This quantity will vary from case to case; but for many animals in which compression is likely to have had a significant effect on the spinal cord, it would be expected that at least 50% of the diameter of the vertebral canal will be filled with herniated material. This amount might then equate to an area of 0.5 cm^2 in many chondrodystrophic dogs and perhaps stretch over about 1.0 cm, suggesting a total volume of about 0.5 cm^3 (0.5 mL). This volume is considerable. (Think of half the volume contained in a 1-mL syringe in the vertebral canal of a chondrodystrophic dog.) If less than this amount is removed, then it might (well) be that the decompression is incomplete.

A further guide to completeness of decompression can be the position of the spinal cord. When the canal is first opened in dogs with disk herniation, the spinal cord is pushed away from the bone; but as decompression is achieved, the spinal cord expands to fill the area more completely and will also lie flat on the floor of the vertebral canal. Sometimes additional material ventral to the spinal cord can be removed by using fine-gauge hooks to sweep across the floor of the vertebral canal. In cases in which a substantial portion of the herniated material, lies ventral to the spinal cord a ventral (corpectomy) approach will be necessary.

WHAT DO I NEED TO LOOK FOR POSTOPERATIVELY?

In cases in which the spinal cord has been compressed and the compression has been responsible for the clinical signs then it would be expected that functional recovery will occur very rapidly. Many such dogs will recover to walk again within 24 to 48 hours of decompressive surgery. However, much more frequently, contusive injury to the spinal cord is the major cause of spinal cord dysfunction, implying that decompression will have little effect. In these cases, it would be expected that recovery of lost neurologic function might take at least 3 weeks and possibly as long as 3 months or even more.

Recovery of dogs that have had a very severe spinal cord injury, such that they have lost pain perception in the hindquarters, will often take many weeks to months to recover useful function; it is critical that owners are guided as to how long the recovery process might be. They must be supported in looking after the animals while the spinal cord recovers spontaneously because there is nothing that can be done to hasten recovery of the contused spinal cord. Particular attention is required for the bladder because it is very easy for it to become overfull, which can then lead to secondary damage to the upper urinary tract and may even be fatal if there is concurrent infection.

Early recurrence of clinical signs following decompressive surgery is usually a sign that there has been recurrence of herniation at the same site,[64] and this can be prevented by fenestration at the same site as the herniation occurs (see Nick D. Jeffery and Paul M. Freeman's article, "The Role of Fenestration in Management of Type I Thoracolumbar Disk Degeneration," in this issue).

SUMMARY

Once decompressive surgery has been elected, the approach that maximizes the likelihood of gaining access to the herniated material for complete removal should be chosen. In most cases, a procedure that optimizes access to the ventrolateral aspect of the spinal cord will be advantageous but it is important to tailor the details of the surgical procedure to suit individual patients. Decompressive surgery for chronic (type II) herniations will frequently demand a ventral approach with partial corpectomy.

REFERENCES

1. Nashmi R, Fehlings MG. Changes in axonal physiology and morphology after chronic compressive injury of the rat thoracic spinal cord. Neuroscience 2001; 104:235–51.
2. Shi R, Blight AR. Compression injury of mammalian spinal cord in vitro and the dynamics of action potential conduction failure. J Neurophysiol 1996;76:1572–80.
3. Shi R, Pryor JD. Pathological changes of isolated spinal cord axons in response to mechanical stretch. Neuroscience 2002;110:765–77.
4. Kurokawa R, Murata H, Ogino M, et al. Altered blood flow distribution in the rat spinal cord under chronic compression. Spine (Phila Pa 1976) 2011;36:1006–9.
5. Werndle MC, Saadoun S, Phang I, et al. Monitoring of spinal cord perfusion pressure in acute spinal cord injury: initial findings of the injured spinal cord pressure evaluation study. Crit Care Med 2014;42:646–55.
6. al-Mefty O, Harkey HL, Marawi I, et al. Experimental chronic compressive cervical myelopathy. J Neurosurg 1993;79:550–61.
7. Brisson BA. Intervertebral disc disease in dogs. Vet Clin North Am Small Anim Pract 2010;40:829–58.
8. Freeman P, Jeffery ND. Re-opening the window on fenestration as a treatment for acute thoracolumbar intervertebral disc herniation in dogs. J Small Anim Pract 2017;58:199–204.
9. Langerhuus L, Miles J. Proportion recovery and times to ambulation for non-ambulatory dogs with thoracolumbar disc extrusions treated with hemilaminectomy or conservative treatment: a systematic review and meta-analysis of case-series studies. Vet J 2017;220:7–16.

10. Dimar JR, Glassman SD, Raque GH, et al. The influence of spinal canal narrowing and timing of decompression on neurological recovery after spinal cord contusion in a rat model. Spine 1999;24:1623–33.
11. Kubota K, Saiwai H, Kumamaru H, et al. Neurological recovery is impaired by concurrent but not by asymptomatic pre-existing spinal cord compression after traumatic spinal cord injury. Spine (Phila Pa 1976) 2012;37:1448–55.
12. Sukhiani HR, Parent JM, Atilola MA, et al. Intervertebral disk disease in dogs with signs of back pain alone: 25 cases (1986–1993). J Am Vet Med Assoc 1996;209: 1275–9.
13. Nout YS, Beattie MS, Bresnahan JC. Severity of locomotor and cardiovascular derangements after experimental high-thoracic spinal cord injury is anesthesia dependent in rats. J Neurotrauma 2012;29:990–9.
14. Dixon A, Fauber AE. Effect of anesthesia-associated hypotension on neurologic outcome in dogs undergoing hemilaminectomy because of acute, severe thoracolumbar intervertebral disk herniation: 56 cases (2007-2013). J Am Vet Med Assoc 2017;250:417–23.
15. Fenn J, Laber E, Williams K, et al. Associations between anesthetic variables and functional outcome in dogs with thoracolumbar intervertebral disk extrusion undergoing decompressive hemilaminectomy. J Vet Intern Med 2017. http://dx.doi.org/10.1111/jvim.14677.
16. Jeffery ND, Barker AK, Hu HZ, et al. Factors associated with recovery from paraplegia in dogs with loss of pain perception in the pelvic limbs following intervertebral disk herniation. J Am Vet Med Assoc 2016;248:386–94.
17. Piazza M, Schuster J. Timing of surgery after spinal cord injury. Neurosurg Clin N Am 2017;28:31–9.
18. Gutierrez-Quintana R, Edgar J, Wessmann A, et al. The cutaneous trunci reflex for localising and grading thoracolumbar spinal cord injuries in dogs. J Small Anim Pract 2012;53:470–5.
19. Cooper JJ, Young BD, Griffin JF 4th, et al. Comparison between noncontrast computed tomography and magnetic resonance imaging for detection and characterization of thoracolumbar myelopathy caused by intervertebral disk herniation in dogs. Vet Radiol Ultrasound 2014;55:182–9.
20. Prata RG. Neurosurgical treatment of thoracolumbar disks: the rationale and value of laminectomy with concomitant disk removal. J Am Anim Hosp Assoc 1981;17:17–26.
21. Doppman JL, Girtow M. Angiographic study of the effect of laminectomy in the presence of acute anterior epidural masses. J Neurosurg 1976;45:195–202.
22. Forterre F, Gorgas D, Dickomeit M, et al. Incidence of spinal compressive lesions in chondrodystrophic dogs with abnormal recovery after hemilaminectomy for treatment of thoracolumbar disc disease: a prospective magnetic resonance imaging study. Vet Surg 2010;39:165–72.
23. Roach WJ, Thomas M, Weh JM, et al. Residual herniated disc material following hemilaminectomy in chondrodystrophic dogs with thoracolumbar intervertebral disc disease. Vet Comp Orthop Traumatol 2012;25:109–15.
24. Huska JL, Gaitero L, Brisson BA, et al. Presence of residual material following mini-hemilaminectomy in dogs with thoracolumbar intervertebral disc extrusion. Can Vet J 2014;55:975–80.
25. Gage ED, Hoerlein BF. Hemilaminectomy and dorsal laminectomy for relieving compressions of the spinal cord in the dog. J Am Vet Med Assoc 1968;152: 351–9.

26. Funkquist B. Decompressive laminectomy in thoraco-lumbar disc protrusion with paraplegia in the dog. J Small Anim Pract 1970;11:445–51.
27. Moore SA, Early PJ, Hettlich BF. Practice patterns in the management of acute intervertebral disc herniation in dogs. J Small Anim Pract 2016;57:409–15.
28. Jeffery ND. Treatment of acute and chronic thoracolumbar disc disease by 'mini hemilaminectomy'. J Small Anim Pract 1988;29:611–6.
29. Lubbe AM, Kirberger RM, Verstraete FJM. Pediculectomy for thoracolumbar spinal decompression in the dachshund. J Am Anim Hosp Assoc 1994;30:233–8.
30. Moissonnier P, Meheust P, Carozzo C. Thoracolumbar lateral corpectomy for treatment of chronic disk herniation: technique description and use in 15 dogs. Vet Surg 2004;33:620–8.
31. Flegel T, Boettcher IC, Ludewig E, et al. Partial lateral corpectomy of the thoracolumbar spine in 51 dogs: assessment of slot morphometry and spinal cord decompression. Vet Surg 2011;40:14–21.
32. Salger F, Ziegler L, Böttcher IC, et al. Neurologic outcome after thoracolumbar partial lateral corpectomy for intervertebral disc disease in 72 dogs. Vet Surg 2014;43:581–8.
33. Medl SC, Reese S, Medl NS. Individualized mini-hemilaminectomy-corpectomy (iMHC) for treatment of thoracolumbar intervertebral disc herniation in large breed dogs. Vet Surg 2017;46:422–32.
34. Sharp NJH, Wheeler SJ. Thoracolumbar disc disease. In: Sharp NJH, Wheeler SJ, editors. Small animal spinal disorders: diagnosis and surgery. Chapter 8. 2nd edition. London: Elsevier Mosby; 2005. p. 121–60.
35. Svensson G, Simonsson US, Danielsson F, et al. Residual spinal cord compression following hemilaminectomy and mini-hemilaminectomy in dogs: a prospective randomized study. Front Vet Sci 2017;4:42.
36. Morgan JP, Atilola M, Bailey CS. Vertebral canal and spinal cord mensuration: a comparative study of its effect on lumbosacral myelography in the dachshund and German shepherd dog. J Am Vet Med Assoc 1987;191:951–7.
37. Braund KG, Taylor TK, Ghosh P, et al. Lateral spinal decompression in the dog. J Small Anim Pract 1976;17:583–92.
38. Yturraspe DJ, Lumb WV. A dorsolateral muscle-separating approach for thoracolumbar intervertebral disk fenestration in the dog. J Am Vet Med Assoc 1973;162: 1037–40.
39. Redding RW. Laminectomy in the dog. Am J Vet Res 1951;12:123–8.
40. Mortera-Balsa V, van Oostrom H, Yeamans C, et al. Suspected air embolism through the thoracic ventral internal vertebral plexus during hemilaminectomy in dogs. J Small Anim Pract 2017;58:355–8.
41. Toombs JP, Waters DJ. Intervertebral disk disease. In: Slatter D, editor. Textbook of small animal surgery. Philadelphia: Saunders; 2003. p. 1193–209.
42. Parker AJ, Smith CW. Functional recovery from spinal cord trauma following incision of spinal meninges in dogs. Res Vet Sci 1974;16:276–9.
43. Parker AJ, Smith CW. Functional recovery following incision of spinal meninges in dogs. Res Vet Sci 1972;13:418–21.
44. Teague HD, Brasmer TH. Midline myelotomy of the clinically normal canine spinal cord. Am J Vet Res 1978;39:1584–90.
45. Malik Y, Spreng D, Konar M, et al. Laser-Doppler measurements of spinal cord blood flow changes during hemilaminectomy in chondrodystrophic dogs with disk extrusion. Vet Surg 2009;38:457–62.

46. Blaser A, Lang J, Henke D, et al. Influence of durotomy on laser-Doppler measurement of spinal cord blood flow in chondrodystrophic dogs with thoracolumbar disk extrusion. Vet Surg 2012;41:221–7.
47. Loughin CA, Dewey CW, Ringwood PB, et al. Effect of durotomy on functional outcome of dogs with type I thoracolumbar disc extrusion and absent deep pain perception. Vet Comp Orthop Traumatol 2005;18:141–6.
48. Phang I, Papadopoulos MC. Intraspinal pressure monitoring in a patient with spinal cord injury reveals different intradural compartments: injured spinal cord pressure evaluation (ISCoPE) study. Neurocrit Care 2015;23:414–8.
49. Saadoun S, Werndle MC, Lopez de Heredia L, et al. The dura causes spinal cord compression after spinal cord injury. Br J Neurosurg 2016;30:582–4.
50. Phang I, Werndle MC, Saadoun S, et al. Expansion duroplasty improves intraspinal pressure, spinal cord perfusion pressure, and vascular pressure reactivity index in patients with traumatic spinal cord injury: injured spinal cord pressure evaluation study. J Neurotrauma 2015;32:865–74.
51. Saadoun S, Chen S, Papadopoulos MC. Intraspinal pressure and spinal cord perfusion pressure predict neurological outcome after traumatic spinal cord injury. J Neurol Neurosurg Psychiatry 2016;88:452–3.
52. Shores A. Spinal trauma. Pathophysiology and management of traumatic spinal injuries. Vet Clin North Am Small Anim Pract 1992;22:875.
53. Jeffery ND. Vertebral fracture and luxation in small animals. Vet Clin North Am Small Anim Pract 2010;40:809–28.
54. Vizcaíno Revés N, Bürki A, Ferguson S, et al. Influence of partial lateral corpectomy with and without hemilaminectomy on canine thoracolumbar stability: a biomechanical study. Vet Surg 2012;41:228–34.
55. Hartmann F, Janssen C, Böhm S, et al. Biomechanical effect of graded minimal-invasive decompression procedures on lumbar spinal stability. Arch Orthop Trauma Surg 2012;132:1233–9.
56. Forterre F, Spreng D, Rytz U, et al. Thoracolumbar dorsolateral laminectomy with osteotomy of the spinous process in fourteen dogs. Vet Surg 2007;36:458–63.
57. Coates JR, Wininger FA. Canine degenerative myelopathy. Vet Clin North Am Small Anim Pract 2010;40:929–50.
58. Zeng R, Coates JR, Johnson GC, et al. Breed distribution of SOD1 alleles previously associated with canine degenerative myelopathy. J Vet Intern Med 2014;28:515–21.
59. Smith PM, Jeffery ND. Histological and ultrastructural analysis of white matter damage after naturally-occurring spinal cord injury. Brain Pathol 2006;16:99–109.
60. Crawford AH, De Decker S. Clinical presentation and outcome of dogs treated medically or surgically for thoracolumbar intervertebral disc protrusion. Vet Rec 2017;180:569.
61. Ferrand FX, Moissonnier P, Filleur A, et al. Thoracolumbar partial lateral corpectomy for the treatment of chronic intervertebral disc disease in 107 dogs. Ir Vet J 2015;68:27.
62. McKee WM, Downes CJ. Vertebral stabilisation and selective decompression for the management of triple thoracolumbar disc protrusions. J Small Anim Pract 2008;49:536–9.
63. Brisson BA, Holmberg DL, Parent J, et al. Comparison of the effect of single-site and multiple-site disc fenestration on the rate of recurrence of thoracolumbar disc

extrusion in dogs; a prospective, randomized, controlled study. J Am Vet Med Assoc 2011;238:1593–600.
64. Hettlich BF, Kerwin SC, Levine JM. Early reherniation of disk material in eleven dogs with surgically treated thoracolumbar intervertebral disk extrusion. Vet Surg 2012;41:215–20.

The Role of Fenestration in Management of Type I Thoracolumbar Disk Degeneration

Nick D. Jeffery, BVSc, MSc, PhD, FRCVS[a,*],
Paul M. Freeman, MA, VetMB, CertSAO[b]

KEYWORDS

- Therapeutic fenestration • Intervertebral disk fenestration
- Thoracolumbar intervertebral disk herniation • Decompressive surgery

KEY POINTS

- Fenestration offers the advantages of prophylaxis without the need for specialized instrumentation and imaging.
- Currently there is a lack of equipoise regarding the efficacy of fenestration relative to decompression for treatment of acute canine intervertebral disk herniation; most veterinary spinal surgeons do not consider the 2 procedures equivalently efficacious.
- Therapeutic fenestration should perhaps be given greater consideration, especially if advanced imaging shows only mild to moderate spinal cord compression or there are restrictions on the duration of surgery, when it might be better to spend the time on fenestration rather than decompression.

INTRODUCTION

Intervertebral disk fenestration has an interesting history in veterinary medicine. When first introduced as a surgical treatment of thoracolumbar intervertebral disk herniation (IVDH) in the 1950s it was described as a means by which the clinical signs—both pain and paresis—could be alleviated.[1] During the 1980s and early 1990s, fenestration became popular and widely practiced and was associated with good clinical outcomes.[2–6] Since then it has lost popularity, particularly as a treatment option, whereas decompressive surgery has become more widely adopted. Prophylactic fenestration has continued to be used by some veterinary surgeons, buoyed by findings that strongly support its prophylactic effect in dogs with previous episodes of symptomatic IVDH.[7–9]

The authors have nothing to disclose.

[a] Department of Small Animal Clinical Sciences, Texas A&M University, 4474 TAMU, College Station, TX 77843, USA; [b] Department of Veterinary Medicine, University of Cambridge, Cambridge CB3 0ES, UK

* Corresponding author.

E-mail address: njeffery@cvm.tamu.edu

Vet Clin Small Anim 48 (2018) 187–200
http://dx.doi.org/10.1016/j.cvsm.2017.08.012 vetsmall.theclinics.com

Its waning popularity as a treatment coincided with increased veterinary access to cross-sectional imaging of the vertebral column, which made it clear that the spinal cord is often grossly deformed after IVDH, thus suggesting the need for decompression, which cannot be attained through fenestration alone. Contemporaneously, experimental evidence that decompression after contusion and compression improved functional outcome became available,[10] and there were numerous reports of rapid recovery after spinal cord decompression in clinically affected dogs.[11] This weight of evidence led to the current widely held view that fenestration is useful for prophylaxis but should not be considered a useful therapy for canine IVDH.[8,12]

Despite this point of view there are several questions that remain unanswered regarding the value of decompressive spinal surgery for Hansen type I IVDH. For instance, dogs can have severe spinal cord compression, including that resulting from disk herniation, while showing minimal neurologic deficits.[13] There is also poor correlation between severity of compression and severity of dysfunction or prognosis.[14] Moreover, several investigators have detected residual compressive material after decompressive surgery and, in some dogs, large compressive volumes,[15] raising the possibility that decompression may not be essential for functional recovery after symptomatic disk herniation. Furthermore, the current assumption that the spinal cord requires decompression suggests that previous reports that implied the effectiveness of fenestration must be incorrect. Is it possible that the reports of its apparent efficacy were erroneous and that numerous surgeons were misled?

In an attempt to answer these questions, we recently re-examined the available published data to compare outcomes between the different available therapies for symptomatic Type I thoracolumbar IVDH.[11] Surprisingly, the analysis suggests that fenestration is an effective therapy, with a total of 951 dogs across a total of 11 publications showing an overall recovery rate of 94% for dogs with intact pain sensation in the hindquarters and 45% for dogs that had lost deep pain perception before surgery. These results compare well with reported recovery rates after decompressive surgery. This article explores further what this finding implies about treatment of Type I thoracolumbar IVDH in dogs, after first summarizing what is known about fenestration as prophylaxis.

PROPHYLACTIC FENESTRATION

Evidence of Effect

Traditionally, disk fenestration describes the procedure in which a window is cut into the lateral aspect of the annulus fibrosus and the nucleus is removed with a variety of sharp and blunt manual instruments,[1,2,16] often dental instruments. Although the technique was originally used as a means of promoting functional recovery, it is currently most commonly used for prophylaxis against further herniations in the same region. Even this effect has been controversial and discussion of the risks and benefits continue to the present day.[12,17,18] The underlying problem is that it is known that IVDH is a body-wide condition in many affected animals and those that have symptomatic disease at 1 site are at high risk for recurrence at another.[19] Approximately 90% of thoracolumbar Type I IVDH occur between T11 and L3,[7,20] meaning that it is possible to target susceptible areas for prophylaxis. The usefulness of fenestration as an adjunct to decompressive surgery has traditionally been most controversial mainly because it is not straightforward to compare outcomes from series in which decompression was or was not accompanied by fenestration. Despite this, fenestration has been suspected of reducing the risk of recurrence for many decades[21–23] and more recent studies continue to support this viewpoint.[7,24]

Comparison of recurrence between the large group of dogs reported by Mayhew and colleagues[25] that did not receive prophylactic fenestration and the large group reported by Brisson and colleagues[26] that were fenestrated strongly suggested a protective effect of fenestration (recurrence rates of 19% vs 5%). A subsequent well-designed prospective trial reported by Brisson and colleagues[9] compared the recurrence rate in dogs that underwent decompressive surgery for symptomatic disk herniation and were either fenestrated at a single site (of symptomatic disk herniation) or all disks between T11 and L3. There was a substantial reduction in risk of recurrence in the multifenestrated group (7% vs 17%) strongly confirming the previous tentative conclusions from observational studies. This same trial also confirmed that 87% of recurrences occur adjacent to the site of previous herniation.[9]

Other investigators have suggested that disk calcification is a risk factor for recurrence[25] and it is undoubtedly associated with disk degeneration.[20,27] Because fenestration of all disks from T11 through L3, especially when combined with hemilaminectomy, is an invasive and time-consuming procedure, the judgment of many surgeons is to fenestrate the affected disk plus those immediately adjacent to it, particularly if those disks are calcified on imaging studies. Nevertheless, even this is a difficult decision to justify, bearing in mind that disks that appear radiographically normal at one time point may appear calcified within a short period of time afterward[28] and that there is reason to suppose that noncalcified disks are just as likely to undergo extrusion.[27] It has also been noted that calcification may disappear with age,[19,20,28] implying that it cannot be used as a reliable indicator of sites of irreversible progression to herniation (**Fig. 1**).

Further Questions

Risk-benefit ratio

The remaining discussion around the prophylactic benefits of fenestration centers on the risk-benefit ratio.[18] It is true that there are many possible adverse effects of the procedure, including pneumothorax, increased surgical time, and inadvertent spinal cord or nerve damage as well as the more general risks of surgical infection.[12,17,29] Such adverse effects seem uncommon, with only a small percentage of treated dogs developing these complications, many of which are self-limiting and need no further intervention to resolve.[22,26,29] A more difficult, philosophic, question centers on whether it is appropriate to treat a certain number of dogs to prevent a much smaller number from developing recurrence.[18] (Based on data from Brisson and colleagues,[9] on average 10 dogs are treated to prevent 1 recurrence within 2–3 years.)

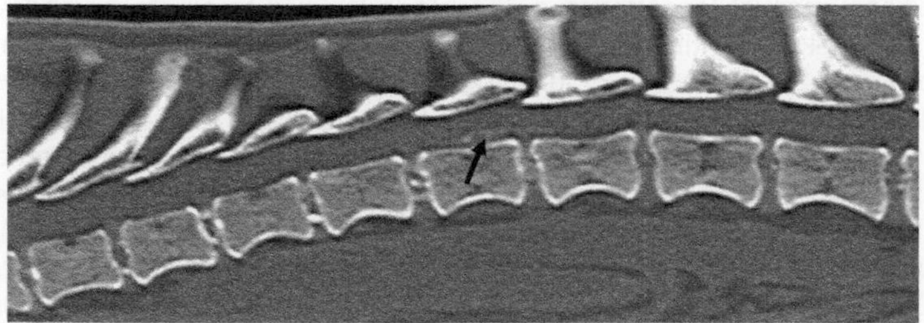

Fig. 1. Reconstructed midsagittal CT scan of the thoracolumbar junction of a 5-year-old dachshund. There is evidence of recent disk herniation (*arrow*) but there is also mineralization in every other intervertebral disk, providing evidence of widespread intervertebral disk degeneration in this individual.

The answer probably is different for each dog owner but there is a real risk (of unknown magnitude) of owners not pursuing any further treatment if their dog suffers recurrence; anecdotally, such affected dogs are sometimes euthanized, although how commonly this occurs is currently unknown.

Completeness of nuclear removal

Other than efficacy in preventing recurrence, the most contentious aspect of prophylactic fenestration is probably the amount of material that must be removed for the procedure to be efficacious. The original purpose of fenestration was to eliminate the dynamic component of disk herniation,[1] so it could be argued that simply making a scalpel incision through the annulus might suffice because, in experimental animals, this is sufficient to allow escape of large volumes of nucleus into the surrounding tissues.[30,31] It has also been found, however, that the incision in the annulus rapidly heals and there is replacement of the nucleus with fibrocartilage,[31,32] leading to suggestions that complete evacuation of the nucleus may be required for optimal results.[33]

Air-powered burs,[33] cavitron ultrasonic surgical aspirator (CUSA),[34] and a vacuum-assisted device[35] can all augment removal of nucleus and have been used safely in clinical patients. However, none of these techniques has been shown to have outcome benefits superior to those achieved through manual fenestration alone and there is evidence that no technique will completely evacuate the nucleus nor that it is essential for effective prophylaxis.[24] Therefore, the question as to whether removal of more nucleus corresponds to a greater prophylactic benefit has not yet been answered. As a related question, it has been suggested that making a smaller hole in the annulus might also be beneficial[34]—because the disk space will not then collapse to the same degree but, again, although this is entirely plausible there currently is no evidence in support of this effect.

Surgical Approach

Many veterinary surgeons continue to use the dorsal approach[36] to the thoracolumbar vertebrae for decompressive surgery, although access for hemilaminectomy, minihemilaminectomy, and pediculectomy is often more easily, and less traumatically, achieved via dorsolateral[37] or lateral[38] approaches. There are many benefits to the more lateral approaches, such as the reduced requirement for muscle trauma or detachment from bone, but also the dorsolateral approach[37] provides much better access for multilevel fenestration and was designed for this purpose. More recently, the various techniques have been compared for their provision of access for fenestration and the dorsolateral approach seems optimal (the lateral approach provides a smaller window).[39]

In traditional manual fenestration a #11 blade is used to create a window in the annulus. The disk is identified by locating either the transverse process or rib head and following these structures cranially and slightly dorsally until the disk can be palpated with a needle or blade. Sometimes it can be useful to use gauze held in hemostats to dry the region so as to be able to clearly see the dorsoventral striations in the annulus. The neurovascular bundle together with adjacent muscle is then retracted cranially to protect it from the sharp instruments used to cut the annulus. After incising the annulus, nuclear material is removed with the use of a dental scraper, House curette, 16-gauge hypodermic needle, or similar implements. It has been postulated that recurrence after fenestration may in some cases be due to remaining nuclear material that is not removed because of unfavorable access to the disk governed by the surgical approach,[39] but this has not yet been shown to be a clinically significant factor.

Percutaneous laser disk ablation has been adopted from human medicine as a minimally invasive procedure that could provide the same potential prophylactic benefits as traditional surgical fenestration. An initial report demonstrated that this procedure is safe and efficacious,[40] and more recently reported data strongly suggest a useful prophylactic effect.[41] In this procedure, fluoroscopy is used to guide percutaneous placement of needles into a series of intervertebral disks (**Fig. 2**). A fine fiberoptic cable is passed through the needle and positioned in the center of the disk; the laser is activated for a 40-second period and ablates the nuclear material. In a large series of cases (n = 277) there was a very low complication rate (5 dogs; <2%) and only 1 dog that showed neurologic signs afterward (of a total of 3) required surgery for resolution (and it is probable that this was a developing lesion when the laser procedure was carried out).[40] In a second report examining recurrence of clinical signs at a minimum of 3 years after laser fenestration there were 60 of 303 (20%) dogs suspected of having recurrence, but recurrence was only confirmed by imaging or surgery in 11 of 303 (3.6%) dogs.[41]

There is some doubt about whether this procedure may be dangerous to the spinal cord if there is rupture of the annulus, and current recommendations are only to perform laser fenestration 6 weeks or more after recovery from an IVDH episode to allow time for the annulus to heal. This, therefore, requires a further procedure under general anesthesia. Sensitive owner counseling along with accurate reporting of recurrence rates of IVDH may be necessary for some owners to be willing to agree to this, but it is likely to be worthwhile for many dogs suffering an acute severe episode of IVDH. The low rate of complications and evidence suggestive of high efficacy when

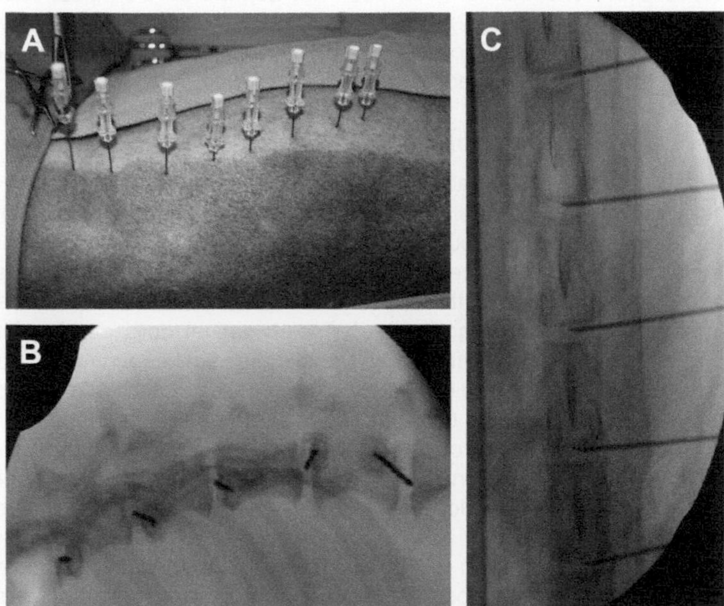

Fig. 2. Percutaneous laser-assisted fenestration after aseptic preparation in lateral recumbency spinal needles are placed into the targeted intervertebral disks under fluoroscopic guidance (*A*); lateral (*B*) and ventrodorsal (*C*) radiographs showing needle tips accurately positioned in the centers of the intervertebral disks. (*Courtesy of* Dr Danielle Dugat, Oklahoma State University, Stillwater, OK.)

contrasted with the high risk of disk herniation in some breeds[42,43] suggest that it is worth exploring its use as routine prophylaxis in young nonsymptomatic chondrodystrophic dogs when they undergo other routine health care, such as spaying and neutering.

FENESTRATION AS THERAPY

When fenestration was first used as therapy for intervertebral disk herniation, the rationale was that it would reduce intradiscal pressure and eliminate the presumed dynamic lesion by reducing the pressure applied from within the disk to communicate with the epidural space.[1,6] There is good evidence for the first proposition: reduction of intradiscal pressure would be expected to reduce pain because it would eliminate nociceptive activation associated with stretching of the annulus in the degenerate disk.[44,45] There is direct evidence of pain from a stretched annulus in human low back pain patients: discography (injection of a low volume of contrast into the disk nucleus) is a well-established diagnostic method because the consequent increase in intradiscal pressure evokes a painful response from the affected disk.[46] Fenestration remains the first choice of surgery for some veterinary neurosurgeons for dogs with Type I IVDH that show pain alone.[47]

On the other hand, the notion that relief of intradiscal pressure might aid spinal cord decompression nowadays is regarded by most spinal surgeons as a little fanciful. Nevertheless, as we recently summarized,[11] there is still the inconvenient finding that, according to the available data, the functional recovery rate after fenestration seem similar to that after decompressive surgery. There are several explanations, including (1) recovery of spinal function does not depend on a surgical intervention to decompress the spinal cord, (2) the original data were flawed in some way, and (3) relief of intradiscal pressure does alleviate the pressure on the spinal cord and so allows recovery of function. Each of these is considered in turn.

Does Recovery Depend upon Decompression?

Although not a currently widely accepted viewpoint, partly because there is such obvious distortion of spinal cord shape in cross-sectional images, there is evidence that functional recovery after acute IVDH does not depend on decompression. Notably, there is plentiful evidence that a majority of dogs that suffer acute Type I IVDH recover with conservative therapy alone.[11] This clinical evidence seems at odds with experimental data suggesting that early spinal cord decompression is important for recovery.[10] The difficulty in translating such experimental results is that it is impossible to create in the laboratory the unique combination of compression and contusion that occurs in each clinical case of acute thoracolumbar IVDH and the timescale in which experimental decompression is completed may not be readily achievable in the clinic. Often clinicians cannot even be sure how long the spinal cord has been compressed, let alone accomplish decompression within 6 hours to 8 hours.

Furthermore, there is imaging evidence that the material that causes cord compression after IVDH can disappear with time.[48,49] A potential explanation of this observation is that the material that causes the compression is often composed of a not-very-dense mixture of blood and fragmented herniated material. Initially, this may perhaps be repulsed by spinal cord pulsations in a similar way to that proposed to occur with fragments of bone in the vertebral canal after fractures.[50] During subsequent stages the extruded material can be cleared by phagocytosis.

On the other hand, it is a recurrent theme that the recovery rate after conservative therapy is not thought to be as good as that after surgery, especially for the more severely affected cases, and this conclusion is supported by a recent meta-analysis.[51] One problem with such meta-analysis is that it is dependent on the data that are available. For instance, the period over which conservatively treated dogs are followed up is, in many case series, not equivalent to that for surgical cases. In some studies, for instance, dogs were taken to surgery if they deteriorated or failed to recover within a period of up to 1 month,[52] meaning that the outcome with conservative therapy alone is not known. For dogs that have severe spinal cord injury, the conclusion has to be even more circumspect because there are so few dogs with loss of pain perception (ie, deep pain negative) and treated conservatively for which outcomes have been reported. On the other hand, perhaps it is possible that compression plays a more important role if the initial contusive lesion is more severe.

Another viewpoint is that because, in most cases, loss of function after IVDH can largely be attributed to the contusion injury,[53] for which there is no effective therapy, there may well not be a difference between decompression and fenestration because the spinal cord must recover spontaneously (or not) after either procedure (**Fig. 3**). This

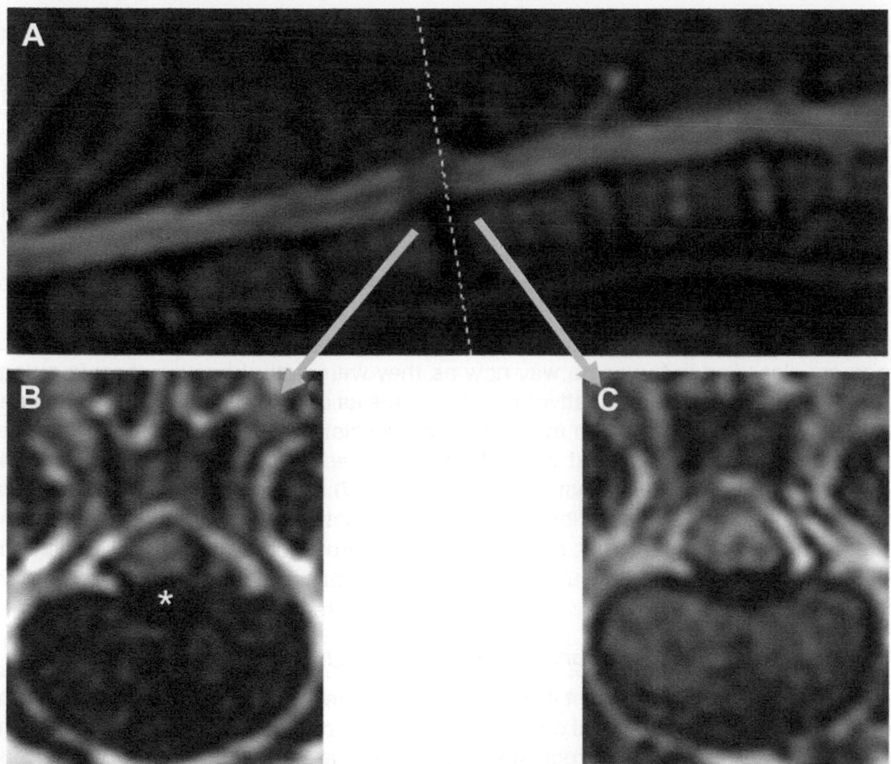

Fig. 3. Not all acute intervertebral disk herniations are associated with clinically important spinal cord compression. The sagittal T2-weighted MRI scan (*A*) identifies a region of mild cord distortion overlying an intervertebral disk; transverse scans just cranial (*B*) and caudal (*C*) to the epicenter confirm minimal spinal cord compression associated with nuclear herniation (*asterisk*). Such a case may be appropriate for fenestration alone rather than attempted decompressive surgery.

provides an explanation for why fenestration may be beneficial compared with conservative therapy: it prevents more material from extruding into the epidural space thereby preventing worsened compression,[6] which then allows the spinal cord to recover as well as if it had been decompressed.

It is also possible that the decompressive procedures in previously published series were suboptimal, meaning that the spinal cord of many animals that undergo the procedure remain compressed, and there is evidence for residual compression in a large proportion of reimaged cases.[54] This potentially reduces the recovery rates associated with decompressive surgery and may provide another reason for the similar recovery rate after fenestration alone. Because loss of function can largely be attributed to contusion injury, it might be that suboptimal decompression is not important, meaning that fenestration and decompression then become equivalent procedures. In articles on decompression, the focus is usually on whether the animal recovers or not rather than the quality of recovery; it is possible that there might be a need for complete decompression to allow full recovery. Similarly, for both fenestration and decompression there are few data on swiftness of recovery. Decompressive surgery is often stated as leading to a quicker and more complete recovery than medical treatment. Nevertheless, both propositions remain speculative at present because there are no published data to support these assertions.

Did Original Fenestration Reports Suggest an Unduly Positive Outcome?

In the process of examining the literature reporting the results of treatment of acute IVDH with fenestration alone, we made every effort to treat these articles in the same way as those reporting the results of decompressive surgery. The bulk of the literature reporting the results of lateral fenestration comes from the late 1970s, 1980s, and early 1990s, with some more recent publications also reporting on other ways of performing fenestration, such as percutaneously or via a ventral approach. There are some large case series, with good detail on inclusion criteria, neurologic status before surgery, and outcome; there seems little reason to consider them inferior to the comparative decompression articles and no reason to suppose that those investigators were untruthful about their outcomes. What may be in question is whether the dogs are classified in the same way now as they were many decades ago: is a dog designated as "deep pain negative" now the same as a deep pain negative dog diagnosed in the 1950s? If modern methods of diagnosis have improved, perhaps more recent series include dogs that would have been designated deep pain negative in previous decades, meaning that earlier series (which focused more on fenestration) might contain a greater proportion of more mildly affected dogs. From the current vantage point, it is unlikely that this question can be addressed adequately, meaning that the only definitive answer would come from a randomized trial to compare the 2 interventions.

Does Fenestration Actively Improve Spinal Cord Function?

As a final explanation, perhaps it is plausible to consider that fenestration does work in some way to alleviate the spinal cord damage caused by acute IVDH. This explanation suggests that Olsson[1] was correct: fenestration eliminates a dynamic effect of the herniated disk, which then allows recovery. A possible mechanism could be that fenestration causes—as a side effect of the surgical approach and procedure itself—muscle spasm around the affected area that then stabilizes the region. Similar effects on paraspinal musculature have been proposed as mechanisms for increased stiffness in the cervical vertebral column after laminectomy.[55,56] The elimination of the dynamic effect might then be proposed to promote recovery of the injured spinal cord.

CAN THE COMPRESSION THAT IS VISIBLE ON CROSS-SECTIONAL IMAGING BE IGNORED?

For most dogs affected by acute thoracolumbar IVDH, cross-sectional images provide an almost irresistible reason to decompress the spinal cord. And, as discussed previously, there seems to be laboratory evidence in support of decompression as therapy.[10,57,58] Even so, it is difficult to be sure that it is reasonable to translate the inferences made in experimental rat spinal cord injury with short follow-up periods and comparatively early decompression into clinical IVDH in dogs. Most experimental compression and decompression studies are carried out in rats within a period of 8 hours—which is rarely achieved in dogs—and, clinicians rarely know how long the spinal cord has been compressed. Extensive compression commonly affects other parts of the nervous system, such as brain tumors or cervical disk herniations and does not always require urgent decompression. On the other hand, rapidly accumulating small compressing volumes, such as subdural hematoma, are recognized as highly dangerous and warrant emergency interventions.

Clinical studies in dogs provide some evidence that spinal cord compression after thoracolumbar IVDH need not necessarily be an emergency. For instance, in a study on dogs that had lost hindquarter pain perception, there was no apparent benefit to early surgery in promoting recovery of locomotion,[59] although there are also other data suggesting the opposite conclusion.[60] If it is assumed, however, that late surgery is just as effective, perhaps that means that no decompression is also just as effective? On the other hand, there is indirect evidence that failure to remove material from within the vertebral canal might, at least in some individuals, risk the development of persistent spinal pain.[13] Unfortunately, there is insufficient current information to know how commonly this occurs.

For clinical cases undergoing routine investigation, perhaps it might be preferable to pose the question other way round—if compression can be seen on cross-sectional images, why would decompressive surgery be foregone? Although this must be a decision made by each individual veterinary spinal surgeon, perhaps it is worth considering the following:

- The time that is spent on decompression might perhaps be better used doing other procedures. Currently, many surgeons carry out decompressive surgery but then do not fenestrate. It is established that this means that many of these cases remain at relatively high risk for recurrence,[9] and some of these might be euthanized by their owners if they develop a second symptomatic episode. Optimally, the treatment of each affected dog is decompression and multilevel fenestration but, if a choice is made of 1 or the other (perhaps because of time budgeting), then it could be argued that fenestration might be the better option.
- Many owners find that the cost of cross-sectional imaging and surgery is prohibitive, so they decline surgery, and, sometimes, dogs are euthanatized as a result. Such an outcome is depressing because a large proportion of these cases, no matter how severely affected at presentation, still recover with conservative therapy alone.[11] It is important to stress to owners that decompressive surgery is not imperative, but, if they are able to afford fenestration, there is evidence that it will accomplish as much as decompressive surgery for dogs that present with intact pain sensation.
- Therapeutic fenestration may extend owner access to effective spinal surgery. Fenestration does not require much specialized equipment and there is minimal need for preoperative imaging (because the site of herniation does not need to be accurately diagnosed). In many early studies on fenestration, plain radiographs alone were used to rule out bone destructive lesions (mainly discospondylitis

or neoplasia) before the surgery. Other differential diagnoses to consider in small chondystrophic dogs with acute-onset thoracolumbar pain or paraparesis are infectious or inflammatory diseases that are routinely diagnosed using cerebrospinal fluid and blood analyses. In practice, most cases presented for potential decompression of acute IVDH have typical history and signalment that suggest a high likelihood of acute IVDH. Many primary care veterinarians have access to appropriate equipment to carry out fenestration and offer this option to owners with financial or travel limitations.

A factor mentioned against fenestration is the risks involved[17,18]; many surgeons do not believe the risk is worth the benefit. Certainly, it can be technically demanding procedure, particularly in larger dogs and in the thoracic region. Theoretic risks include creation of pneumothorax when fenestrating the more cranial thoracic intervertebral disks, iatrogenic damage to the neurovascular bundle or even the spinal cord through inadvertent entry into the spinal canal via the intervertebral foramen, and severe hemorrhage due to iatrogenic penetration of the aorta.[17] Currently available data suggest that, in practice, the risks of fenestration are very low.[7,22,26,29]

SUMMARY AND RECOMMENDATIONS

There is clear and strong evidence to use prophylactic fenestration to reduce the risk of future Type I IVDH.[7,9] When a dog presents with acute intervertebral disk herniation, the choice initially is between surgical and medical management; if the decision is made to go ahead with decompressive surgery, then consideration should be given to performing concurrent prophylactic fenestration. The choice is then of how many disks to fenestrate; performing the procedure on 5 disks (T11 to L3) may be considered optimal because this treats the disks involved in 90% of acute IVDH[7] but inevitably prolongs surgical time and carries increased, albeit still low, risk of morbidity. Basing the decision on imaging findings may be worthy of consideration but needs further investigation before definitive conclusions may be drawn. If only the disk affected by the episode of herniation is fenestrated, then it may be anticipated that the chances of delayed recovery due to further herniation or recurrence associated with that disk should be significantly reduced. However, because recurrences of symptomatic Type I IVDH more than after 1 month from the initial surgery are a result of of herniation at another site,[61] fenestrating just the affected disk is unlikely to have much effect on the long-term recurrence rate. Because recurrence can be a devastating event for many owners leading perhaps to greater consideration of euthanasia of the affected animal, fenestration of at least the disks adjacent to the affected one should always be considered.

Therapeutic fenestration offers the advantages of prophylaxis without the need for specialized instrumentation and imaging but currently there is a lack of equipoise regarding the efficacy of fenestration relative to decompression for treatment of acute canine IVDH: most veterinary spinal surgeons do not consider the 2 procedures equivalently efficacious for reversing clinical signs after acute disk herniation. However, therapeutic fenestration should perhaps be given greater consideration, especially if advanced imaging shows only mild to moderate spinal cord compression or there are restrictions on the duration of surgery, when it might be better to spend the time on fenestration rather than decompression. There also remains the possibility that, because there is no guarantee that herniated material in the vertebral canal will disappear with time, therapeutic fenestration may not eliminate the risk of long-term spinal pain.

Laser disk ablation seems safe and effective for removal of the nucleus pulposus and reduces risk of future herniation. Currently it has limited availability but in the future it may become more widely available and could perhaps be used for more generalized prophylaxis.

REFERENCES

1. Olsson SE. Observations concerning disc fenestration in dogs. Acta Orthop Scand 1951;20:349–56.
2. Flo GL, Brinker WO. Lateral fenestration of thoracolumbar discs. J Am Anim Hosp Assoc 1975;11:619–26.
3. Denny HR. The lateral fenestration of canine thoracolumbar disc protrusions: a review of 30 cases. J Small Anim Pract 1978;19:259–66.
4. Funkquist B. Investigations of the therapeutic and prophylactic effects of disc evacuation in cases of thoraco-lumbar herniated discs in dogs. Acta Vet Scand 1978;19:441–57.
5. Knapp DW, Pope ER, Hewett JE, et al. A retrospective study of thoracolumbar fenestration in dogs using a ventral approach: 160 cases (1976-1986). J Am Anim Hosp Assoc 1990;26:543–9.
6. Butterworth SJ, Denny HR. Follow-up study of 100 cases with thoracolumbar disc protrusions treated by lateral fenestration. J Small Anim Pract 1991;32:443–7.
7. Aikawa T, Fujita H, Kanazono S, et al. Long-term neurologic outcome of hemilaminectomy and disk fenestration for treatment of dogs with thoracolumbar intervertebral disk herniation: 831 cases (2000-2007). J Am Vet Med Assoc 2012;241:1617–26.
8. Brisson BA. Intervertebral disc disease in dogs. Vet Clin North Am Small Anim Pract 2010;40:829–58.
9. Brisson BA, Holmberg DL, Parent J, et al. Comparison of the effect of single-site and multiple-site disc fenestration on the rate of recurrence of thoracolumbar disc extrusion in dogs; a prospective, randomized, controlled study. J Am Vet Med Assoc 2011;238:1593–600.
10. Dimar JR, Glassman SD, Raque GH, et al. The influence of spinal canal narrowing and timing of decompression on neurological recovery after spinal cord contusion in a rat model. Spine 1999;24:1623–33.
11. Freeman P, Jeffery ND. Re-opening the window on fenestration as a treatment for acute thoracolumbar intervertebral disc herniation in dogs. J Small Anim Pract 2017;58:199–204.
12. Brisson BA. Pros and cons of prophylactic fenestration: arguments in favor. Chapter 35. In: Fingeroth JM, Thomas WB, editors. Advances in intervertebral disc disease in dogs and cats. 1st edition. Ames (IA): Wiley & Sons Inc; ACVS Foundation; 2015. p. 259–63.
13. Sukhiani HR, Parent JM, Atilola MA, et al. Intervertebral disk disease in dogs with signs of back pain alone: 25 cases (1986-1993). J Am Vet Med Assoc 1996;209:1275–9.
14. Penning V, Platt SR, Dennis R, et al. Association of spinal cord compression seen on magnetic resonance imaging with clinical outcome in 67 dogs with thoracolumbar intervertebral disk extrusion. J Small Anim Pract 2006;47:644–50.
15. Roach WJ, Thomas M, Weh JM, et al. Residual herniated disc material following hemilaminectomy in chondrodystrophic dogs with thoracolumbar intervertebral disc disease. Vet Comp Orthop Traumatol 2012;25:109–15.

16. Sharp NJH, Wheeler SJ. Thoracolumbar disc disease. Chapter 8. In: Sharp NJH, Wheeler SJ, editors. Small animal spinal disorders. 2nd edition. London: Elsevier Mosby; 2005. p. 121–60.
17. Fingeroth JM. Fenestration: pros and cons. Probl Vet Med 1989;1:445–66.
18. Forterre F, Fingeroth JM. Pros and cons of prophylactic fenestration: the potential arguments against. Chapter 36. In: Fingeroth JM, Thomas WB, editors. Advances in intervertebral disc disease in dogs and cats. 1st edition. Ames (IA): Wiley & Sons Inc; ACVS Foundation; 2015. p. 264–7.
19. Smolders LA, Bergknut N, Grinwis GC, et al. Intervertebral disc degeneration in the dog. Part 2: chondrodystrophic and non-chondrodystrophic breeds. Vet J 2013;195:292–9.
20. Hansen HJ. A pathologic-anatomical study on disc degeneration in dog, with special reference to the so-called enchondrosis intervertebralis. Acta Orthop Scand Suppl 1952;11:1–117.
21. Levine SH, Caywood DD. Recurrence of neurological deficits in dogs treated for thoracolumbar disc disease. J Am Anim Hosp Assoc 1984;20:889–94.
22. Black AP. Lateral spinal decompression in the dog: a review of 39 cases. J Small Anim Pract 1988;29:581–8.
23. McKee WM. A comparison of hemilaminectomy (with concomitant disc fenestration) and dorsal laminectomy for the treatment of thoracolumbar disc protrusion in dogs. Vet Rec 1992;130:296–300.
24. Forterre F, Konar M, Spreng D, et al. Influence of intervertebral disc fenestration at the herniation site in association with hemilaminectomy on recurrence in chondrodystrophic dogs with thoracolumbar disc disease: a prospective MRI study. Vet Surg 2008;37:399–405.
25. Mayhew PD, McLear RC, Ziemer LS, et al. Risk factors for recurrence of clinical signs associated with thoracolumbar intervertebral disk herniation in dogs: 229 cases (1994-2000). J Am Vet Med Assoc 2004;225:1231–6.
26. Brisson BA, Moffatt SL, Swayne SL, et al. Recurrence of thoracolumbar intervertebral disk extrusion in chondrodystrophic dogs after surgical decompression with or without prophylactic fenestration: 265 cases (1995-1999). J Am Vet Med Assoc 2004;224:1808–14.
27. Rohdin C, Jeserevic J, Viitmaa R, et al. Prevalence of radiographic detectable intervertebral disc calcifications in dachshunds surgically treated for disc extrusion. Acta Vet Scand 2010;52:24.
28. Jensen VF, Arnbjerg J. Development of intervertebral disk calcification in the dachshund: a prospective longitudinal radiographic study. J Am Anim Hosp Assoc 2001;37:274–82.
29. Bartels KE, Creed JE, Yturraspe DJ. Complications associated with the dorsolateral muscle-separating approach for thoracolumbar disk fenestration in the dog. J Am Vet Med Assoc 1983;183:1081–3.
30. Smith JW, Walmsley R. Experimental incision of the intervertebral disc. J Bone Joint Surg Br 1951;33:612–25.
31. Wagner SD, Ferguson HR, Leipold H, et al. Radiographic and histologic changes after thoracolumbar disc curettage. Vet Surg 1987;16:65–9.
32. Shores A, Cechner PE, Cantwell HD, et al. Structural changes in thoracolumbar disks following lateral fenestration. A study of radiographic, histologic and histochemical changes in the chondrodystrophic dog. Vet Surg 1985;14:117–23.
33. Holmberg DL, Palmer NC, Vanpelt D, et al. A comparison of manual and power-assisted thoracolumbar disc fenestration in dogs. Vet Surg 1990;19:323–7.

34. Forterre F, Dickomeit M, Senn D, et al. Microfenestration using the CUSA excel ultrasonic aspiration system in chondrodystrophic dogs with thoracolumbar disk extrusion: a descriptive cadaveric and clinical study. Vet Surg 2011;40:34–9.
35. Thomovsky SA, Packer RA, Lambrechts NE, et al. Canine intervertebral disc fenestration using a vacuum-assisted tissue resection device. Vet Surg 2012; 41:1011–7.
36. Redding RW. Laminectomy in the dog. Am J Vet Res 1951;12:123–8.
37. Yturraspe DJ, Lumb WV. A dorsolateral muscle-separating approach for thoracolumbar intervertebral disk fenestration in the dog. J Am Vet Med Assoc 1973;162: 1037–40.
38. Braund KG, Taylor TK, Ghosh P, et al. Lateral spinal decompression in the dog. J Small Anim Pract 1976;17:583–92.
39. Morelius M, Bergadano A, Spreng D, et al. Influence of surgical approach on the efficacy of the intervertebral disk fenestration: a cadaveric study. J Small Anim Pract 2007;48:87–92.
40. Bartels KE, Higbee RG, Bahr RJ, et al. Outcome of and complications associated with prophylactic percutaneous laser disk ablation in dogs with thoracolumbar disk disease: 277 cases (1992-2001). J Am Vet Med Assoc 2003;222:1733–9.
41. Dugat DR, Bartels KE, Payton ME. Recurrence of disk herniation following percutaneous laser disk ablation in dogs with a history of thoracolumbar intervertebral disk herniation: 303 cases (1994-2011). J Am Vet Med Assoc 2016;249: 1393–400.
42. Bergknut N, Egenvall A, Hagman R, et al. Incidence of intervertebral disk degeneration-related diseases and associated mortality rates in dogs. J Am Vet Med Assoc 2012;240:1300–9.
43. Lappalainen AK, Mäki K, Laitinen-Vapaavuori O. Estimate of heritability and genetic trend of intervertebral disc calcification in dachshunds in Finland. Acta Vet Scand 2015;23(57):78.
44. von Düring M, Fricke B, Dahlmann A. Topography and distribution of nerve fibers in the posterior longitudinal ligament of the rat: an immunocytochemical and electron-microscopical study. Cell Tissue Res 1995;281:325–38.
45. Freemont AJ, Peacock TE, Goupille P, et al. Nerve ingrowth into diseased intervertebral disc in chronic back pain. Lancet 1997;350:178–81.
46. Manchikanti L, Glaser SE, Wolfer L, et al. Systematic review of lumbar discography as a diagnostic test for chronic low back pain. Pain Physician 2009;12: 541–59.
47. Moore SA, Early PJ, Hettlich BF. Practice patterns in the management of acute intervertebral disc herniation in dogs. J Small Anim Pract 2016;57:409–15.
48. Hong J, Ball PA. Resolution of lumbar disk herniation without surgery. N Engl J Med 2016;374:1564.
49. Zhong M, Liu JT, Jiang H, et al. Incidence of spontaneous resorption of lumbar disc herniation: a meta-analysis. Pain Physician 2017;20:E45–52.
50. Dai L-Y. Remodeling of the spinal canal after thoracolumbar burst fractures. Clin Orthop Relat Res 2001;382:119–23.
51. Langerhuus L, Miles J. Proportion recovery and times to ambulation for non-ambulatory dogs with thoracolumbar disc extrusions treated with hemilaminectomy or conservative treatment: a systematic review and meta-analysis of case-series studies. Vet J 2017;220:7–16.
52. Levine JM, Levine GJ, Johnson SI, et al. Evaluation of the success of medical management for presumptive thoracolumbar intervertebral disk herniation in dogs. Vet Surg 2007;36:482–91.

53. Jeffery ND, Levine JM, Olby NJ, et al. Intervertebral disk degeneration in dogs: consequences, diagnosis, treatment, and future directions. J Vet Intern Med 2013;27:1318–33.
54. Forterre F, Gorgas D, Dickomeit M, et al. Incidence of spinal compressive lesions in chondrodystrophic dogs with abnormal recovery after hemilaminectomy for treatment of thoracolumbar disc disease: a prospective magnetic resonance imaging study. Vet Surg 2010;39:165–72.
55. Panjabi MM, Pelker R, Crisco JJ, et al. Biomechanics of healing of posterior cervical spinal injuries in a canine model. Spine (Phila Pa 1976) 1988;13:803–7.
56. Büff HU, Panjabi MM, Sonu CM, et al. Functional stability of the canine cervical spine after injury. A three-month in vivo study. Spine (Phila Pa 1976) 1990;15:1040–6.
57. Delamarter RB, Sherman J, Carr JB. Pathophysiology of spinal cord injury. Recovery after immediate and delayed decompression. J Bone Joint Surg Am 1995;77:1042–9.
58. Shields CB, Zhang YP, Shields LB, et al. The therapeutic window for spinal cord decompression in a rat spinal cord injury model. J Neurosurg Spine 2005;3:302–7.
59. Jeffery ND, Barker AK, Hu HZ, et al. Factors associated with recovery from paraplegia in dogs with loss of pain perception in the pelvic limbs following intervertebral disk herniation. J Am Vet Med Assoc 2016;248:386–94.
60. Brown NO, Helphrey ML, Prata RG. Thoracolumbar disk disease in the dog: a retrospective analysis of 187 cases. J Am Anim Hosp Assoc 1977;13:665–72.
61. Dhupa S, Glickman N, Waters DJ. Reoperative neurosurgery in dogs with thoracolumbar disc disease. Vet Surg 1999;28:421–8.

Acupuncture for Small Animal Neurologic Disorders

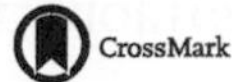

Patrick Roynard, DVM, MRCVS[a,b],
Lauren Frank, DVM, MS, CVA, CVCH, CCRT[c], Huisheng Xie, DVM, PhD, MS[d],
Margaret Fowler, DVM, MS[e,f,*]

KEYWORDS

- Traditional Chinese veterinary medicine (TCVM) • Acupuncture
- Electroacupuncture (EA) • Herbal • Dog • Intervertebral disk disease (IVDD)
- Cervical spondylomyelopathy (CSM) • Pain

KEY POINTS

- Research in neuroscience is progressively unveiling the different mechanisms of action of traditional Chinese veterinary medicine (TCVM) and allowing the modern clinician to understand it as a several millennia–old metaphor.
- Scientific literature demonstrates the efficacy of TCVM for many small animal neurologic disorders, including intervertebral disk disease (IVDD), other myelopathies, and painful conditions.
- TCVM, including acupuncture and herbals, is overall innocuous and easy to implement clinically.
- TCVM can be used as an adjunct or occasionally as an alternative to conventional treatment, and can improve functional outcome and pain management.

 **Video content accompanies this article at http://www.vetsmall.theclinics.com.**

Disclosure: Dr H. Xie is one of the owners of Chi Institute of Traditional Chinese Veterinary Medicine and Jing Tang Herbal, Inc. Drs P. Roynard, L. Frank and M. Fowler have nothing to disclose.

[a] Neurology/Neurosurgery Department, Long Island Veterinary Specialists, 163 South Service Road, Plainview, NY 11803, USA; [b] Fipapharm, 26 rue du marais, Mont-Saint-Aignan 76130, France; [c] Physical Rehabilitation and Acupuncture Service, Long Island Veterinary Specialists, 163 South Service Road, Plainview, NY 11803, USA; [d] Department of Small Animal Clinical Sciences, University of Florida, 2089 Southwest 16th Avenue, Gainesville, FL 32608, USA; [e] Acupuncture and Holistic Veterinary Services, 105 Lilith Lane, Summerville, SC 29485, USA; [f] The Chi Institute of Traditional Chinese Veterinary Medicine, 9650 West Highway 318, Reddick, FL 32686, USA

* Corresponding author. Acupuncture and Holistic Veterinary Services, 105 Lilith Lane, Summerville, SC 29485.
E-mail address: drmpfowler@gmail.com

Vet Clin Small Anim 48 (2018) 201–219
http://dx.doi.org/10.1016/j.cvsm.2017.08.003

INTRODUCTION

Traditional Chinese medicine (TCM), such as acupuncture and administration of Chinese herbal formulas, has been used for thousands of years to effectively treat many conditions, including pain and neurologic issues.[1,2] The first known text about TCM, *Huangdi Neijing* (Yellow Emperor's Classic of Internal Medicine) is estimated from approximately the period 475 BC to 225 BC.[3] Traditional Chinese veterinary medicine (TCVM) started in Chinese agricultural culture and is often associated with an equine practitioner known as Bo Le.[4–6] Bo Le's techniques were recorded in what many consider to be the first TCVM text, *Bo Le Zhen Jing* (*Bo Le*'s Canon of Veterinary Acupuncture).[7] Western interest in TCM/TCVM started in the 1970s, and in the past 40 years has mushroomed in popularity, both clinically and in research (**Fig. 1**). Although TCVM has long been overlooked by some practitioners, modern neuroscience has shed some light on the mechanism of action of acupuncture.[8–10] Despite the perception that TCVM presents the clinician with an entirely different way of approaching a patient, parallels with "Western" medicine are numerous, especially for those familiar with neurophysiology and neurologic disorders.

Due to the paucity of clinical studies in veterinary acupuncture, much of the data available are human or laboratory based, and indicate evidence for its effectiveness. This is further supported by a few veterinary clinical trials and case reports. This review is meant to help guide the use of TCVM for neurologic disorders in small animals, based on available information and recommendations from experienced TCVM practitioners.

TRADITIONAL CHINESE VETERINARY MEDICINE TREATMENT MODALITIES

Acupuncture is defined as the stimulation of specific point(s) on the surface of the body by insertion of a needle, resulting in a therapeutic or homeostatic effect.[11] From a TCVM standpoint, the aim is to allow *Qi* (energy) to flow harmoniously, which for a Western practitioner can be seen as a stimulation of the nervous system. TCVM defines 2 important concepts that are opposites, *Yin* and *Yang*, whose functioning

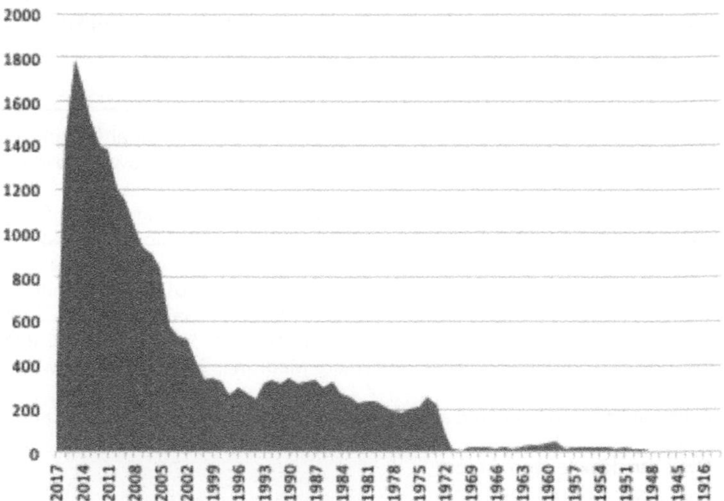

Fig. 1. PubMed search results for the word "acupuncture" by year. (*Data from* www.ncbi.nlm.nih.gov/pubmed. Accessed April 20, 2017.)

relationship can be paralleled to anabolism and catabolism or to the parasympathetic and sympathetic components of the autonomic nervous system.[12] Although TCVM presents the acupoints as areas where *Qi* is concentrated in the body, modern studies have revealed that acupuncture points are located in areas of sensitive neuroimmune modulation.[13,14] Histologically, acupuncture points are found in areas with a high density of mast cells, lymphatics, and arteriovenous plexi, in addition to regions of concentrated innervation.[13,14] This dense innervation consists of somatic afferent/efferent fibers, autonomic norepinephrine (NE) sympathetic fibers and cholinergic acetylcholine (Ach) parasympathetic fibers, with an increased ratio of myelinated to unmyelinated fibers compared with nonacupuncture points.[14] Along this parallel, TCVM describes the acupoints as organized along several meridians portrayed as channels, similar to rivers where *Qi* flows, often following peripheral nerve pathways (eg, the pericardium [PC] meridian and the median nerve, the gallbladder [GB] meridian and the sciatic nerve). New research allows us to better understand TCM/TCVM theory as a several millennia–old metaphor, with the nervous system as a cornerstone of its mechanisms of action.

Acupuncture has been used effectively for the treatment of neurologic disorders, such as intervertebral disk disease (IVDD)[15] and spinal cord injury.[16–18] Stimulation of acupuncture points with a needle produces analgesia, and other physiologic effects through neural, neurohumoral, neuromuscular, and musculoskeletal mechanisms.[19] It has been demonstrated that certain acupoints can regulate proinflammatory factors, such as interleukin-6 (IL-6), cyclooxygenase-2 (COX-2), tumor necrosis factor-α (TNF-α), and many others.[8,10,20–22] One of acupuncture's most studied mechanisms is the stimulation of production of β-endorphins, promoting a profound and long-term analgesic effect.[22,23] Moreover, certain acupoints can reduce the damage of free radicals and improve microcirculation.[24,25] These events may contribute to the efficacy of acupuncture for the neurologic diseases discussed here.

Stimulation of acupoints can be achieved by various techniques: dry needle (DN), electroacupuncture (EA), aqua-acupuncture (AA), and moxibustion (**Fig. 2**). DN is the most commonly used technique in veterinary acupuncture, and involves the insertion of fine, sterile needles into acupoints. EA, the modern practice of stimulating inserted needles with electricity, has been shown to have more profound effects compared with other techniques. It is used in many cases because of its rapid onset of pain relief and its ability to stimulate peripheral nerves. It is especially useful for neuralgia, nervous system injury, and persistent pain.[8–10] AA is the injection of sterile liquids (eg, vitamin B-12) into acupuncture points, which may result in a prolonged stimulus. Moxibustion involves heating of an acupoint (directly or over a needle) with moxa, a type of bundled herb consisting primarily of *Artemisia* (mugwort). The mechanisms of moxibustion mainly relate to the thermal and nonthermal radiation, and pharmacologic effects of moxa and its combustion products acting on a specific acupoint.[26]

In general, herbal medicine is also used in TCVM as an adjunct to acupuncture. However, the review of this topic other than *Yunnan Baiyao* use is beyond the scope of this article.

EPILEPSY/SEIZURE DISORDERS

From a TCVM standpoint, seizures are Internal Wind or "Wind in the Sea in Marrow"; the text *Huangdi Neijing* considered the brain, encased in a bony skull, as a reservoir of bone marrow, the "Sea of Marrow." A recent review from the Cochrane Library concluded that there is not enough current evidence to support the use of acupuncture

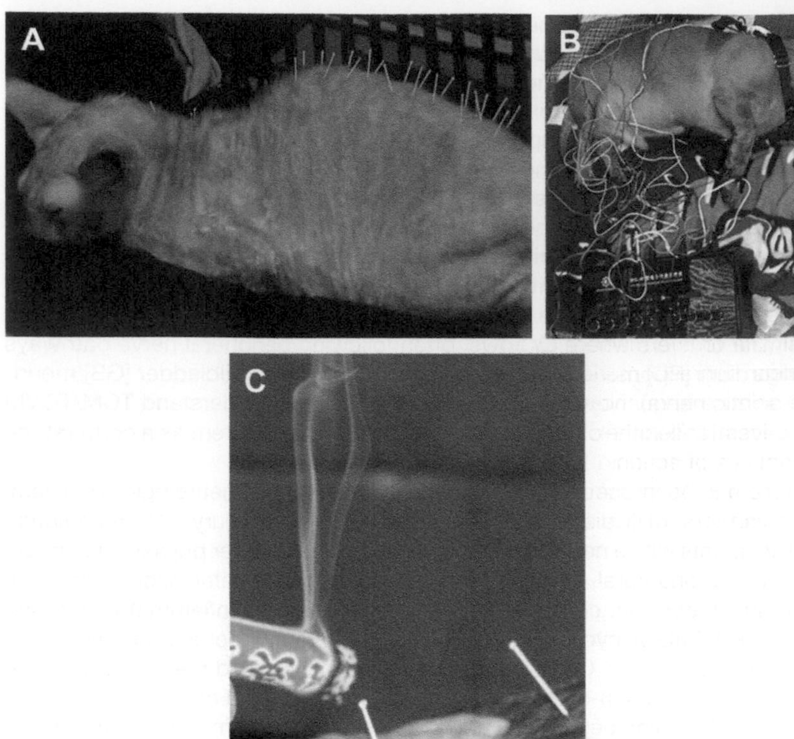

Fig. 2. Different acupuncture techniques used in patients with multifocal IVDD: (*A*) DN technique on a 12-year-old Devon rex cat. (*B*) Electroacupuncture technique on a 7-year-old dachshund. (*C*) Moxibustion technique. The stick of moxa is held close to the needles to provide warming *Qi*.

for human epilepsy, but it also noted that both DN and catgut implantation at acupoints may be effective in achieving at least 50% reduction in seizure frequency when compared with valproate and antiepileptic drugs in several trials.[27] Better quality of life after treatment was also reported in the acupuncture groups.[27] Although the use of EA has traditionally not been recommended in seizure disorders (due to a suspected but unverified pro-epileptic effect), recent research has shown beneficial effects of EA in several models of epilepsy, without however a consensus on acupoints and frequency to use. While using stimulation points outside the brain, the use of EA for seizures/epilepsy is somewhat similar in concept to the different intracranial or vagus nerve stimulation techniques in human refractory epilepsy (as EA may suppress seizures by parasympathetic activation and generation of similar neurotransmitters as intracranial electrical stimulation).[28] As an example, it has been suggested that response to EA could predict therapeutic effect of hippocampal high-frequency electrical stimulation in patients with pharmacoresistant temporal lobe epilepsy[29] and of anterior nucleus thalamus high-frequency electrical stimulation in medically refractory epilepsy.[30] A study in rats found that both low-frequency (10 Hz/1 mA) and high-frequency (100 Hz/1 mA) EA at select acupoints significantly ($P<.05$ compared with control) reduced epileptic seizures, with greater control at the high frequency.[31] Further research has shown that low-frequency (10 Hz) EA at bilateral gallbladder 20 (GB-20) suppressed pilocarpine-induced focal epilepsy by action on the μ, δ, and κ opioid receptors of the central nucleus of amygdala.[28] Furthermore, EA at stomach-36 (ST-36) +/− stomach-37 (ST-37) reduced spontaneous seizures and can decrease epileptogenesis by elevating the expression of GAD(67) mRNA in the dentate gyrus granule cell layer,[32] and by reducing mossy fiber sprouting and COX-2 levels in the hippocampus.[33,34]

Few clinical data are available regarding the antiepileptic effect of acupuncture in dogs, but 3 separate studies/case series reported success. One study using 2-mm to 3-mm gold wire pieces implanted at multiple acupoints reported a 50% or more reduction in the seizure frequency of 9 (60%) of 15 dogs with idiopathic epilepsy.[35] Another case series describes the use of small subcutaneous gold implants placed over the calvaria on the Bladder (BL), Governing Vessel (GV), and GB meridians in 5 epileptic dogs nonresponsive to anticonvulsants, with 5 of 5 dogs experiencing decrease in seizure frequency after treatment.[36] As gold implants can create significant signal loss and other susceptibility artifacts on MRI, Clemmons[37] used 1.0 × 0.5-mm polylactic acid beads inserted at multiple acupoints using a modified 16-gauge needle in 10 dogs with refractory epilepsy (unsatisfactory seizure control despite 2 anticonvulsant medications within therapeutic range). He reported significant reduction in amplitude of electroencephalogram activity, reduction of seizures by more than 50% in 9 (90%) of 10 dogs, and change in seizure characteristics from cluster seizures to singular seizures.[37] This may represent a promising new method to help control canine refractory epilepsy.

DISORDERS OF THE SPINAL CORD/MYELOPATHIES

Spinal Cord Injury

From a TCVM standpoint, spinal cord injuries (SCIs) are due to *Qi* and *Blood* stagnation, and acupuncture has long been used for various disorders of the spinal cord. Modern neuroscience has established the importance of secondary injury in SCI, with calcium entry in neurons and glial cells resulting in a cascade of cytokine and free radical release by activated microglia and damaged mitochondrial membranes.[38,39] Of special interest are the roles of proinflammatory cytokines and mediators, such as TNF-α, interleukin-1β (IL-1β), matrix metalloprotease-9 (MMP-9), and nitric oxide (NO). Such factors promote the inflammatory cascade, and neuronal and oligodendrocyte damage, which leads to demyelination of axons and progressive disruption of nervous tissue. Long-term consequences of neuronal inflammation are associated with the development of astrocytosis, glial scar formation, and syringohydromyelia.[39,40] Although there is currently no proven pharmacologic protocol protective from these secondary damages available to veterinary patients, recent research has shed some light on how acupuncture may fill this void. An experimental study of SCI in rats with sham/placebo control showed that DN treatment significantly ($P<.01$) improved functional recovery after SCI compared with control groups. Acupuncture treatment resulted in significantly attenuated microglial activation and significantly reduced expression of TNF-α, IL-1β, IL-6, MMP-9, NO synthase, and COX-2, providing neuroprotection and reducing apoptotic cell death of both neurons and oligodendrocytes. A significantly decreased size of lesion and axonal loss were also confirmed on histology and immune-histochemical staining.[8] Interestingly, another study in a rat model of cerebral ischemic stroke showed that these benefits of acupuncture in SCI may extend to brain injury, as EA treatment reduced the motor impairment following middle cerebral artery occlusion, via inhibition of microglia-mediated neuro-inflammation and significantly decreased levels of TNF-α, IL-1β, and IL-6 in both sensorimotor cortex tissue and blood serum.[41]

Intervertebral Disk Disease

Acupuncture has been shown to accelerate recovery of motor function and improve analgesia in dogs affected with IVDD,[42–47] and TCVM for IVDD is documented in the veterinary literature.[45] In a randomized controlled study in rats, EA inhibited Wnt-β-catenin, which may contribute to its effect in delaying the degenerative process of the cervical intervertebral disks.[48] Acupuncture also can reduce the amount of type I collagen in the nucleus pulposus while promoting the production of type II collagen, changes necessary for the proper hydration of proteoglycans leading to compression resistance,[49] thus improving the ability of degenerated disks to repair.[50] EA also increased blood flow in the vertebrae and increased micro-vessel density compared with control rats.[51] The number of normal neurons in the spinal cord and pelvic limb motor function were also increased.[51]

Some clinical research suggests that EA may have a success rate of 83% in treating canine thoracolumbar (TL) IVDD.[44,47] In one study by Hayashi and colleagues,[43] 50 dogs with signs of TL IVDD were classified with a scale of neurologic deficits from grades 1 to 5 (**Table 1**). Dogs were separated into 2 groups, either receiving conventional medical treatment alone or conventional medical treatment with EA. In grades 3 or 4, the time to recover ambulation was significantly (P = .0341) less (10.10 ± 6.49 days) in the group receiving EA than without EA (20.83 ± 11.99 days). The success rate, defined as the ability to walk without assistance, for grades 3 or 4 was significantly (P = .047) higher with EA (10/10) than without EA (6/9). The overall success rate was significantly (P = .015) higher with EA (23/26; 88.5%) than without EA (14/24; 58.3%). Although this study presented methodological flaws and researcher bias (groups not matched, evaluator not blinded), EA combined with conventional medical treatment was more effective than conventional medication alone and resulted in a shorter time to recover ambulation (**Fig. 3**).[43]

In a retrospective study, the outcome of 80 dogs with paraplegia and intact nociception from TL IVDD (grade 4) treated with EA and prednisone versus prednisone alone were compared. The combination of EA with prednisone was significantly (P = .01) more effective than prednisone alone to recover ambulation, allowed faster

Table 1
Neurologic grading scale in canine intervertebral disk disease and suggested recommendation for use of traditional Chinese veterinary medicine (TCVM)

0	Normal
1	Cervical or thoracolumbar pain, hyperesthesia: TCVM as an *adjunct or alternative* to standard management (cage rest and analgesics)
2	Ataxia, paresis, decreased proprioception, ambulatory: TCVM as an *adjunct* to standard management (cage rest and analgesics) including rehabilitation
3	Paresis with absent proprioception, nonambulatory: TCVM as an *adjunct* to standard management with recommendation for advanced imaging ± decompressive surgery and rehabilitation
4	Paralysis, nociception present: TCVM as an *adjunct* to standard management with recommendation for advanced imaging ± decompressive surgery and rehabilitation
5	Paralysis, absent nociception: TCVM as an *adjunct* to decompressive surgery and rehabilitation

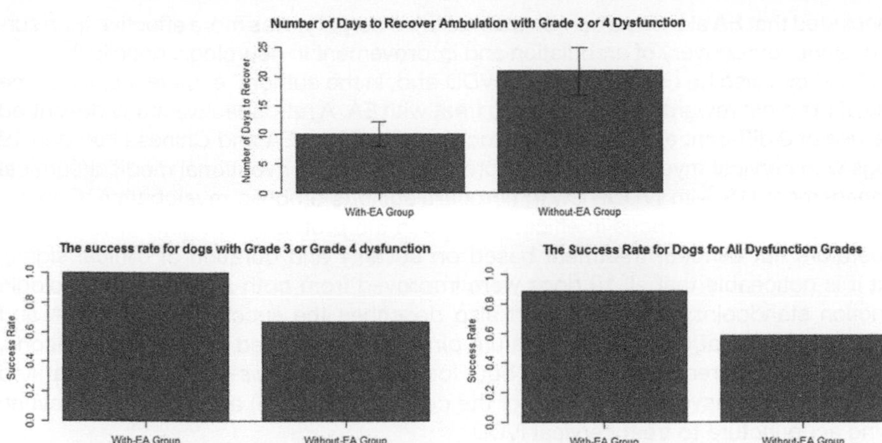

Fig. 3. Effect of EA on IVDD in dogs. (*Data from* Hayashi A, Matera J, Fonseca Pinto A. Evaluation of electroacupuncture treatment for thoracolumbar intervertebral disk disease in dogs. J Am Vet Med Assoc 2007;231:913–8.)

return to ambulatory status (*P* = .011), relieved back pain (*P* = .001), and decreased relapse rate (*P* = .031).[52] Another study compared EA, hemilaminectomy, and hemilaminectomy + EA in 40 dogs with more than 48 hours of severe neurologic deficits due to IVDD (only grades 4 and 5) confirmed by diagnostic imaging (MRI, computed tomography [CT], myelography). "Clinical success," defined as a patient initially classified grade 4 or 5 being classified as grade 1 or 2 within 6 months of treatment, was significantly (*P*<.05) higher for dogs that received EA alone (15/19 or 79%) or EA and surgery (8/11 or 73%) than for dogs that had surgery alone (4/10 or 40%) (**Fig. 4**). Thus, it was

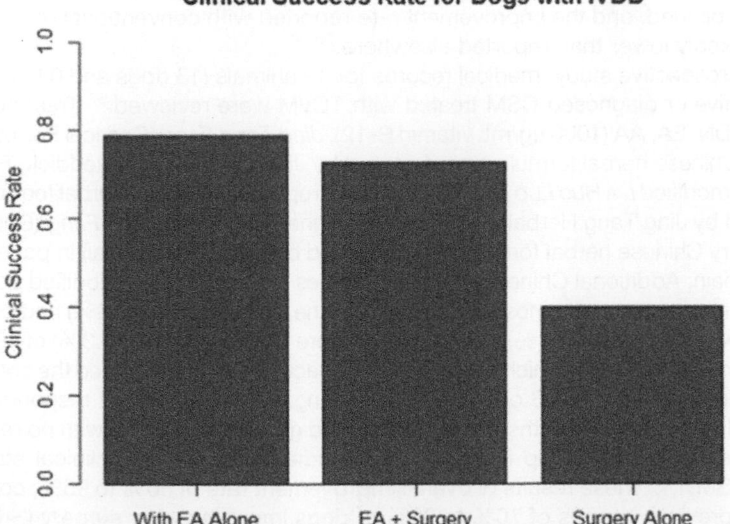

Fig. 4. Effect of EA on IVDD in dogs. (*Data from* Joaquim J, Luna S, Brondani J, et al. Comparison of decompression surgery, electroacupuncture, and decompressive surgery followed by electroacupuncture for the treatment of dogs with intervertebral disk disease with long-standing severe neurologic deficits. J Am Vet Med Assoc 2010;236:1225–9.)

concluded that EA alone or a combination of EA + surgery, was more effective than surgery alone for recovery of ambulation and improvement in neurologic deficits.[42]

TCVM can also be used for cervical IVDD and, in the authors' experience, it may be one of the most rewarding conditions to treat with EA. A retrospective study described the use of 3 different acupuncture protocols using DN ± EA and Chinese herbs in 19 dogs with cervical myelopathy having previously failed conventional medical/surgical management (18 with IVDD, 1 with fibrocartilaginous embolic myelopathy). Conclusions regarding differences in efficacy between the protocols are difficult to surmise (operators not blinded; treatment based on severity and duration of clinical signs), but it is noticeable that all 19 dogs were improved from both a pain and neurologic function standpoint.[53] A case report also describes the successful use of EA and herbals for IVDD at C3-C4 in a miniature pinscher.[45] As noted in these publications, the investigators recommend using both local points (*Jing-jia-ji*, located dorsal and ventral to the transverse processes of the cervical vertebrae) and distal points when using acupuncture to treat cervical IVDD.

Although the authors still recommend advanced imaging and decompressive surgery when indicated for cases of presumptive IVDD, these results justify offering EA as an adjunct to conventional treatment. A suggested recommendation for the use of TCVM based on grading of neurologic deficits is included in **Table 1**.

Cervical Spondylomyelopathy

A clinical trial of 40 dogs with presumptive or diagnosed cervical spondylomyelopathy (CSM) was conducted over 3 years to evaluate the efficacy of standard treatment (medical and surgical) versus standard treatment + EA. EA resulted in pain relief quickly, often after the first session, with proprioceptive deficits being slower to respond. The overall efficacy of EA was 85%, whereas surgery and conventional medications resulted in a low 20% efficacy in this trial.[54] However, these results should be interpreted cautiously, as a number of dogs were only presumptively diagnosed with CSM, the method of randomization between the 2 groups was not clear, the assessors were not blinded, and the improvement rate reported with conventional management was markedly lower than reported elsewhere.[55,56]

In a retrospective study, medical records for 19 animals (13 dogs and 6 horses) with presumptive or diagnosed CSM treated with TCVM were reviewed.[57] Treatment consisted of DN, EA, AA (1000 μg/mL vitamin B-12), *Jing Tong Fang* (Cervical Formula; Proprietary Chinese herbal formula manufactured by Jing Tang Herbal, Reddick, FL) for all patients, modified *Da Huo Luo Dan* (Double P II; Proprietary Chinese herbal formula manufactured by Jing Tang Herbal) in grades 2 or higher, and *Shen Tong Fang* (Body Sore; Proprietary Chinese herbal formula manufactured by Jing Tang Herbal) in patients with cervical pain. Additional Chinese herbal medicines were given and modified according to the Chinese pattern diagnosis at the time. Of the 19 cases, 10 (52.6%) had complete clinical recovery and 8 (42.1%) improved 1 or more grade(s). Only 1 (5.3%) of 19 had no improvement, a horse for which poor tolerance of acupuncture precluded the completion of treatment, resulting in 13 of 13 dogs improving. All 18 cases that responded were observed for at least 6 months and demonstrated good quality of life with no relapse.

Despite shorter follow-up in these 2 EA studies than in other clinical studies of canine CSM,[55,56] these results of overall improvement rate of 80% to 95%, compared with the previous reports of 70% to 90% of dogs improved after surgery (~50% for conventional medical treatment) and warrant further clinical trials of management of CSM with TCVM. Furthermore, there were no cases of worsening with TCVM, making it a viable adjunct or alternative to conventional medicine and surgery, specifically early in the course of the disease. As for IVDD, the authors still recommend advanced imaging and surgery (if indicated) for presumptive cases of CSM, but also recommend integrating TCVM for ideal pain management and functional recovery (**Fig. 5**, Video 1).

TRADITIONAL CHINESE VETERINARY MEDICINE FOR PAINFUL NEUROLOGIC CONDITIONS/MISCELLANEOUS: ACUPUNCTURE AND PAIN

Numerous human clinical trials, many with low to moderate evidence, have been evaluated in large systematic reviews and meta-analyses, and acupuncture has proven effective for different types of pain associated with neurologic conditions, including postoperative, headaches, sciatica, diabetic neuropathy,[58,59] cervical, and lumbar.[60–62] Acupuncture acts on all levels of the pain pathway, with many of the bioactive chemicals involved in inflammatory pain models decreasing with acupuncture,[20,63] and also a modulatory effect on endogenous adenosine, cannabinoids, corticosterone, and opioids. Other mechanisms at the spinal cord level include serotoninergic, catecholaminergic, dopaminergic, substance P, and glutamate-receptor-driven pathways.[10]

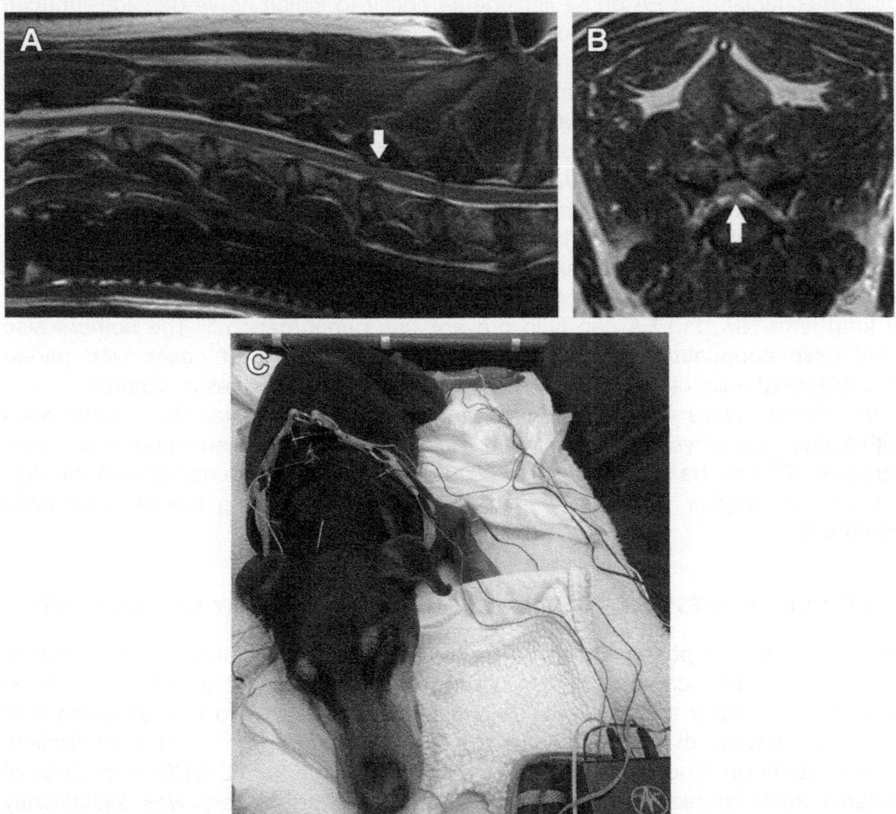

Fig. 5. (*A*) Sagittal and (*B*) transverse MRI of a 9-year-old female spayed (FS) Doberman presented for tetraplegia, diagnosed with disk-associated CSM at C5-C6 (*arrow*). A ventral slot was performed at C5-C6. (*C*) Patient receiving electroacupuncture in local (*Jing-jia-ji*) and distal points postoperatively. Herbal treatment was also used with Cervical Formula (proprietary Chinese herbal formula manufactured by Jing Tang Herbal) and *Buyang Huanwu*. The patient recovered ambulatory status within 1 month (see Video 1).

In neuropathic pain (NP) models, acupuncture effects have been primarily studied at the spinal cord level. Low-frequency EA (2–10 Hz) has been associated with a more robust, longer-lasting endogenous opioid response than higher frequencies (100 Hz), which correlates with a vast quantity of research indicating that low-frequency EA inhibits NP more effectively, although both showed a positive response.[10] It has been proposed that very low-frequency EA (2 Hz) triggers prolonged synaptic depression in the dorsal horn of rats, leading to an increased duration of analgesia.[64] In tactile allodynia, non-nociceptive fibers Aβ (faster than C and Aδ fibers associated with pain) become involved in the pain signal.[65–67] These changes, along with the gate theory[68] and with the ability of EA to recruit Aα and Aβ before Aδ and C fibers,[69] is another explanation for the ability of acupuncture to relieve NP.

NP and inflammatory pain share some similarities, such as the stimulation of N-methyl-D-aspartate receptors, which gives EA the ability to target both based on its ability to activate α2-adrenoceptors and 5-HT1Ars and inhibit GluN1.[10,70] EA's analgesic effects are at least partially due to the inhibition of excitatory amino acids, such as glutamate, and stimulation of inhibitory amino acids, such as GABA.[10,71–76] Other mechanisms of EA on NP include its ability to inhibit nerve-damage–induced upregulation of glial fibrillary acidic protein, OX-42, MMP-9, MMP-2, TNF-α, IL-6, IL-1β, and microglia activation in the spinal cord.[77,78]

Clinical veterinary studies evaluating acupuncture's effectiveness for NP are lacking, but the authors have used acupuncture successfully in many cases, specifically early in the course of the disease. In cases of painful radiculopathy/"nerve root signature" (eg, foraminal IVDD, cervical or at L7-S1 with resulting sciatica), EA can be extremely rewarding and result in a fast improvement. It is unclear if the sharp, acute pain encountered in these cases is a true form of NP or nociceptive/inflammatory pain due to involvement of the local *nervi nervorum*,[79,80] but clinicians should not underestimate the role of the *nervi nervorum* in subsequent development of long-term NP, and EA can help prevent this phenomenon.[81] The authors also have used acupuncture successfully in the management of cases with paresthesia/dysesthesia of unclear etiology (eg, feline hyperesthesia syndrome). For more chronic cases with central nervous system NP (eg, Chiari-like malformation with syringohydromyelia), the lack of efficacy of acupuncture mentioned by some investigators[82] may be related to central sensitization but also remodeling of the dorsal horn and higher centers of pain processing, emphasizing the need for early treatment.

TRADITIONAL CHINESE VETERINARY MEDICINE AND VETERINARY NEUROSURGERY

Several studies on postoperative pain after abdominal procedure in small animals have shown that acupuncture can decrease the dosage of anesthetic agent(s) required for surgery and can provide analgesia comparable to that achieved with injectable opioids or nonsteroidal anti-inflammatory drugs.[83–85] In a controlled, blinded study on 15 dogs undergoing hemilaminectomy for TL IVDD, total dose of fentanyl administered during the first 12 hours after surgery was significantly ($P = .04$) lower in the group receiving EA than in the control group. Pain score ($P = .018$) was significantly lower in the EA group than in the control group 36 hours after surgery.[86] Another study indicated that EA combined with low-dosage morphine suppressed postoperative pain better than either one did individually.[87] One human clinical study on preoperative EA indicated significantly decreased amount of morphine required during the first 24 hours postoperatively and

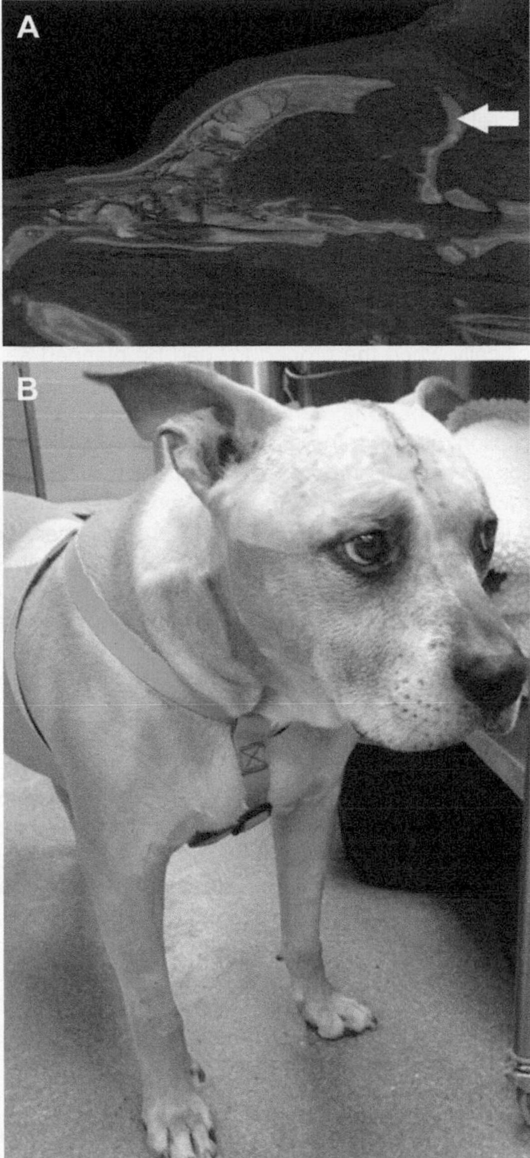

Fig. 6. (*A*) Sagittal CT image of a 9-year-old male neutered (MN) Pitbull presented for a large mass in the occipital area (*arrow*). The osteolytic mass invades the occipital, parietal, and temporal bones of the calvaria bilaterally. Biopsy was consistent with an osteosarcoma of high grade and surgical removal was elected. As perioperative hemorrhage was expected to be significant, the patient was treated with *Yunnan Baiyao* for a week before surgery. (*B*) Surgical removal was uneventful, with minimal blood loss and no transfusion required. Patient 3 days postoperative, with normal neurologic examination (see Video 2A and B).

significantly reduced incidence of nausea and dizziness during the same period compared with sham EA.[88] The authors routinely use EA as part of the postoperative pain management of every spinal surgery, ideally with bilateral stimulation because it is associated with better analgesic effect.[89]

Yunnan Baiyao (literally "the white medicine from the province of Yunnan") is an herbal formulation of relative innocuity, and is easily implemented with many potential benefits in veterinary neurology/neurosurgery. Although its complete formula is owned and kept partially secret by the government of the People's Republic of China, recent research has proven numerous benefits: as an antihemorrhagic agent, but also as an analgesic and antineoplastic supplement.[90] In recent human clinical publications, *Yunnan Baiyao* has been associated with significantly decreased intraoperative blood loss,[91] significantly decreased postoperative C-reactive protein and IL-6,[92] and significantly decreased postoperative inflammation and swelling,[93] with no allergic reactions, thromboembolic events, or other side effects reported. One of the authors (PR) is now routinely using *Yunnan Baiyao* preoperatively for every patient undergoing neurosurgery, specifically when the procedure can be planned several days ahead and if intraoperative hemorrhage is expected to be significant in volume (eg, craniectomy for multilobular tumor of bone, combined suboccipital and rostrotentorial craniectomy with occlusion of the transverse sinus, cervical dorsal laminectomy in large-breed dogs) or in terms of impact on visualization of the nervous tissue (eg, ventral slot) (see **Fig. 5**; **Figs. 6** and **7**, Video 2). *Yunnan Baiyao* is commercialized in capsules of 250 mg (16 regular capsules + 1 small "emergency red pill" in the middle of the blister) and other forms, such as paste, patches, powder, and aerosol. Suggested dosage is 1 capsule/10 kg by mouth once to twice daily for dogs (the "emergency red pill" can be given preoperatively), and 0.5 to 1 capsule by mouth twice daily for cats.

DISCUSSION/CONTROVERSIES ABOUT THE USE OF TRADITIONAL CHINESE VETERINARY MEDICINE

Although advances in neuroscience are slowly explaining the TCM/TCVM theory and the metaphor it constitutes, much remains to be discovered (eg, specificity of action of certain acupoints, role of the different frequencies used in EA). Before this is achieved, it is the authors' opinion that TCVM is most successful when an experienced practitioner makes an accurate Chinese pattern diagnosis, then chooses the appropriate acupuncture and herbal prescriptions. Although often effective in straightforward simpler cases, "cook-booking" or using a predetermined routine set of acupoints may not be as effective in more complicated cases.

Similar to conventional operator-dependent disciplines, such as neurosurgery, acupuncture treatments can be heavily dependent on practitioner expertise and a higher level might reflect on a better outcome for the patient, but also for the overall cohort in controlled studies. This may explain the discrepancy in the perceived benefits of acupuncture among clinicians and when comparing studies, as one's assessment of his or her own performance is influenced by skill/capabilities level,[94] the perceived difficulty of the task performed,[95] and the self-relevance of the task.[96] These could be some of the contributing factors to why there are few scientifically valid clinical studies on veterinary acupuncture, resulting in skepticism in some of the scientific community, but also raises the question of the role of formal education in the veterinary curriculum. Although nearly 25% of recent graduates face questions regarding the potential benefits of TCVM on a frequent basis, a lack in formal scholar training exists, with only 1 (3%) of 34 American Veterinary Medical Association–accredited colleges offering a required course in complementary and alternative veterinary medicine and 15 (44%) of 34 offering an elective course.[97,98] There remains a need for an evidence-based, unbiased scholar training of acupuncture and TCVM modalities in the veterinary curriculum.[98]

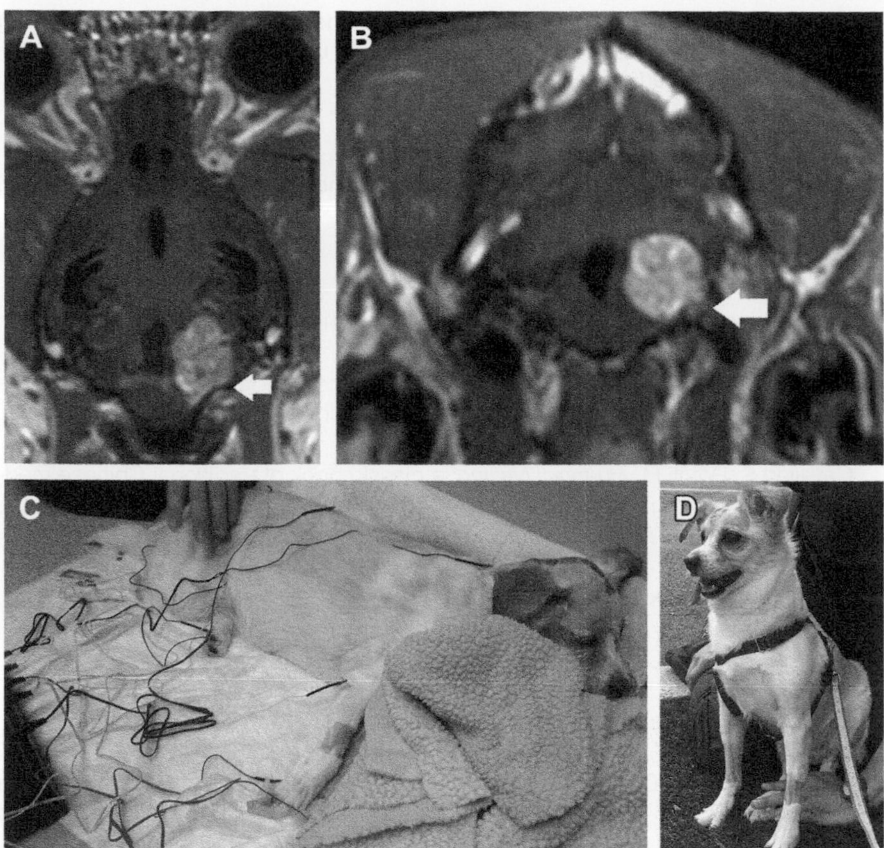

Fig. 7. (*A*) Dorsal and (*B*) transverse postcontrast brain MRI of a 5-year-old FS mixed breed dog. A large contrast-enhancing mass is seen at the level of the right cerebello-ponto-medullary angle (*arrow*), consistent with a choroid plexus tumor. Before surgery, the patient was treated with *Yunnan Baiyao* to help hemostasis. Gross total resection was achieved through a combined suboccipital and right rostro-tentorial craniectomy, with occlusion of the right transverse sinus. (*C*) The patient suffered neurologic worsening postoperatively, with nonambulatory tetraparesis, right facial paralysis, and severe right head tilt, and received extensive rehabilitation/EA with marked improvement of all deficits and recovery of ambulatory status (*D*).

SUMMARY

As research unveils the different mechanisms of action of acupuncture and Chinese herbals, TCVM can be better understood by Western practitioners. The laboratory models and limited clinical research available are supportive for the use of TCVM in the management of neurologic conditions in small animals, specifically in cases of IVDD, other myelopathies, and painful conditions. The relative innocuity of TCVM modalities (specifically acupuncture) make them easy to implement in a clinical setting, and provide a useful adjunct or occasionally alternative to conventional management. TCVM is best used in conjunction with a proper conventional diagnosis and can result in faster recovery and better pain control in neurologic conditions, whether the patient is managed medically or surgically (eg, IVDD). There remains a need for larger randomized controlled trials before further indications can be fully validated, along with an evidence-based approach to TCVM to reach unbiased conclusions in veterinary education and medical recommendations.

SUPPLEMENTARY DATA

Supplementary data related to this article can be found online at http://dx.doi.org/10.1016/j.cvsm.2017.08.003.

REFERENCES

1. Xie H, Priest V. Xie's veterinary acupuncture. Ames (IA): Blackwell Publishing; 2007. p. xii, 247, 260–261, 335.
2. Xie H, Wedemeyer L, Chrisman C, et al. Practical guide to traditional Chinese veterinary medicine small animal practice. Reddick, (FL): Chi Institute Press; 2014. 2014: 241-250, 924–930.
3. Cavalieri S, Rotoli M. *Huangdi Neijing*: a classic book of traditional Chinese medicine. Recenti Prog Med 1997;88:541–6 [in Italian].
4. Yu C. History. In: Traditional Chinese veterinary medicine. Beijing (China): China Agricultural Press; 1987. p. 1–6 [in Chinese].
5. Zhou JZ. Bo Le. In: Chen LF, editor. China agricultural encyclopedia: traditional Chinese veterinary medicine volume. Beijing (China): China Agricultural Press; 1991. p. 25–6 [in Chinese].
6. Yu C. Introduction. In: Traditional Chinese veterinary acupuncture and moxibustion. Beijing (China): China Agricultural Press; 1995. p. 1–6 [in Chinese].
7. Zhou JZ. Fan Mu Cuan Yan Fang. In: Chen LF, editor. China agricultural encyclopedia: traditional Chinese veterinary medicine volume. Beijing (China): China Agricultural Press; 1991. p. 73 [in Chinese].
8. Choi D, Lee J, Moon Y, et al. Acupuncture-mediated inhibition of inflammation facilitates significant functional recovery after spinal cord injury. Neurobiol Dis 2010;39:272–82.
9. Liu H, Qian X, An J, et al. Analgesic effects and neuropathology changes of electroacupuncture on curing a rat model of brachial plexus neuralgia by cobra venom. Pain Physician 2016;19:E435–48.
10. Zhang R, Lao L, Ren K, et al. Mechanisms of acupuncture-electroacupuncture on persistent pain. Anesthesiology 2014;120:482–503.
11. Campbell A. History of medical acupuncture. In: Filshie J, White A, Cummings M, editors. Medical Acupuncture: a Western scientific approach. 2nd edition. Philadelphia: Elsevier; 2016. p. 11–20.
12. Jaggar D. History and basic introduction to veterinary acupuncture. Probl Vet Med 1992;4:1–11.
13. Langevin H, Yandow J. Relationship of acupuncture points and meridians to connective tissue planes. Anat Rec 2002;269:257–65.
14. Li A, Zhang J, Xie W. Human acupuncture points mapped in rats are associated with excitable muscle/skin-nerve complexes with enriched nerve endings. Brain Res 2004;1012:154–9.
15. Erol G. The clinical effectiveness and application of veterinary acupuncture. Amer J Trad Chin Vet Med 2008;3:8–9.
16. Shin B, Lee M, Kong J, et al. Acupuncture for spinal cord injury survivors in Chinese literature: a systematic review. Complement Ther Med 2009;17:316–27.

17. Dorsher P, McIntosh P. Acupuncture's effects in treating the sequelae of acute and chronic spinal cord injuries: a review of allopathic and traditional Chinese medicine literature. Evid Based Complement Alternat Med 2011;2011:428108.
18. Tangjitjaroen W. Acupuncture for the treatment of spinal cord injuries. Amer J Trad Chin Vet Med 2011;6:37–43.
19. Steiss J. The neurophysiological basis of acupuncture. In: Schoen A, editor. Veterinary acupuncture: Ancient art to modern medicine. 2nd edition. St Louis (MO): Mosby; 2001. p. 342–3.
20. Su T, Zhao Y, Zhang L, et al. Electroacupuncture reduces the expression of proinflammatory cytokines in inflamed skin tissues through activation of cannabinoid CB2 receptors. Eur J Pain 2012;16:624–35.
21. Lee J, Jang K, Lee Y, et al. Electroacupuncture inhibits inflammatory edema and hyperalgesia through regulation of cyclooxygenase synthesis in both peripheral and central nociceptive sites. Am J Chin Med 2006;34:981–8.
22. Anand P, Whiteside G, Fowler C, et al. Targeting CB2 receptors and the endocannabinoid system for the treatment of pain. Brain Res Rev 2009;60:255–66.
23. Skarda R, Tejwani G, Muir W. Cutaneous analgesia, hemodynamic and respiratory effects, and β-endorphin concentration in spinal fluid and plasma of horses after acupuncture and electroacupuncture. Am J Vet Res 2002;63:1435–42.
24. Hong J, Liu J, Zhang C, et al. Acupuncture-moxibustion at *Jiaji* points for intervertebral disc herniation: a systematic review. J Acupunct Tuina Sci 2015;13:217–21.
25. Liu R, Jiang Y. Analgesic mechanism of *Huatuo Jiaji* points. Zhongguo Zhongyi Jichu Yixue Zazhi 2008;14:943–4 [in Chinese].
26. Deng H, Shen X. The mechanism of moxibustion: ancient theory and modern research. Evid Based Complement Alternat Med 2013;2013:379291.
27. Cheuk D, Wong V. Acupuncture for epilepsy. Cochrane Database Syst Rev 2014;(5):CD005062.
28. Yi P, Lu C, Jou S, et al. Low-frequency electroacupuncture suppresses focal epilepsy and improves epilepsy-induced sleep disruptions. J Biomed Sci 2015; 7:49.
29. Meng F, Kao C, Zhang H, et al. Using electroacupuncture at acupoints to predict the efficacy of hippocampal high-frequency electrical stimulation in pharmacoresistant temporal lobe epilepsy patients. Med Hypotheses 2013;80:244–6.
30. Yan N, Chen N, Lu J, et al. Electroacupuncture at acupoints could predict the outcome of anterior nucleus thalamus high-frequency electrical stimulation in medically refractory epilepsy. Med Hypotheses 2013;81:426–8.
31. Kang X, Shen X, Xia Y. Electroacupuncture-induced attenuation of experimental epilepsy: a comparative evaluation of acupoints and stimulation parameters. Evid Based Complement Alternat Med 2013;2013:149612.
32. Guo J, Liu J, Fu W, et al. The effect of electroacupuncture on spontaneous recurrent seizure and expression of GAD(67) mRNA in dentate gyrus in a rat model of epilepsy. Brain Res 2008;10:165–72.
33. Liu C, Lin Y, Hsu H, et al. Electroacupuncture at ST36-ST37 and at ear ameliorates hippocampal mossy fiber sprouting in kainic acid-induced epileptic seizure rats. Biomed Res Int 2014;2014:756019.
34. Liao E, Tang N, Lin Y, et al. Long-term electrical stimulation at ear and electroacupuncture at ST36-ST37 attenuated COX-2 in the CA1 of hippocampus in kainic acid-induced epileptic seizure rats. Sci Rep 2017;7:472.
35. Goiz-Marquez G, Caballero S, Solis H, et al. Electroencephalographic evaluation of gold wire implants inserted in acupuncture points in dogs with epileptic seizures. Res Vet Sci 2009;86(1):152–61.

36. Klide A, Farnbach G, Gallagher S. Acupuncture therapy for the treatment of intractable, idiopathic epilepsy in five dogs. Acupunct Electrother Res 1987;12: 71–4.
37. Clemmons R. PLA Bead treatment of refractory epilepsy in dogs. 2015 ACVIM Forum Research Reports Program. J Vet Intern Med 2015;29:1257–83.
38. Olby N. The pathogenesis and treatment of acute spinal cord injuries in dogs. Vet Clin North Am Small Anim Pract 2010;40:791–807.
39. Jeffery N, Levine J, Olby N, et al. Intervertebral disk degeneration in dogs: consequences, diagnosis, treatment, and future directions. J Vet Intern Med 2013;27: 1318–33.
40. Olby N, Jeffery N. Pathogenesis and physiology of central nervous system disease and injury. In: Tobias KM, Johnston SA, editors. Veterinary surgery: small animal. 1st edition. Saint Louis (MO): Elsevier; 2012. p. 374–87.
41. Liu W, Wang X, Yang S, et al. Electroacupuncture improves motor impairment via inhibition of microglia-mediated neuroinflammation in the sensorimotor cortex after ischemic stroke. Life Sci 2016;151:313–22.
42. Joaquim J, Luna S, Brondani J, et al. Comparison of decompression surgery, electroacupuncture, and decompressive surgery followed by electroacupuncture for the treatment of dogs with intervertebral disk disease with long-standing severe neurologic deficits. J Am Vet Med Assoc 2010;236:1225–9.
43. Hayashi A, Matera J, Fonseca Pinto A. Evaluation of electroacupuncture treatment for thoracolumbar intervertebral disk disease in dogs. J Am Vet Med Assoc 2007;231:913–8.
44. Janssens L, De Prins E. Treatment of thoracolumbar disk disease in dogs by means of acupuncture: a comparison of two techniques. J Am Anim Hosp Assoc 1989;25:169–74.
45. Hayashi A, Matera J, da Silva T, et al. Electro-acupuncture and Chinese herbs for treatment of cervical intervertebral disk disease in a dog. J Vet Sci 2007;8:95–8.
46. Janssens LA. Acupuncture for the treatment of thoracolumbar and cervical disc disease in the dog. Probl Vet Med 1992;4:107–16.
47. Janssens LA. Acupuncture treatment for canine thoracolumbar disk protrusions. Vet Med Small Anim Pract 1983;10:1580–5.
48. Jun L, Qiaoyu X, Le Z, et al. Effects of electro-acupuncture on Wnt-B-catenin signal pathway in annulus fibrous cells in intervertebral disc in rats with cervical spondylosis. Zhongguo Zhen Jiu 2014;34:1203–7 [in Chinese].
49. Innes JF, Melrose J. Embryology, innervation, morphology, structure, and function of the canine intervertebral disc. In: Fingeroth JM, Thomas WB, editors. Advances in intervertebral disc disease in dogs and cats. 1st edition. Ames (IA): Wiley Blackwell; 2015. p. 3–7.
50. Wang X, Li Y, Ma X, et al. Effect of acupuncture at cervical *Huatuo Jiaji* on type I and II collagen and pulpiform nucleus ultrastructure in rat degenerative cervical intervertebral discs. Shanghai Zhenjiu Zazhi 2009;28:674–7 [in Chinese].
51. Jiang D, Lu Z, Li G, et al. Electroacupuncture improves microcirculation and neuronal morphology in the spinal cord of a rat model of intervertebral disc extrusion. Neural Regen Res 2015;10:237–43.
52. Han H, Yoon H, Kim J, et al. Clinical effect of additional electroacupuncture on thoracolumbar intervertebral disc herniation in 80 paraplegic dogs. Am J Chin Med 2010;38:1015–25.
53. Liu C, Chang F, Lin C. Retrospective study of the clinical effects of acupuncture on cervical neurological diseases in dogs. J Vet Sci 2016;17:337–45.

54. Sumano H, Bermudez E, Obregon K. Treatment of wobbler syndrome in dogs with electroacupuncture. Dtsch Tierarztl Wochenschr 2000;107:231–5 [in German].
55. Dewey C, da Costa RC. Myelopathies: disorders of the spinal cord. In: Dewey C, da Costa RC, editors. Practical guide to canine and feline neurology. 3rd edition. Ames (IA): Wiley Blackwell; 2015. p. 345–53.
56. da Costa R, Parent J, Holmberg D, et al. Outcome of medical and surgical treatment in dogs with cervical spondylomyelopathy: 104 cases (1988-2004). J Am Vet Med Assoc 2008;233:1284–90.
57. Xie H, Rimar F. Effect of a combination of acupuncture and herbal medicine on wobbler syndrome in dogs and horses. In: Yang Z, Xie H, editors. Traditional Chinese veterinary medicine-empirical techniques to scientific validation. Reddick (FL): Jing-tang Pub; 2010. p. 101–12.
58. Zhang C, Ma Y, Yan Y. Clinical effects of acupuncture for diabetic peripheral neuropathy. J Tradit Chin Med 2010;30:13–4.
59. Garrow A, Xing M, Vere J, et al. Role of acupuncture in the management of diabetic painful neuropathy (DPN): a pilot RCT. Acupunct Med 2014;32:242–9.
60. Bartosz C. Acupuncture: evidence-based medicine. In: 2003 consensus statement WHO official position. 2014. Available at: http://www.evidencebasedacupuncture.org/who-official-position/. Accessed April 20, 2017.
61. Kelly R. Acupuncture for pain. Am Fam Physician 2009;80:481–4.
62. Hopton A, MacPherson H. Acupuncture for chronic pain: is acupuncture more than an effective placebo? A systematic review of pooled data from meta-analyses. Pain Pract 2010;10:94–102.
63. Ozaktay A, Kallakuri S, Takebayashi T, et al. Effects of interleukin-1 beta, interleukin-6, and tumor necrosis factor on sensitivity of dorsal root ganglion and peripheral receptive fields in rats. Eur Spine J 2006;15:1529–37.
64. Sun R, Wang H, Wang Y. Effect of electroacupuncture with different frequencies on neuropathic pain in a rat model. Zhongguo Ying Yong Sheng Li Xue Za Zhi 2002;18:128–31 [in Chinese].
65. Campbell J, Raja S, Miyer R, et al. Myelinated afferents signal the hyperalgesia associated with nerve injury. Pain 1988;32:89–94.
66. Koltzenburg M, Torebjork H, Wahren L. Nociceptor modulated central sensitization causes mechanical hyperalgesia in acute chemogenic and chronic neuropathic pain. Brain 1994;117:579–91.
67. Torebjork H, Lundberg L, LaMotte R. Central changes in processing of mechanoreceptive input capsaicin-induced secondary hyperalgesia in humans. J Physiol 1992;448:765–80.
68. Melzack R, Wall P. Pain mechanisms: a new theory. Science 1965;150:971–9.
69. Barlas P, Lundeberg T. Transcutaneous electrical nerve stimulation and acupuncture. In: McMahon SB, Koltzenburg M, editors. Wall and Melzack's textbook of pain. 5th edition. Philadelphia: Elsevier; 2006. p. 583–91.
70. Xu Q, Yaksh TL. A brief comparison of the pathophysiology of inflammatory versus neuropathic pain. Curr Opin Anaesthesiol 2011;24:400–7.
71. Yan L, Wu X, Yin Z, et al. Effect of electroacupuncture on the levels of amino acid neurotransmitters in the spinal cord in rats with chronic constrictive injury. Zhen Ci Yan Jiu 2011;36:353–6, 379.
72. Ma C, Li CX, Yi JL, et al. Effects of electroacupuncture on glutamate and aspartic acid contents in the dorsal root ganglion and spinal cord in rats with neuropathic pain. Zhen Ci Yan Jiu 2008;33:250–4 [in Chinese].

73. Park J, Han J, Kim S, et al. Spinal GABA receptors mediate the suppressive effect of electroacupuncture on cold allodynia in rats. Brain Res 2010;1322:24–9.
74. Vidal-Torres A, Carceller A, Zamanillo D, et al. Evaluation of formalin-induced pain behavior and glutamate release in the spinal dorsal horn using in vivo microdialysis in conscious rats. J Pharmacol Sci 2012;120:129–32.
75. Choi I, Cho J, An C, et al. 5-HT(1B) receptors inhibit glutamate release from primary afferent terminals in rat medullary dorsal horn neurons. Br J Pharmacol 2012;167:356–67.
76. Li X, Eisenach JC. α2A-adrenoceptor stimulation reduces capsaicin-induced glutamate release from spinal cord synaptosomes. J Pharmacol Exp Ther 2001;299:939–44.
77. Gim G, Lee J, Park E, et al. Electroacupuncture attenuates mechanical and warm allodynia through suppression of spinal glial activation in a rat model of neuropathic pain. Brain Res Bull 2011;86:403–11.
78. Choi D, Lee J, Lim E, et al. Inhibition of ROS-induced p38MAPK and ERK activation in microglia by acupuncture relieves neuropathic pain after spinal cord injury in rats. Exp Neurol 2012;236:268–82.
79. Ashbury A, Fields H. Pain due to peripheral nerve damage: a hypothesis. Neurology 1984;34:1587–90.
80. Bove G, Light A. The nervi nervorum: missing link for neuropathic pain? Pain Forum 1997;6:181–90.
81. Teixeira M, Almeida D, Yeng L. Concept of acute neuropathic pain. The role of nervi nervorum in the distinction between acute nociceptive and neuropathic pain. Rev Dor Sao Paulo 2016;17:S5–10.
82. Lindley S. Acupuncture in veterinary medicine. In: Filshie J, White A, Cummings M, editors. Medical acupuncture: a Western scientific approach. 2nd edition. Philadelphia: Elsevier; 2016. p. 651–63.
83. Zuo B, Jin-hua W, Jia L, et al. The regulatory effect of different amount of zoletil combined acupuncture anesthesia on canine stress hormones-catecholamine. Chin J Vet Sci 2013;33:1750–3.
84. Ruas de SousaI N, LunaI SPL, Buffo de Cápua ML II, et al. Analgesia of preemptive pharmacopuncture with meloxicam or aqua-acupuncture in cats undergoing ovariohysterectomy. Ciência Rural 2012;42:1231–6 [in Spanish].
85. Coletto-Freitas PM, Wangles P, Simões JR, et al. Electroacupuncture and morphine on cardiorespiratory parameters on cat elective ovariohysterectomy. Rev Bras Sande Prod 2011;12:961–9 [in Spanish].
86. Laim A, Jaggy A, Forterre F, et al. Effects of adjunct electroacupuncture on severity of postoperative pain in dogs undergoing hemilaminectomy because of acute thoracolumbar disk disease. J Am Vet Med Assoc 2009;234:1141–6.
87. Zhang R, Lao L, Wang L, et al. Involvement of opioid receptors in electroacupuncture-produced anti-hyperalgesia in rats with peripheral inflammation. Brain Res 2004;1020:12–7.
88. Lin JG, Lo MW, Wen YR, et al. The effect of high and low frequency electroacupuncture in pain after lower abdominal surgery. Pain 2002;99:509–14.
89. Cassu RN, Luna SP, Clark RM, et al. Electroacupuncture analgesia in dogs: is there a difference between uni and bi-lateral stimulation? Vet Anaesth Analg 2008;35:52–61.
90. Yang B, Xu ZQ, Zhang H, et al. The efficacy of *Yunnan Baiyao* on hemostasis and antiulcer: a systematic review and meta-analysis of randomized controlled trials. Int J Clin Exp Med 2014;7:461–82.

91. Tang ZL, Wang X, Yi B, et al. Effects of the preoperative administration of *Yunnan Baiyao* capsules on intraoperative blood loss in bimaxillary orthognathic surgery: a prospective, randomized, double-blind, placebo-controlled study. Int J Oral Maxillofac Surg 2009;38:261–6.
92. Tang ZL, Wang X, Yi B, et al. Evaluation of *Yunnan Baiyao* capsules for reducing postoperative swelling after orthognathic surgery. Zhonghua Yi Xue Za Zhi 2008; 88:2339–42 [in Chinese].
93. Tang ZL, Wang X, Yi B. Reverse-engineering-based quantitative three-dimensional measurement of facial swelling after administration of *Yunnan Baiyao* following orthognathic surgery. Zhonghua Yi Xue Za Zhi 2008;88:2482–6 [in Chinese].
94. Kruger J, Dunning D. Unskilled and unaware of it: how difficulties in recognizing one's own incompetence lead to inflated self-assessments. J Pers Soc Psychol 1999;77:1121–34.
95. Burson KA, Larrick RP, Klayman J. Skilled or unskilled, but still unaware of it: how perceptions of difficulty drive miscalibration in relative comparisons. J Pers Soc Psychol 2006;90:60–77.
96. Kim YH, Chiu CY, Bregant J. Unskilled and don't want to be aware of it: the effect of self-relevance on the unskilled and unaware phenomenon. PLoS One 2015; 10(6):e0130309.
97. Memon M, Sprunger LK. Survey of colleges and schools of veterinary medicine regarding education in complementary and alternative veterinary medicine. J Am Vet Med Assoc 2011;239:619–23.
98. Memon M, Shmalberg J, Adair H, et al. Integrative veterinary medical education and consensus guidelines for an integrative veterinary medicine curriculum within veterinary colleges. Open Vet J 2016;6:44–56.

Three-Dimensional Printing Role in Neurologic Disease

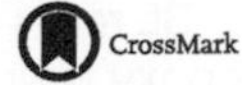

Adrien-Maxence Hespel, DVM, MS

KEYWORDS

- Three-dimensional printing • Rapid prototyping • Presurgical planning
- Stereolithography • Fused deposition modeling

KEY POINTS

- Most commonly in veterinary medicine, 3-dimensional (3D) printing involves the acquisition of raw data using computed tomography MRI or ultrasound. The raw data are processed through different software to create the 3D models.
- Different 3D printing technologies employ various material offering an array of options and cost depending on the purpose of the print.
- 3D printing is used for educational, research and pre-surgical planning purposes.
- 3D printing is becoming a versatile and accessible tool for the clinical floor.

This article, after briefly reviewing the different types of 3-dimensional (3D) printing technologies available and the processes involved in the creation of a prototype, focuses on the applications of 3D models in both human and veterinary neurosurgery.

Currently, 3D images can be created almost instantaneously with the use of advanced imaging technologies such as computed tomography (CT), 4-dimensional ultrasound scan, or MRI. These 3D representations are displayed on computer screens in a 2-dimensional environment but are found to improve surgical planning and the learning experience.[1]

Three-dimensional printing, also known as rapid prototyping, emerged in human medicine in the 1980s. All 3D printing techniques are grouped under the category of additive technologies and are based on the construction of models by addition of successive layers of material on top of the one before. This process could be compared with the construction of toy models using building blocks. The initial additive technology used was a process called *stereolithography* (SL, also known as SLA). Since then, numerous new technologies have emerged and currently include selective laser sintering, multijet modeling, and fused deposition modeling (FDM).[2] This article reviews 2 of the technologies that are most commonly encountered: SL and FDM.

Conflicts of Interest: The author has nothing to disclose.

University of Tennessee, 2407 River Drive, Knoxville, TN 37991, USA
E-mail address: ahespel@utk.edu

Vet Clin Small Anim 48 (2018) 221–229
http://dx.doi.org/10.1016/j.cvsm.2017.08.013
0195-5616/18/Published by Elsevier Inc.

SL relies on the use of an ultraviolet laser to solidify a liquid acrylic photopolymer, or epoxy resin, contained in a tank. The hardened acrylic is anchored on a build plate, which is lowered at the end of each completed layer so that uncured material remains at the surface to create the upcoming layer. At the time of completion of the model, the build plate is raised, and the surrounding unexposed liquid material is drained. Finally, the model is fully cured in an ultraviolet oven.[3] Selective laser sintering relies on a similar principle, but the raw material is in a powdered form and is being sintered by a high-power laser. The substrate can be plastic, metal, glass, or ceramic and does not require ultraviolet curing.[3]

FDM printers are probably the most widely known, advertised, and accessible printers. They use a roll of raw thermoplastic, commonly polylactic acid (PLA) or acrylonitrile butadiene styrene, which is being fed into a heated extrusion nozzle. When passed in the nozzle, the plastic is melted into a hairlike thin filament, which is then deposited on the build plate 1 layer at a time.

From the data acquisition to the production of the 3D models, there are 4 essential steps.[4]

In the medical field, the data are initially obtained through advanced imaging technologies such as CT, MRI, or ultrasound scan. These techniques are referred to as *transmissive*, and allow the evaluation and reproduction of both the surface and inner structures of an object.[4] In other domains, such as engineering or architectural design, nontransmissive techniques are more common and rely on the use of laser scanners and triangulation. These techniques allow only the surface of an object to be reproduced.[4]

Studies evaluating the ideal parameters for CT acquisition found that data acquired with 2-mm slice thickness, 25% to 75% overlap, and a pitch of 1.5 were adequate for the creation of 3D models.[5–7] However, in the author's experience and in a more recent publication,[8] and with the progression of CT and printer technologies, thinner slices such as 0.65 to 1 mm, provide much more detailed and accurate models. MRI was also evaluated as a way to acquire 3D data but the models created were smaller, more likely to contain artifacts, rougher, and more likely to have a discontinued appearance when compared with models created from CT.[8]

The second step on the path to 3D printing involves the importation and processing of the raw data in a 3D software program. These programs come in a variety of prices and abilities (eg, Mimics, Materialise, Leuven, Belgium and OsiriX, Bernex, Switzerland). After importation, the data to be reproduced are identified and selected based on their density (thresholding) and/or topography (segmentation).[6] These processes allow the elimination of nondesirable information, such as electrocardiogram leads or feces. At this point, a digital 3D mesh is created within the software and is the representation of the structure to be printed under the form of numerous continuous and contiguous polygons (**Fig. 1**).[9] The number of polygons directly influences the resolution of the model; an increase in the number of polygons results in an improvement in resolution. However, this improvement also results in an increase in computational power needs.

The third step is focused on optimization and depends on the prototype's purpose and the printer's potential limitations. The most common alterations are edge smoothing and reducing the object's size to fit the printer's build envelope. After being created, the mesh is exported as a CAD (computer-aided design) or an STL (surface tessellation language) file.

Lastly, the CAD or STL file is imported into a software program that is able to communicate with the 3D printer such as Makerware (Makerbot, Brooklyn, NY), ReplicatorG (open source) or Cura (Ultimaker, Geldermalsen, Netherlands). In this step,

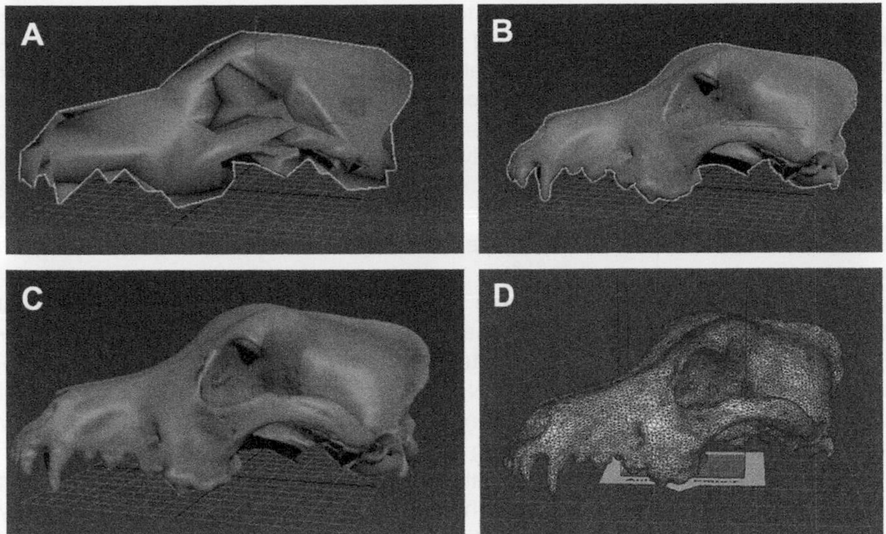

Fig. 1. (*A–D*) Computer rendering of the skull of a skeletally mature dog. Note the increase in resolution from the image A to C. The number of polygons increase from 1000 (*A*), 10,000 (*B*), and 60,000 (*C*). The intricacy of the polygonal mesh is visible (*D*).

the print settings are defined (ie, layer height, temperature of extrusion), the type of material is chosen, and the object is printed.

An inclusive, descriptive tutorial on how to create a 3D model from the CT data acquisition to the final printing step is available online and could be used as a guideline.[9]

From an economical perspective, 3D printers are available in a range of prices. Many of the current consumer grade FDM printers vary between $500 and $2000. Industrial-grade SL printers can reach prices up to $500,000. When considering the purchase of a printer, one needs to consider the type of technology, the size of the building plate, the resolution, and the type of material used to print. SL or selective laser sintering printers represent a higher investment cost, and a higher overall use and maintenance cost, when compared with FDM printers. However, they have the advantage of allowing for the use of a wider range of materials, some of them being Us Food and Drug Administration approved. They also do not always require support material to build the prototype and usually have an overall smoother finish when compared with FDM. On the other hand, FDM printers are more available, easier to use and maintain, and do not require extensive expertise for optimal results.

Printing resolution is commonly as high as 25 to 100 μm. One could think that the higher the printer resolution the better; however, for medical applications, the best currently available clinical CTs have detectors measuring between 500 and 650 μm. Therefore, the CT data are often the limiting factor in the case of rapid prototyping resolution.

It should also be mentioned that multiple companies that specialize in rapid prototyping also offer the services of creating, printing, and shipping the models for a fee.

In human medicine, including neurosurgery, 3 main uses for rapid prototyping have been explored: creation of tailored anatomic models for clinical surgical planning and educational and research prototypes.[10]

Patient-specific models have been extensively used and studied in cases of cerebral aneurysm.[11–20] Those studies found that the models were anatomically accurate when compared with the anatomy visually[16,18,19] and were precise to the millimeter level when analyzed.[18] The use of prototypes allowed for decreased intraoperative time for cases of arteriovenous malformations in pediatric patients.[18] Models have also been used for hemodynamic analysis[13] and flow prediction and for surgical training.[16]

In cases of brain and spinal tumors, 3D models have been used to evaluate the association between neoplastic and adjacent healthy tissues to help delineate margins (osseous, nervous, and vascular).[21,22]

Rapid prototyping has also been used and evaluated for the management of spinal trauma. In trauma cases, it was found that 3D models allowed better and faster identification of complex fractures of the vertebral column when compared with 3D computer renderings and 2D CT images.[23] Neurosurgical guides have been created and evaluated for the placement of screws in the pedicle of thoracic vertebrae with very high accuracy and a deviation averaging less than 1 mm.[24]

Training devices have been created to practice technically challenging surgeries such as the transnasal sphenoid endoscopic approach to pituitary neoplasia[25,26] and also have the potential to be combined with surgical navigation systems.[26,27]

In veterinary medicine to date and to the author's best knowledge, there are no scientific studies focused on the neurosurgical applications of rapid prototyping. However, in the author's experience, multiple uses have been beneficial clinically for neurologic patients and for research purposes.

Spinal applications are aimed at presurgical planning for cases such as atlanto-axial subluxation and spinal fractures. Atlanto-axial subluxation is a challenge to surgically correct in dogs; the patients are usually toy breeds, leaving little room to place stabilizing implants. Many techniques have been described for stabilization of these cases and complications described.[28–34] In the cases that the author experienced, it was the preference of the neurosurgeon to use 2 small plates secured by screws to bridge along the ventral aspect of the atlas and axis (**Fig. 2**). Our protocol

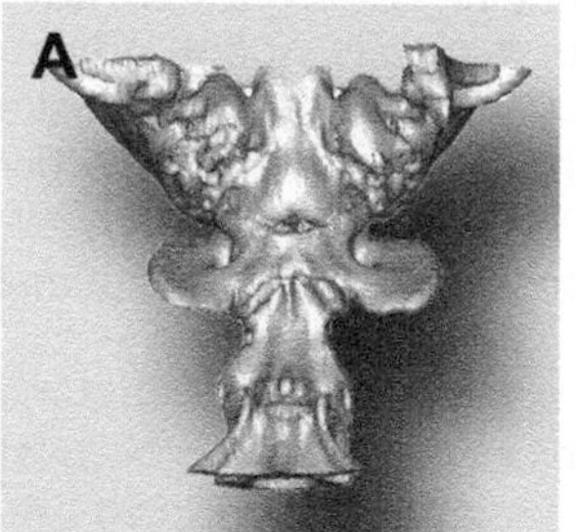

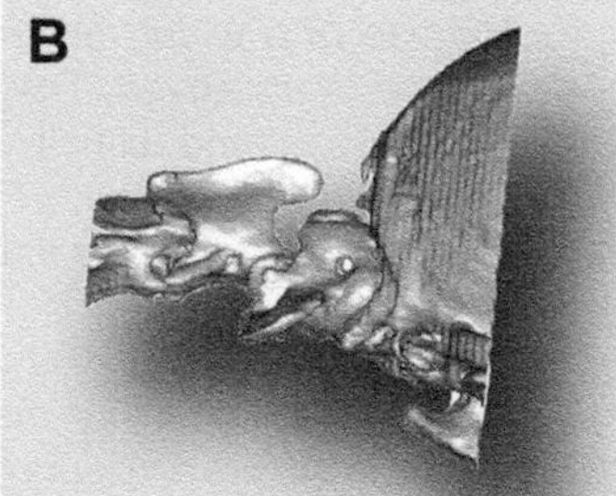

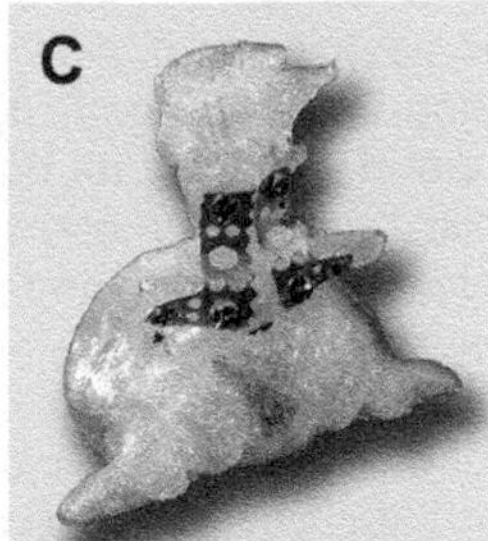

Fig. 2. (*A–C*) Computer-rendered illustrations of a cervical spine affected by atlanto-axial luxation including the caudal aspect of the skull and the cranial aspect of C3, dorsoventral projection (*A*), and right lateral projection (*B*). Dorsoventral view (*C*) of a model of the same cervical spine. Note the 2 bent plates and surgical screws anchored on the ventral aspect of the vertebral bodies of C1 and C2. These plates were used as template for the contouring of the actual surgical plates. Model printed using transparent PLA on a Replicator 2 (Makerbot) with a resolution of 200 μm.

is as follows: the patient undergoes a CT scan of the cervical area, with 0.65-mm slice thickness and pitch of 1.5, and the images are reconstructed in a sharp kernel. After being exported, the model is made based on bone thresholding and segmentation of the spine, including the caudal aspect of the skull and extending caudally up to the midbody of C3. This focused approach allows for a relatively fast printing time, making the technology more clinically available (60–90 min). The models are usually printed in multiple copies. Based on the prototype, the surgical plates or surgical plate templates can be bent to shape and screws chosen and measured to have the optimal length, maximizing bone purchase while avoiding violation of the spinal canal. The evaluation of screw placement can be done directly, as one can visually assess the lumen of the spinal canal of the model. The prototype also allows for surgical training of junior surgeons, surgical practice, and delineation of potential landmarks, to decrease the actual surgery time. Based on personal experience, the surgery time was decreased by 25% to 33% when a neurosurgeon with more than 20 years of experience was provided with the models ahead of surgery.

At the author's current institution, there is research in the development of surgical guides to correct for atlanto-axial instability. The guides are custom made based on the patient's anatomy, sterilized, and used in surgery to guide accurate placement of the surgical implants (**Fig. 3**). The ventral aspect of the guide conforms to the ventral aspect of the vertebral body of C1 and C2. Pipes are created through these guides to provide guidance for surgical pin placement. The pins are later bridged using a resin such as polymethyl methacrylate.

Similar uses can be found in cases of vertebral fractures (**Fig. 4**) or congenital spinal abnormalities that require surgical correction. The model can also be used to determine whether potential surgery is appropriate based on the involved anatomy. Specifically, in a case of comminuted fractures of the axis that was scheduled to undergo surgical fixation, it was deemed that the risks of the surgery outweighed its potential benefits once the model had been examined and the surgical options considered and practiced.

Neuro-oncology applications for 3D printing have also been discovered. A protocol was developed to print brain tumors using a combination of MRI and CT. There were

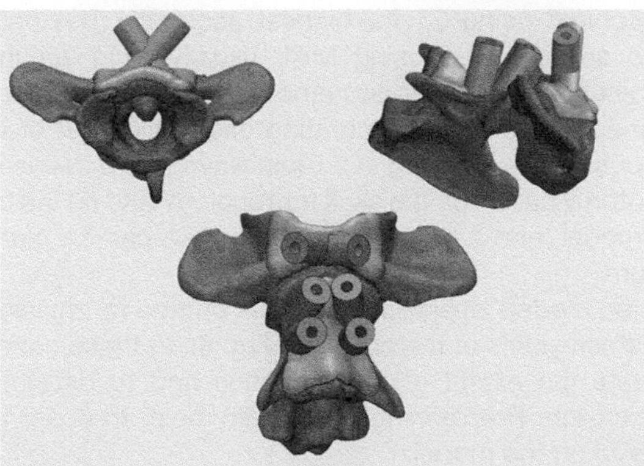

Fig. 3. Computer-rendered illustrations of a cervical spine and the created guide for surgical pins placement. The guides are custom made based on the patient's specific anatomy to contour the ventral aspect of the vertebral bodies. The directions of the tunnels are determined to provide a safe corridor for pin placement. (*Courtesy of* Dr Kyle Snowdon, University of Tennessee, Knoxville, TN.)

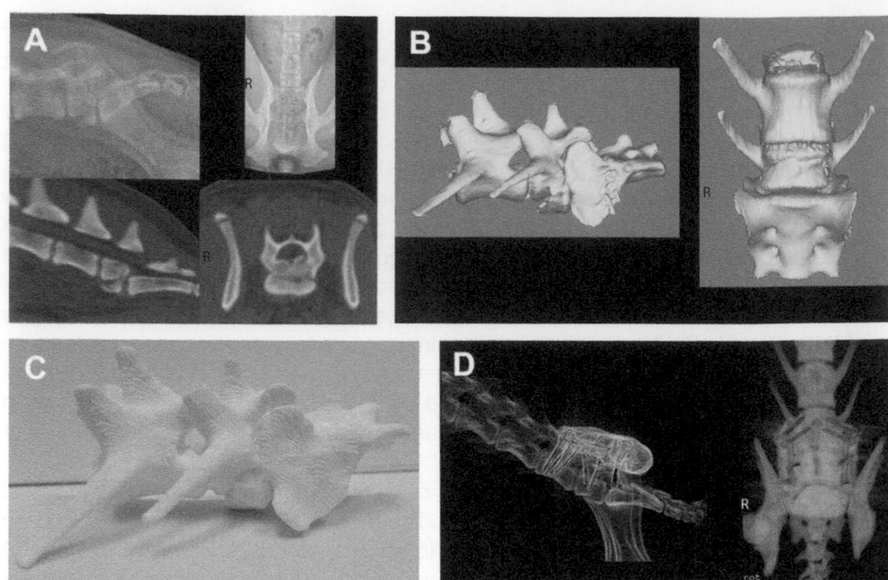

Fig. 4. (*A*) Lateral and ventrodorsal radiographs and multiplanar reconstruction CT images of the lumbar spine of a dog. (*B*) The caudoventral aspect of L6 is fractured and displaced ventrally and cranially. Computer-rendered illustrations of the same spine after 3D rendering. (*C*) Three-dimensional prototype made for presurgical planning, printed with PLA at 200 μm on a Replicator 2. (*D*) Computer-rendered 3D illustration of the postsurgical CT examination. The pins are displayed in pink and are embedded dorsally in polymethyl methacrylate. (*Courtesy of* Dr Kelsey Cline, University of Auburn, Auburn, AL.)

benefits to using this combined modality approach. As brain tumors are not necessarily visible on CT images, and studies have found that MRI tends to create models of reduced size and with more artifacts,[5] a combination of the 2 modalities provides the best compromise. The data pertaining to the osseous structures (ie, cranium, falx cerebri) are acquired using CT for highest accuracy. The data delineating the neoplastic process are acquired using MRI, usually a T1-weighted postcontrast sequence, in combination with other sequences. The 2 data sets are extracted and interpolated into one another (**Fig. 5**), creating one unified set of data. The models created are used for surgical planning in 2 main ways: (1) to delineate potential landmarks for the craniotomy based on the skull morphology and (2) the craniotomy can be performed on the model, and a surgical mesh or plate can be planned to cover the defect in the cranium.

In a similar manner, models of skulls have been printed for multilobular osteochondrosarcoma and osteomyelitis of the cranium (**Fig. 6**). In these cases, the prototypes are used to delineate the extent of the condition and to determine the extent of possible surgical excision. Preplanning of metallic mesh to cover the skull defect is also performed based on the model.

Finally, rapid prototyping technology has been used for research purposes. For example, at the University of Auburn, a research project was conducted to evaluate osseous anomalies of cats affected with gangliosidosis. The models were used to perform measurement of the bones and to compare with healthy specimens at different ages.

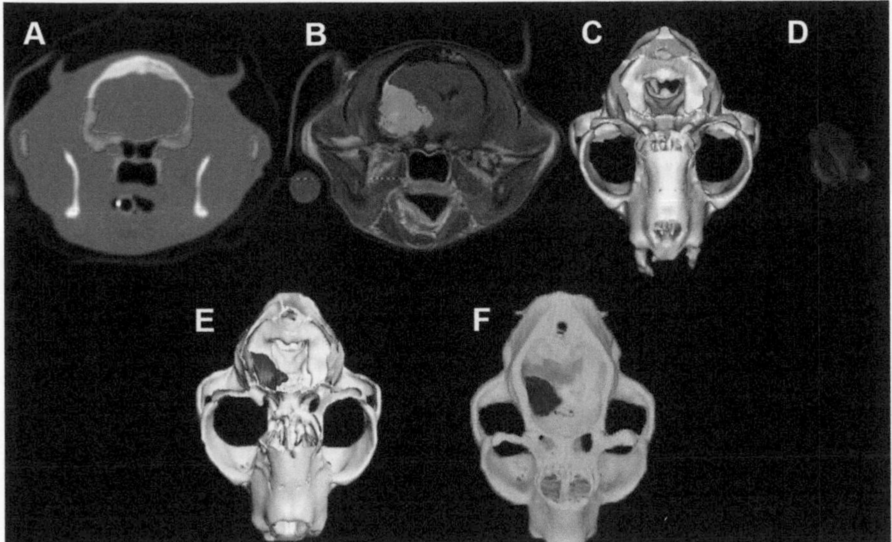

Fig. 5. (*A*) Transverse CT image of the skull of cat at the level of the midbrain. The highlighted in pink parts of the skull are the parts that have been segmented. (*B*) Transverse T1 postcontrast MRI image of the brain of the same cat. The highlighted part in green represents the meningioma as segmented based on the contrast enhancement. (*C*) Computer-rendered 3D illustration of the cranium as delineated in (*A*). (*D*) Computer-rendered 3D illustration of the meningioma as delineated in (*B*). (*E*) The 2 sets of data are interpolated into one another to create a computer-rendered 3D illustration including the skull and the neoplastic tissue accurately. The tumor is displayed in red. (*F*) Three-dimensional printed model of the cranium and extra-axial mass for surgical planning. Model printed using white and red PLA on a Big Builder (Builder 3D, Netherlands); resolution 200 μm.

The advantages of 3D printing are numerous, and its overall low cost is making it an ideal tool to be used clinically and for educational and research purposes. The future of 3D printing will likely be clinical application of printed cells and tissues for reconstructive surgeries, but this process is still in its infancy.

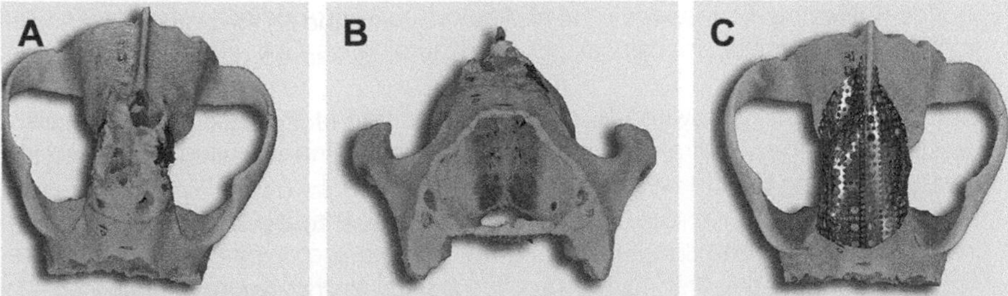

Fig. 6. (*A, B*) Three-dimensional model of a dog affected with osteomyelitis secondary to a bite wound. The surgical landmarks for debridement have been delineated. (*C*) A metallic mesh template was created to conform to the ostectomy needed to remove the osteomyelitis.

REFERENCES

1. Hespel AM, Wilhite R, Hudson J. Invited review-applications for 3d printers in veterinary medicine. Vet Radiol Ultrasound 2014;55(4):347–58.
2. Liew Y, Beveridge E, Demetriades AK, et al. 3D printing of patient-specific anatomy: a tool to improve patient consent and enhance imaging interpretation by trainees. Br J Neurosurg 2015;29(5):712–4.
3. McGurk M, Amis A, Potamianos P, et al. Rapid prototyping techniques for anatomical modelling in medicine. Ann R Coll Surg Engl 1997;79(3):169.
4. Corney J, Hieu L, Zlatov N, et al. Medical rapid prototyping applications and methods. Assemb Autom 2005;25(4):284–92.
5. Hopper KD, Pierantozzi D, Potok PS, et al. The quality of 3D reconstructions from 1.0 and 1.5 pitch helical and conventional CT. J Comput Assist Tomogr 1996; 20(5):841–7.
6. Barker T, Earwaker W, Lisle D. Accuracy of stereolithographic models of human anatomy. J Med Imaging Radiat Oncol 1994;38(2):106–11.
7. Lill W, Solar P, Ulm C, et al. Reproducibility of three-dimensional CT-assisted model production in the maxillofacial area. Br J Oral Maxillofac Surg 1992; 30(4):233–6.
8. White D, Chelule K, Seedhom B. Accuracy of MRI vs CT imaging with particular reference to patient specific templates for total knee replacement surgery. Int J Med Robot 2008;4(3):224–31.
9. Doney E, Krumdick LA, Diener JM, et al. 3D printing of preclinical x-ray computed tomographic data sets. J Vis Exp 2013;(73):e50250.
10. Randazzo M, Pisapia JM, Singh N, et al. 3D printing in neurosurgery: a systematic review. Surg Neurol Int 2016;7(Suppl 33):S801.
11. Abla AA, Lawton MT. Three-dimensional hollow intracranial aneurysm models and their potential role for teaching, simulation, and training. World Neurosurg 2015; 83(1):35–6.
12. Thawani JP, Pisapia JM, Singh N, et al. Three-dimensional printed modeling of an arteriovenous malformation including blood flow. World Neurosurg 2016;90: 675–83.e2.
13. Anderson JR, Thompson WL, Alkattan AK, et al. Three-dimensional printing of anatomically accurate, patient specific intracranial aneurysm models. J Neurointerv Surg 2016;8(5):517–20.
14. Ionita CN, Mokin M, Varble N, et al. Challenges and limitations of patient-specific vascular phantom fabrication using 3D Polyjet printing. Proc SPIE Int Soc Opt Eng 2014;9038:90380M.
15. Kondo K, Nemoto M, Masuda H, et al. Anatomical reproducibility of a head model molded by a three-dimensional printer. Neurol Med Chir (Tokyo) 2015;55(7): 592–8.
16. Mashiko T, Otani K, Kawano R, et al. Development of three-dimensional hollow elastic model for cerebral aneurysm clipping simulation enabling rapid and low cost prototyping. World Neurosurg 2015;83(3):351–61.
17. Namba K, Higaki A, Kaneko N, et al. Microcatheter shaping for intracranial aneurysm coiling using the 3-dimensional printing rapid prototyping technology: preliminary result in the first 10 consecutive cases. World Neurosurg 2015;84(1): 178–86.
18. Weinstock P, Prabhu SP, Flynn K, et al. Optimizing cerebrovascular surgical and endovascular procedures in children via personalized 3D printing. J Neurosurg Pediatr 2015;16(5):584–9.

19. Wurm G, Tomancok B, Pogady P, et al. Cerebrovascular stereolithographic biomodeling for aneurysm surgery: technical note. J Neurosurg 2004;100(1):139–45.
20. Xu W-H, Liu J, Li M-L, et al. 3D printing of intracranial artery stenosis based on the source images of magnetic resonance angiograph. Ann Transl Med 2014;2(8):74.
21. Oishi M, Fukuda M, Yajima N, et al. Interactive presurgical simulation applying advanced 3D imaging and modeling techniques for skull base and deep tumors: clinical article. J Neurosurg 2013;119(1):94–105.
22. Spottiswoode B, Van den Heever D, Chang Y, et al. Preoperative three-dimensional model creation of magnetic resonance brain images as a tool to assist neurosurgical planning. Stereotact Funct Neurosurg 2013;91(3):162–9.
23. Li Z, Li Z, Xu R, et al. Three-dimensional printing models improve understanding of spinal fracture—A randomized controlled study in China. Sci Rep 2015;5: 11570.
24. Sugawara T, Higashiyama N, Kaneyama S, et al. Multistep pedicle screw insertion procedure with patient-specific lamina fit-and-lock templates for the thoracic spine: clinical article. J Neurosurg Spine 2013;19(2):185–90.
25. Inoue D, Yoshimoto K, Uemura M, et al. Three-dimensional high-definition neuroendoscopic surgery: a controlled comparative laboratory study with two-dimensional endoscopy and clinical application. J Neurol Surg A Cent Eur Neurosurg 2013;74(06):357–65.
26. Waran V, Menon R, Pancharatnam D, et al. The creation and verification of cranial models using three-dimensional rapid prototyping technology in field of transnasal sphenoid endoscopy. Am J Rhinol Allergy 2012;26(5):e132–6.
27. Waran V, Pancharatnam D, Thambinayagam HC, et al. The utilization of cranial models created using rapid prototyping techniques in the development of models for navigation training. J Neurol Surg A Cent Eur Neurosurg 2014; 75(01):012–5.
28. Beaver DP, Ellison GW, Lewis DD, et al. Risk factors affecting the outcome of surgery for atlantoaxial subluxation in dogs: 46 cases (1978–1998). J Am Vet Med Assoc 2000;216(7):1104–9.
29. Havig ME, Cornell KK, Hawthorne JC, et al. Evaluation of nonsurgical treatment of atlantoaxial subluxation in dogs: 19 cases (1992–2001). J Am Vet Med Assoc 2005;227(2):257–62.
30. Platt SR, Chambers JN, Cross A. A modified ventral fixation for surgical management of atlantoaxial subluxation in 19 dogs. Vet Surg 2004;33(4):349–54.
31. Sanders SG, Bagley RS, Silver GM, et al. Outcomes and complications associated with ventral screws, pins, and polymethyl methacrylate for atlantoaxial instability in 12 dogs. J Am Anim Hosp Assoc 2004;40(3):204–10.
32. Schulz KS, Waldron DR, Fahie M. Application of ventral pins and polymethylmethacrylate for the management of atlantoaxial instability: results in nine dogs. Vet Surg 1997;26(4):317–25.
33. Sorjonen D, SHIRES PK. Atlantoaxial instability: a ventral surgical technique for decompression, fixation, and fusion. Vet Surg 1981;10(1):22–9.
34. Thomas WB, Sorjonen DC, Simpson ST. Surgical management of atlantoaxial subluxation in 23 dogs. Vet Surg 1991;20(6):409–12.

Printed and bound by CPI Group (UK) Ltd, Croydon, CR0 4YY

07/10/2024

01040502-0007